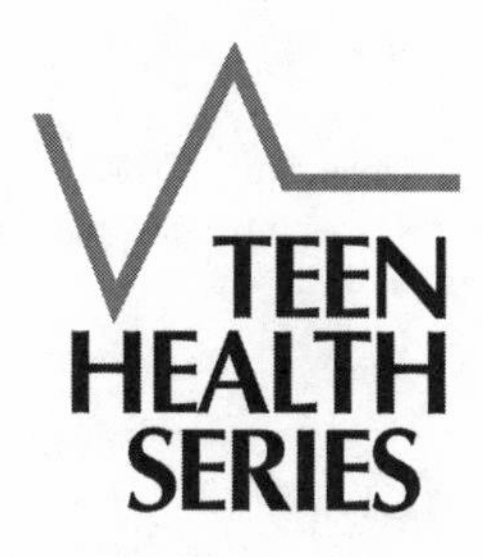

Third Edition

Mental Health Information for Teens

Health Tips about Mental Wellness and Mental Illness

Including Facts about Mental and Emotional Health, Depression and Other Mood Disorders, Anxiety Disorders, Behavior Disorders, Self-Injury, Psychosis, Schizophrenia, and More

Edited by Karen Bellenir

Omnigraphics

P.O. Box 31-1640, Detroit, MI 48231

Bibliographic Note

Because this page cannot legibly accommodate all the copyright notices, the Bibliographic Note portion of the Preface constitutes an extension of the copyright notice.

Edited by Karen Bellenir

Teen Health Series

Karen Bellenir, *Managing Editor*
David A. Cooke, M.D., *Medical Consultant*
Elizabeth Collins, *Research and Permissions Coordinator*
Cherry Edwards, *Permissions Assistant*
EdIndex, Services for Publishers, *Indexers*

* * *

Omnigraphics, Inc.
Matthew P. Barbour, *Senior Vice President*
Kevin M. Hayes, *Operations Manager*

* * *

Peter E. Ruffner, *Publisher*

ISBN 978-0-7808-1087-7

Library of Congress Cataloging-in-Publication Data

Mental health information for teens : health tips about mental wellness and mental illness including facts about mental and emotional health, depression and other mood disorders, anxiety disorders, behavior disorders, self-injury, psychosis, schizophrenia, and more / edited by Karen Bellenir. -- 3rd ed.

p. cm.

Summary: "Provides basic consumer health information for teens about mental illness and treatment, along with tips for maintaining mental and emotional health. Includes index, resource information and recommendations for further reading"--Provided by publisher.

Includes bibliographical references and index.

ISBN 978-0-7808-1087-7 (hardcover : alk. paper) 1. Teenagers--Mental health. 2. Adolescent psychology. 3. Child mental health. I. Bellenir, Karen.

RJ499.M419 2010

613'.0433--dc22

2010000806

This book is printed on acid-free paper meeting the ANSI Z39.48 Standard. The infinity symbol that appears above indicates that the paper in this book meets that standard.

Printed in the United States

Table of Contents

Part Three: Behavioral, Personality, And Psychotic Disorders

Part Four: Getting Help For Mental Illness

Part Five: Other Issues Related To Mental Health In Teens

Part Six: If You Need More Information

Preface

About This Book

While many young people recognize that physical fitness is important for maintaining a healthy body, the importance of mental fitness for maintaining a healthy mind and emotions is sometimes overlooked. Statistics suggest that nearly one out of every five teens struggles with a mental health concern, and one in ten suffers from a mental disorder severe enough to cause some level of impairment, including poor academic performance, loss of friends, family conflict, faulty body image, and difficulty making decisions. Compounding the problem is that fact that many young people experience a long delay—sometimes decades—between the onset of their symptoms and when they eventually seek treatment.

Mental Health Information for Teens, Third Edition offers updated information about maintaining mental wellness and coping with a host of problems that commonly occur during the adolescent years, including self-esteem issues, stress overload, family problems, heartbreak, and grief. It describes the warning signs that may accompany mental health disorders such as depression, bipolar disorder, anxiety disorders, phobias, behavioral disorders, personality disorders, psychoses, and schizophrenia. It also discusses the types of treatment most commonly used by mental health professionals. Facts about alternative approaches to mental health care are included, and the book concludes with directories of resources for help and support and suggestions for additional reading.

How To Use This Book

This book is divided into parts and chapters. Parts focus on broad areas of interest; chapters are devoted to single topics within a part.

Part One: Maintaining Mental Wellness defines the concept of mental health and offers information about the need to integrate many facets of life, including how a person thinks, feels, and acts in varying situations. This includes responding to challenges, making decisions, building self-esteem, handling stress, and developing relationships.

Part Two: Mood And Anxiety Disorders explains mental disorders characterized by abnormal variations in the emotional responses of sadness, enthusiasm, worry, and fear. Individual chapters describe risk factors, symptoms, and treatments for these disorders, which include depression, bipolar disorder, panic disorder, obsessive-compulsive disorder, and phobias.

Part Three: Behavioral, Personality, and Psychotic Disorders discusses the kinds of mental disorders that influence how a person behaves, relates to others, or perceives reality. Disorders that affect behavior include adjustment disorders, eating disorders, and disorders associated with an inability to control impulsive urges. Personality disorders include paranoid, narcissistic, antisocial, and dependent personalities, and psychotic disorders are those that include such components as hallucinations, delusions, and interruptions in consciousness while awake.

Part Four: Getting Help For Mental Illness offers suggestions for locating appropriate services from mental health professionals, and it describes what to expect during treatment. Various forms of counseling and therapy are explained, and a chapter on medications discusses commonly used mood stabilizers, antipsychotics, and other psychiatric medications. Alternative approaches to mental health care are also discussed.

Part Five: Other Issues Related To Mental Health In Teens offers suggestions for coping with common experiences and other disorders that may have a direct impact on adolescent mental well-being. These include the experience of abuse and violence, learning disabilities, and the often-confusing changes that may accompany puberty.

Part Six: If You Need More Information provides a list of helplines for people in crisis, a directory of mental health organizations, and suggestions for additional reading.

Bibliographic Note

This volume contains documents and excerpts from publications issued by the following government agencies: Centers for Disease Control and Prevention; Health Resources and Services Administration; National Center for Complementary and Alternative Medicine; National Center for Injury Prevention and Control; National Institute of Mental Health; National Institute of Neurological Disorders and Stroke; National Institute on Drug Abuse; National Institutes of Health; National Library of Medicine; National Mental Health Information Center; National Women's Health Information Center; National Youth Violence Prevention Resource Center; Office of Minority Health; Office on Women's Health; Substance Abuse and Mental Health Services Administration; U. S. Department of Health and Human Services; and the U.S. Department of Justice.

In addition, this volume contains copyrighted documents and articles produced by the following organizations: A.D.A.M., Inc.; American Psychological Association; Anxiety Disorders Association of America; Canadian Mental Health Association; Cincinnati Children's Hospital Medical Center; Cleveland Clinic Foundation; Focus Adolescent Services; Merck & Co., Inc.; NAMI: The Nation's Voice on Mental Illness; National Center for Learning Disabilities; Nemours Foundation; PsychNet-UK; Riverside County Department of Health (California); and the University of Michigan, Department of Psychiatry.

The photograph on the front cover is from Juan Gabriel Estey/iStockphoto.

Full citation information is provided on the first page of each chapter. Every effort has been made to secure all necessary rights to reprint the copyrighted material. If any omissions have been made, please contact Omnigraphics to make corrections for future editions.

Acknowledgements

In addition to the organizations listed above, special thanks are due to Liz Collins, research and permissions coordinator; Cherry Edwards, permissions assistant; Zachary Klimecki, editorial assistant; and Elizabeth Bellenir, prepress technician.

About the *Teen Health Series*

At the request of librarians serving today's young adults, the *Teen Health Series* was developed as a specially focused set of volumes within Omnigraphics' *Health Reference Series*. Each volume deals comprehensively with a topic selected according to the needs and interests of people in middle school and high school.

Teens seeking preventive guidance, information about disease warning signs, medical statistics, and risk factors for health problems will find answers to their questions in the *Teen Health Series*. The *Series*, however, is not intended to serve as a tool for diagnosing illness, in prescribing treatments, or as a substitute for the physician/patient relationship. All people concerned about medical symptoms or the possibility of disease are encouraged to seek professional care from an appropriate health care provider.

If there is a topic you would like to see addressed in a future volume of the *Teen Health Series*, please write to:

Editor
Teen Health Series
Omnigraphics, Inc.
P.O. Box 31-1640
Detroit, MI 48231

A Note about Spelling and Style

Teen Health Series editors use *Stedman's Medical Dictionary* as an authority for questions related to the spelling of medical terms and the *Chicago Manual of Style* for questions related to grammatical structures, punctuation, and other editorial concerns. Consistent adherence is not always possible, however, because the individual volumes within the *Series* include many documents from a wide variety of different producers and copyright holders, and the editor's primary goal is to present material from each source as accurately as is possible following the terms specified by each document's producer. This sometimes means that information in different chapters or sections may follow other guidelines and alternate spelling authorities. For example, occasionally a copyright holder may require that eponymous terms be shown in possessive forms (Crohn's disease *vs.* Crohn disease) or that British spelling norms be retained (leukaemia *vs.* leukemia).

Locating Information within the *Teen Health Series*

The *Teen Health Series* contains a wealth of information about a wide variety of medical topics. As the *Series* continues to grow in size and scope, locating the precise information needed by a specific student may become more challenging. To address this concern, information about books within the *Teen Health Series* is included in *A Contents Guide to the Health Reference Series*. The *Contents Guide* presents an extensive list of more than 15,000 diseases, treatments, and other topics of general interest compiled from the Tables of Contents and major index headings from the books of the *Teen Health Series* and *Health Reference Series*. To access *A Contents Guide to the Health Reference Series*, visit www.healthreferenceseries.com.

Our Advisory Board

We would like to thank the following advisory board members for providing guidance to the development of this *Series*:

Dr. Lynda Baker, Associate Professor of Library and Information Science, Wayne State University, Detroit, MI

Nancy Bulgarelli, William Beaumont Hospital Library, Royal Oak, MI

Karen Imarisio, Bloomfield Township Public Library, Bloomfield Township, MI

Karen Morgan, Mardigian Library, University of Michigan-Dearborn, Dearborn, MI

Rosemary Orlando, St. Clair Shores Public Library, St. Clair Shores, MI

Medical Consultant

Medical consultation services are provided to the *Teen Health Series* editors by David A. Cooke, M.D. Dr. Cooke is a graduate of Brandeis University, and he received his M.D. degree from the University of Michigan. He completed residency training at the University of Wisconsin Hospital and Clinics. He is board-certified in internal medicine. Dr. Cooke currently works as part of the University of Michigan Health System and practices in Ann Arbor, MI. In his free time, he enjoys writing, science fiction, and spending time with his family.

Part One

Maintaining Mental Wellness

Chapter 1

What Is Mental Health?

Mental health means striking a balance in all aspects of your life: social, physical, spiritual, economic and mental. Reaching a balance is a learning process. At times, you may tip the balance too much in one direction and have to find your footing again. Your personal balance will be unique, and your challenge will be to stay mentally healthy by keeping that balance.

This information has been prepared with some suggestions to help you strike and keep your balance.

Build A Healthy Self-Esteem

Self-esteem is more than just seeing your good qualities. It is being able to see all your abilities and weaknesses together, accepting them, and doing your best with what you have. For example, you may not play tennis well enough to be a star, but that should not stop you from enjoying the game.

Activity—Build Confidence: Take a good look at your good points. What do you do best? Where are your skills and interest areas? How would a friend describe you? Now, look at your weak points. What do you have difficulty doing? What things make you feel frustrated? Take a look at this list. Remember that all of us have our positive and negative sides. We let our strengths shine, and we build on our weak points to help us mature and grow.

Receive As Well As Give

Many of us confuse having a realistic view of our good points with conceit. We have trouble accepting kindness from others. We often shrug off a compliment with a, "Yes, but..." and put ourselves down.

Activity—Accept Compliments: The next time someone compliments you, say, "Thank you! I'm glad you think so." Then think about other compliments you have had, and how good they made you feel.

Create Positive Family Relationships

Work on building good family relationships. Learn to value each member's skills and abilities. Learn how to give and accept support.

Activity—Make Time: Make time just to be a family. Schedule time for both serious things and fun. Listen respectfully without interruption to what each person has to say. Do it frequently.

Make Friends Who Count

Friends help you understand that you are not alone. They help you by sharing your ups and downs, and you in turn help them. Together, you and your friends share life's challenges and celebrate life's joys.

Activity—Build A Friendship Tree: Keep in touch—invite a friend to lunch. Encourage new friendships—ask your friend to bring someone you have never met.

✎ What's It Mean?

Mental Health: Mental health is how a person thinks, feels, and acts when faced with life's situations. It is how people look at themselves, their lives, and the other people in their lives, evaluate their challenges and problems, and explore choices. This includes handling stress, relating to other people, and making decisions.

Excerpted from "Mental Health 101," Office of Minority Health, U.S. Department of Health and Human Services, July 8, 2008.

Figure Out Your Priorities

Advertisers try very hard to convince us that we "need" their products and services. Our challenge is to know the difference between our real needs (food, shelter, clothing, transportation) and our "wants" (bigger TV, new CD player, expensive fashions, flashy car), and to find the right balance in our spending. Financial problems cause stress; so it is important to avoid over-spending.

Activity—Create A Meaningful Budget: Write out a budget for yourself. Is it realistic? Have you planned what to do with the money left over for your "wants"? Which "wants" are most important to you?

Get Involved

Being involved in things that really matter to us provides a great feeling of purpose and satisfaction. You should always remember that you make a difference, no matter how big or small your efforts.

Activity—Volunteer, 'Be A Volunteer': Read to children at your local library; visit an elderly person at home or in hospital; serve on a committee of your favorite charity; organize a clean-up of a local park or beach; help a neighbor clean out his/her garage.

Learn To Manage Stress Effectively

Stress is a normal part of life. How you deal with it will depend on your attitude. You may become overwhelmed by things that other people deal with easily. Learning to keep a balance among work, family and leisure is difficult and needs skillful management of your time. Planning helps, and so does staying calm.

Activity—Take A Five-Minute Vacation: Each day, set aside five minutes for a mental health break. Close your door or go into another room, and day-dream about a place, person or idea, or think about nothing at all! You will feel like you have been on a mini-vacation.

Cope With Changes That Affect You

It would be nice to "live happily ever after", but real life keeps "throwing monkey-wrenches" at us. Coping with these unexpected (and often unwanted) changes can be stressful. Children have accidents, parents get ill, jobs disappear—we need to be flexible and learn ways to cope.

Activity—Find Strength In Numbers: Search out a support group that deals with the issues you are facing. By teaming up with people who share your problems, you may find a fresh solution. Try starting a group of your own by using the public service announcements in your local newspaper, radio station, or TV station.

Deal With Your Emotions

We are all challenged to find safe and constructive ways to express and share our feelings of anger, sadness, joy and fear. Your ways of experiencing and expressing emotions are unique because you are unique.

Activity—Identify And Deal With Your Moods: Find out what makes you happy, sad, joyful, or angry. What calms you down? Learn ways to deal with your moods. Share joyful news with a friend; "cry on a shoulder" when you feel blue. Physical exercise can help you deal with your anger. Keep a stack of your favorite funny cartoons or a collection of humorous stories or video tapes for times when you feel the need to laugh.

✔ Quick Tip

If you would like more information about mental health, you can contact a community organization, such as the Canadian Mental Health Association (www.cmha.ca), to help you find what you need to know. The Canadian Mental Health Association is a national voluntary association that exists to promote the mental health of all people. CMHA believes that everyone should have choices so that, when they need to, they can reach out to family, friends, formal services, self-help groups or community-based organizations.

Source: © 2009 Canadian Mental Health Association (www.cmha.ca). Reprinted with permission.

Have A Spirituality To Call Your Own

Learn to be at peace with yourself. Get to know who you are: what makes you really happy, what you are really passionate about. Learn to balance what you are able to change about yourself with what you cannot change. Get to know and trust your inner self.

Activity—Build Your Own "You": Set aside quiet, quality time to be totally alone. Do a breathing exercise—try counting your breaths from one to four, then start at one again. Or do something you love to do, like dancing, going to a baseball game, building a bird house, whatever works for you.

Chapter 2

Coping With Life's Challenges

My life seemed over. My family life was rapidly changing forever and there was nothing I could do to stop it. I never thought that the two people I loved most in the world would want to hurt me like that. How could MY parents of all people be getting a divorce? After the first few months went by, my mom told me we couldn't afford to stay in our home any longer. I didn't know what to say or even how to react. We had been in our house since I was born; my best friend lived next door. Now I had to start all over again and try to make new friends. I couldn't stand the pain I was going through, and felt like running away and hiding in a dark hole.

Dealing With Stressors

There are two ways to cope or deal with stressors: in a positive, or adaptive, way or in a negative, or maladaptive, way. Adaptive coping means dealing with the stressor effectively. Negative, or maladaptive coping, means ineffectively responding to stress, which often results in harm to oneself or others.

There are a variety of coping styles that people use when dealing with stressors. The three most effective styles in dealing with stress are:

- Confrontive coping;
- Supportant coping;
- Optimistic coping.

✤ It's A Fact!!

Coping Examples

Here are some examples of adaptive and maladaptive coping techniques:

Positive Examples Of Adaptive Coping

- Talking to parents or friends
- Exercise/sports
- Yoga/meditation
- Reading
- Problem-solving
- Thinking positive/being optimistic/using humor
- Listening to music
- Hobbies/recreation
- Journal/writing
- Hanging out with friends
- Praying/religious activities
- Social support/asking for help

Negative Examples Of Maladaptive Coping

- Smoking cigarettes
- Spending time alone/isolation/social withdrawal
- Avoiding problems
- Eating comfort foods (Often this is instead of eating a healthy diet or perhaps taking in excessive calories)
- Yelling or lashing out at others
- Physical fights

Coping Styles

There are many coping styles people use when dealing with stressors. Some are more effective than others.

- Using drugs
- Drinking alcohol
- Thrill-seeking (Putting yourself at risk or in danger to get a "high" or thrill)
- Binging/purging/restricting calories/eating disorders
- Physical self-abuse/mutilation (Defined as behaviors that deliberately cause harm to self without meaning to die. These behaviors are not suicidal but can occur with suicidal wishes. Behaviors can include burning, cutting, piercing with sharp objects, or hitting self. It does not include tattoos or socially accepted body piercing.)
- Self-criticism
- Wishful thinking (Energy is spent on wishing yourself out of the problem instead of thinking of ways to solve or respond to it. For instance, wishing you didn't have to go through this, wishing things were like they used to be, wishing you were someone else, or even wishing you were dead.)
- Blaming others (Perhaps as a way of saying you're not accountable if it's not your fault. However, even though you may not be at fault, it's still your responsibility to respond to the problem in a positive way. So, instead of looking for someone/something to blame, figure out what you need to do about it.)
- Resignation (Giving up or quit trying to work things out due to feeling very hopeless or helpless about your situation.)

Source: © 2009 Cincinnati Children's Hospital Medical Center.

Confrontive/Evasive Coping Styles

While talking on her cell phone, Sara accidentally backed her mother's brand new car into a light pole when pulling out of the restaurant parking lot. She is now faced with what to do about this. Below are examples describing the type of coping styles she may use in this situation.

Most Effective, Confrontive Coping: Confronting the problem head on or directly dealing with the problem. This could involve using a problem-solving technique.

Least Effective, Evasive Coping: Avoiding/running from the problem—in this case, Sara may take the car to a friend's house and avoid going home for the weekend.

Other avoidant activities could be: sleeping all the time, being a workaholic or just keeping busy, doing drugs or alcohol, or blaming others as a way to escape the problem or not being accountable. However, the problem really doesn't go away and things often become worse with this style of coping.

Problem-Solving Technique

- State the problem—Mom's brand new car is wrecked.
- Find solutions or ways to respond to problem: Option 1: Lie to mom about what happened; Option 2: Tell the truth about what happened; Option 3: Say nothing and act surprised when mom sees the damage.
- Carefully consider the pros (positive consequences) and cons (negative consequences) of your solution or response to the problem.
    - *Pros And Cons Of Option 1:* Pros—If you lie, maybe mom won't be as angry with you about the damage; you will be able to keep your cell phone; you won't lose driving privileges. Cons—Mom will be angrier with you if she learns the truth and will no longer trust you; you'll feel guilty for lying; you will definitely lose your cell phone and driving privileges if mom discovers the truth.
    - *Pros And Cons Of Option 2:* Pros—If you tell the truth, mom will trust you more for it, you won't feel guilty for lying, you'll feel better about yourself for doing what is right. Cons—You may

lose cell phone or driving privileges, but these punishments are temporary in nature.

- *Pros And Cons Of Option 3:* Pros—If you say nothing, you won't lose your cell phone. Cons—Mom may not believe you and be angrier; you still may lose driving privileges; you will lose mom's trust if she finds out the truth; you would definitely lose cell phone privileges for not being upfront about it.

Decide whether what you plan to do is right or wrong. If uncertain whether what you are doing is right or wrong, then ask yourself if you would still do this if others knew about it. If you wouldn't do it if others knew or found out about it, then don't do it! If your solution or approach is against your values or wrong to do, then don't do it.

Do the right thing. In this case, the only right thing to do is to tell the truth. At least you can earn back your privileges of using the car or you cell phone in time. It is more difficult, though, and may take a lot longer to earn someone's trust after you've betrayed their trust by lying.

Evaluate the outcome of your action. Did things get better? If the approach you are using doesn't work or improve the situation, then try something else. However, sometimes doing the right thing may seem to make things worse in the short run. However, in the long run, things will eventually work out and you will grow in the process. Sometimes, you just have to keep finding the next best thing to do until it finally gets resolved or settled.

Support/Self-Reliant Coping Styles

Katie began cutting herself when she was 12 years old. When her mother discovered this, she took her to see a psychologist who diagnosed her with major depression. She began therapy and was prescribed an antidepressant medication.

However, two years later, Katie began feeling numb and stopped taking her antidepressant medication without telling her parents or doctor. She then began cutting herself and tried to stop on her own, but continued to be tempted daily to do it again. She didn't know how to tell her parents or doctor about it and just wanted to run away to show them how she was feeling.

Most Effective, Supportant Coping

- *Asking for help:* Katie had already been seeing the school nurse for some headaches she had been having at school. This would have been a good time to tell the nurse about how she was feeling numb and stopped taking her medication. The nurse could have helped her talk to her mom about the problem before things became worse.
- *Talking to someone about your problems and feelings (i.e., a trusted adult or friend):* Katie had a good friend who she finally talked to about her thoughts of wanting to die. Her friend was able to convince her to tell someone who could help and offered to go with her to see the school nurse. The school nurse called Katie's mother who then took her to see a professional.
- *Religious activities:* Being actively involved in a youth group at church/synagogue; finding purpose and meaning in your life through your faith.
- *Support groups:* Joining a group of people in your age group who are sharing a similar problem as you. For example, there are support groups for children / teens who are grieving the loss of a loved one, have a drug or alcohol problem, or who have been abused.
- *Seeking professional help:* School nurse or counselor; physician—a family doctor or pediatrician; mental health professional—such as a psychiatrist, psychologist, or psychotherapist; clergy—a minister, rabbi, priest or youth minister.

Least Effective, Self-Reliant Coping

- *Does not work with depression/mental disorders*
- *Trying to "fix" the problem yourself:* Katie thought the medication wasn't helping her so she quit taking the antidepressant. After she quit taking the medication, she began cutting herself and tried to stop on her own. However, she continued to be tempted to cut herself and began feeling more depressed, as well as having thoughts of wanting to die. Her depression was getting worse.
- *Keeping problems/feelings to self:* Katie never told her parents how she felt, but just kept her problems and feelings a secret. Instead of talking to them, she wanted to run away to show them how she was feeling.

Optimistic/Fatalistic Coping Styles

It's important to remain optimistic in a crisis.

Tony, a 16-year-old teen, and two of his friends decided to go squirrel hunting one Saturday afternoon. Tony's friend, Matt, was directly behind him when he saw a squirrel running up a tree. He took a quick shot at it and ended up shooting Tony in the right side of his skull and ear. Tony had massive bleeding from the ear and head. His friends rushed him to the hospital where he was immediately taken to surgery. Tony needed multiple skin grafts to reconstruct the ear and was in a lot of pain. He ended up with permanent hearing loss and a continued loud ringing in the affected ear. Read in the examples below describing how Tony remained optimistic throughout his crisis.

Most Effective, Optimistic Coping

- *Looking at the bright side:* Tony realized he could have been killed or brain damaged if he had moved his head or body to the right when his friend pulled the trigger.
- *Using a sense of humor (Not sarcasm):* Although Tony was in a lot of pain, he joked about it. When asked by others what had happened, he replied, "Oh, my friend thought we were ear hunting." Humor does help people feel better by causing endorphins to be released into the bloodstream. These are the body's natural painkillers, which are also released during exercise.
- *Thinking positive—or being hopeful:* For example, although Tony didn't like the loud ringing in his ear, he was hopeful that he could find ways to adjust. For instance, he discovered the ringing wasn't as noticeable at bedtime when he had the radio on. Another way to be positive is to have an attitude of gratitude. Tony was actually thankful to be alive with no brain damage, which aided in his recovery.

Least Effective, Fatalistic Coping

- *Often used by depressed/suicidal teens.*
- *Pessimistic/negative thinking:* For instance, Tony could be resentful about his hearing loss and just constantly complain about the loud ringing.

He could also think that his life has been ruined because of his impairment. Your body is negatively affected by each negative thought you have. It is important to challenge negative thinking or add supportive statements to them.

- *Thinking there's no way out, feeling hopeless:* For example, Tony could have thought that he can't live the rest of his life with this hearing impairment and, as a result, end up with suicidal behaviors. However, although you may not be able to get out, around, or over a situation, you can always get through it. Often this may be with the help of other people.

Palliative Coping (Trying To Feel Better)

Megan and her mother got into an argument about Megan going to a friend's party. Megan blew up when her mom told her she was going to call and talk to the parents first. Mom then told her she wasn't going anywhere and sent her to her room. While in her room, Megan used various relaxation exercises to calm herself before trying to talk to her mother.

Palliative Coping, Healthy Ways

- *Eating a balanced diet.*
- *Exercise:* This conditions your body to better handle stress. Also, endorphins, the body's natural painkillers, are released when you exercise. This contributes to a sense of well-being. Regular exercise can help reduce feelings of stress, which means getting at least 45 minutes of some form of aerobic activity (dancing, walking briskly, bicycling, skating, dancing, basketball, jumping rope, etc.) four times a week.
- *Getting adequate sleep:* Studies show that teenagers need 9.2 hours of sleep each night. Most teenagers get less than 7.5 hours of sleep, which means most teenagers are sleep deprived. This sleep deprivation cannot be made up over the weekends. Studies show that teenagers who are sleep deprived have more depressive symptoms and more difficulty in schoolwork, as well as more accidents.
- *Using a journal/writing:* Expressing feelings by writing them down in a diary or journal.

- *Relaxing:* That is, listening to music or using techniques such as deep breathing; take a slow deep breath while counting to six, hold it to a count of four, and then breathe out slowly to a count of six; will decrease the urge to yell at someone.
- *Progressive muscle relaxation* (tensing and then relaxing muscle groups): Start with muscle groups below, such as toes and feet, and work up to legs, then buttocks, abdomen, and finally ending with neck and facial muscles. Tense or tighten the muscle group while taking a deep breath, hold until a count of four and then relax and breathe out. Do exercise twice before going to next muscle group. Practice whenever feeling tense or stressed
- *Imagery:* Go to your "happy place." When thinking of a calm, happy place, activate the senses. Imagine what you see, hear, taste and feel while there. If imagining walking on a beach, think how it feels when the waves gently touch your feet, the smell of the ocean, the sound of the ocean's roar, the taste of the salty water, and etc.
- *Meditation* (clearing your thoughts): Start with your body being in a comfortable position and in a quiet area. Practice deep-breathing while focusing on a relaxing word, inspirational verse, a sound (like a hum), or relaxing image to keep other thoughts out. This takes practice, if you detect other thoughts coming in your mind, just focus more intensely on that word, verse, sound, or image you decided upon.

Unhealthy Ways

- *Self-medicating* with drugs/alcohol
- *Self-mutilation:* Defined as behaviors that deliberately cause harm to self without meaning to die. These behaviors are not suicidal but can occur with suicidal wishes. Behaviors can include burning, cutting, piercing with sharp objects or hitting self. It does not include tattoos or socially accepted body piercing.

Emotive Coping

After getting over the shock of hearing the news that their best friend was killed in an accident, John and Ricky became angry. Both boys were outside standing next to John's car and were so upset that they wanted to punch something. They then began to punch John's car. John ended up wearing a cast to the funeral after fracturing his wrist during the episode.

Emotive Coping, Healthy Examples

- *Letting off steam:* The best way to let off steam is to exercise. Running, jogging, working out, and/or weight-training are alternate ways to let off steam. However, safety measures should be used at these times to avoid injury. For example, some safety measures could include having a spotter available when lifting weights or wearing gloves when hitting a punching bag.

Emotive Coping, Unhealthy Examples

- *Yelling*
- *Hitting*
- *Risk-taking:* Road rage is an example of people becoming angry on the highway and taking excessive risks to let off steam.

✔ Quick Tip

The promotion of regular sleep is known as sleep hygiene. The following is a list of sleep hygiene tips which can be used to improve sleep.

1. Avoid caffeinated drinks after lunch.
2. Avoid bright light in the evening.
3. Avoid arousing activities around bedtime (for example, heavy study, text messaging, getting into prolonged conversations).
4. Expose yourself to bright light upon awakening in the morning.
5. While sleeping in on weekends is permissible, it should not be more than 2–3 hours past your usual wake time, to avoid disrupting your circadian rhythm governing sleepiness and wakefulness.
6. Avoid pulling an "all-nighter" to study.

Source: Excerpted from "Sleep Hygiene Tips," Centers for Disease Control and Prevention (www.cdc.gov), September 10, 2007.

Chapter 3

Resilience For Teens: Got Bounce?

The ads make it look so easy to be a teen—everyone seems to be laughing, hanging out with friends, wearing exactly the right clothes. But if you're a young adult, you know that life can be pretty tough sometimes. You may face problems ranging from being bullied to the death of a friend or parent. Why is it that sometimes people can go through really rough times and still bounce back? The difference is that those who bounce back are using the skills of resilience.

The good news is that resilience isn't something you're born with or not—the skills of resilience can be learned. Resilience—the ability to adapt well in the face of hard times; disasters like hurricanes, earthquakes or fires; tragedy; threats; or even high stress—is what makes some people seem like they've "got bounce" while others don't.

What are some tips that can help you learn to be resilient? As you use these tips, keep in mind that each person's journey along the road to resilience will be different—what works for you may not work for your friends.

10 Tips To Build Resilience

1. Get Together: Talk with your friends and, yes, even with your parents. Understand that your parents may have more life experience than you do, even if it seems they never were your age. They may be afraid for you if you're going through really tough times and it may be harder for them to talk about it than it is for you! Don't be afraid to express your opinion, even if your parent or friend takes the opposite view. Ask questions and listen to the answers. Get connected to your community, whether it's as part of a church group or a high school group.

2. Cut Yourself Some Slack: When something bad happens in your life, the stresses of whatever you're going through may heighten daily stresses. Your emotions might already be all over the map because of hormones and physical changes; the uncertainty during a tragedy or trauma can make these shifts seem more extreme. Be prepared for this and go a little easy on yourself, and on your friends.

3. Create A Hassle-Free Zone: Make your room or apartment a "hassle-free zone"—not that you keep everyone out, but home should be a haven free from stress and anxieties. But understand that your parents and siblings may have their own stresses if something serious has just happened in your life and may want to spend a little more time than usual with you.

4. Stick To The Program: Spending time in high school or on a college campus means more choices; so let home be your constant. During a time of major stress, map out a routine and stick to it. You may be doing all kinds of new things, but don't forget the routines that give you comfort, whether it's the things you do before class, going out to lunch, or have a nightly phone call with a friend.

5. Take Care Of Yourself: Be sure to take care of yourself—physically, mentally, and spiritually. And get sleep. If you don't, you may be more grouchy and nervous at a time when you have to stay sharp. There's a lot going on, and it's going to be tough to face if you're falling asleep on your feet.

6. Take Control: Even in the midst of tragedy, you can move toward goals one small step at a time. During a really hard time, just getting out of bed and going to school may be all you can handle, but even accomplishing that can help. Bad times make us feel out of control—grab some of that control back by taking decisive action.

7. Express Yourself: Tragedy can bring up a bunch of conflicting emotions, but sometimes, it's just too hard to talk to someone about what you're feeling. If talking isn't working, do something else to capture your emotions like start a journal, or create art.

8. Help Somebody: Nothing gets your mind off your own problems like solving someone else's. Try volunteering in your community or at your school, cleaning up around the house or apartment, or helping a friend with his or her homework.

9. Put Things In Perspective: The very thing that has you stressed out may be all anyone is talking about now. But eventually, things change and bad times end. If you're worried about whether you've got what it takes to get through this, think back on a time when you faced up to your fears, whether it was asking someone on a date or applying for a job. Learn some relaxation techniques, whether it's thinking of a particular song in times of stress, or just taking a deep breath to calm down. Think about the important things that have stayed the same, even while the outside world is changing. When you talk about bad times, make sure you talk about good times as well.

10. Turn It Off: You want to stay informed—you may even have homework that requires you to watch the news. But sometimes, the news, with its focus on the sensational, can add to the feeling that nothing is going right. Try to limit the amount of news you take in, whether it's from television, newspapers or magazines, or the internet. Watching a news report once informs you; watching it over and over again just adds to the stress and contributes no new knowledge.

You can learn resilience. But just because you learn resilience doesn't mean you won't feel stressed or anxious. You might have times when you aren't happy—and that's OK. Resilience is a journey, and each person will take his or her own time along the way. You may benefit from some of the resilience tips above, while some of your friends may benefit from others. The skills of resilience you learn during really bad times will be useful even after the bad times end, and they are good skills to have every day. Resilience can help you be one of the people who've "got bounce."

✔ Quick Tip

For More Help

Developing resilience is a personal journey. If you're stuck or overwhelmed and unable to use the tips listed above, you may want to consider talking to someone who can help, such as a psychologist or other mental health professional. A psychologist can help you cope with many of life's problems. The American Psychological Association does not provide referral services. For a referral to a psychologist in your area call 1-800-964-2000. The operator will use your zip code to locate and connect you with the referral system in your area.

Turning to someone for guidance may help you strengthen resilience and persevere during times of stress or trauma. Information contained in this chapter should not be used as a substitute for professional health and mental health care or consultation. Individuals who believe they may need or benefit from care should consult a psychologist or other licensed health/mental health professional.

The American Psychological Association Practice Directorate gratefully acknowledges the following contributors to this publication:

Mary K. Alvord, Ph.D., Director, Group Therapy Center at Alvord, Baker, and Associates, LLC, Silver Spring, MD

Robin Gurwitch, Ph.D., University of Oklahoma Health Sciences Center

Jana Martin, Ph.D., private practice, Long Beach, CA; 2003 President of the California Psychological Association.

Ronald S. Palomares, Ph.D., Assistant Executive Director, Practice, American Psychological Association

Chapter 4

Building Healthy Self-Esteem

Introduction

Most people feel bad about themselves from time to time. Feelings of low self-esteem may be triggered by being treated poorly by someone else recently or in the past or by a person's own judgments of him or herself. This is normal. However, low self-esteem is a constant companion for too many people, especially those who experience depression, anxiety, phobias, psychosis, delusional thinking or who have an illness or a disability. If you are one of these people, you may go through life feeling bad about yourself needlessly. Low self-esteem keeps you from enjoying life, doing the things you want to do, and working toward personal goals.

You have a right to feel good about yourself. However, it can be very difficult to feel good about yourself when you are under the stress of having symptoms that are hard to manage, when you are dealing with a disability, when you are having a difficult time, or when others are treating you badly. At these times, it is easy to be drawn into a downward spiral of lower and lower self-esteem. For instance, you may begin feeling bad about yourself when someone insults you, you are under a lot of pressure, or you are having

About This Chapter: Text in this chapter is excerpted from "Building Self-Esteem: A Self-Help Guide," Substance Abuse and Mental Health Services Administration (SAMHSA), 2002. Reviewed for currency by David A. Cooke, MD, FACP, October 2009.

a difficult time getting along with someone in your family. Then you begin to give yourself negative self-talk, like "I'm no good." That may make you feel so bad about yourself that you do something to hurt yourself or someone else. The ideas in this chapter will discuss things you can do to feel better about yourself—to raise your self-esteem.

As you begin to work on improving your self-esteem, you may notice that you have some feelings of resistance to positive feelings about yourself. This is normal. Don't let these feelings stop you from feeling good about yourself. They will diminish as you feel better and better about yourself.

Self-Esteem, Depression And Other Illnesses

Before you begin to consider strategies and activities to help raise your self-esteem, it is important to remember that low self-esteem may be due to depression. Low self-esteem is a symptom of depression. To make things even more complicated, the depression may be a symptom of some other illness.

✎ What's It Mean?

Self-Confidence: Self-confidence is having a positive and realistic opinion of yourself and being able to accurately measure your abilities. Self-confidence is also an important part of feeling good about yourself. Self-confidence is that little voice inside of you that tells you that you are okay, that you are a good person, and that you know how to deal with things in good times and in bad.

Self-Esteem: Self-esteem describes the value and respect you have for yourself. If you have a healthy self-esteem, you feel good about yourself as a person and are proud of what you can do. However, it is normal to feel down sometimes. Having a healthy or high self-esteem can help you to think positively, deal better with stress, and boost your drive to work hard. Having low self-esteem can cause you to feel uneasy and may get in the way of doing things you might enjoy. For some, low self-esteem can contribute to serious problems such as depression, drug and alcohol use, and eating disorders.

Source: Excerpted from "Your Emotions," U.S. Department of Health and Human Services (www.girlshealth.gov), June 11, 2008.

✤ It's A Fact!!

Part of being a teen is having thoughts and feelings about different parts of your life, such as how you feel about your friends and other kids your age, how you are doing in school and in other activities, your parents, or the way you look.

While having these new feelings, many changes are also taking place in your body. It is normal to feel self-conscious or shy about the changes in your body and emotions but there are also changes to celebrate. Some cultures even have celebrations to recognize these changes. For example, the Western Apaches have the Sunrise Dance or "Na'ii'ees" and the Jewish community has the Bar/Bat Mitzvah. Even though it might seem tough sometimes, remember that you are absolutely great!

Source: Excerpted from "Your Emotions," U.S. Department of Health and Human Services (www.girlshealth.gov), June 11, 2008.

Have you felt sad consistently for several weeks but don't know why you are feeling so sad, that is nothing terribly bad has happened, or maybe something bad has happened but you haven't been able to get rid of the feelings of sadness? Is this accompanied by other changes, like wanting to eat all the time or having no appetite, wanting to sleep all the time or waking up very early and not being able to get back to sleep?

If you answered yes to either question, there are two things you need to do:

- See your doctor for a physical examination to determine the cause of your depression and to discuss treatment choices.
- Do some things that will help you to feel better right away like eating well, getting plenty of exercise and outdoor light, spending time with good friends, and doing fun things like going to a movie, painting a picture, playing a musical instrument, or reading a good book.

✔ Quick Tip

Test Your Self-Esteem

If you have high or healthy self-esteem, you will agree with the following statements:

- I feel good about who I am.
- I am proud of what I can do, but I do not show off.
- I know there are some things that I am good at and some things I need to improve.
- I am responsible for the things I do and say, both good and bad.
- It is okay if I win or if I lose.
- Before I do something, I usually think "I can do it."

If you have low or poor self-esteem, you might agree with the following statements:

- I can't do anything right.
- I am ugly or dumb.
- I do not have any friends.
- I do not like to try new things.
- It really upsets me to make mistakes.
- I do not think I am as nice, pretty, or smart as the other people in my class.
- I have a hard time making friends.
- I have a hard time making friends because I end up getting angry and fighting with people.
- It makes me uncomfortable when people say nice things about me.
- Sometimes I feel better if I say mean things to other people.

Source: Excerpted from "Your Emotions," U.S. Department of Health and Human Services (www.girlshealth.gov), June 11, 2008.

Things You Can Do Right Away—Every Day—To Raise Your Self-Esteem

Pay attention to your own needs and wants. Listen to what your body, your mind, and your heart are telling you. For instance, if your body is telling you that you have been sitting down too long, stand up and stretch. If your heart is longing to spend more time with a special friend, do it. If your mind is telling you to clean up your room, listen to your favorite music, or stop thinking bad thoughts about yourself, take those thoughts seriously.

Take very good care of yourself. As you have been growing up you may not have learned how to take good care of yourself. In fact, much of your attention may have been on taking care of others, on just getting by, or on "behaving well." Begin today to take good care of yourself. Treat yourself as a wonderful parent would treat a small child or as one very best friend might treat another. If you work at taking good care of yourself, you will find that you feel better about yourself. Here are some ways to take good care of yourself:

- Eat healthy foods and avoid junk foods.
- Exercise.
- Do personal hygiene tasks that make you feel better about yourself.
- Have a physical examination every year to make sure you are in good health.
- Plan fun activities for yourself. Learn new things every day.

Take time to do things you enjoy. You may be so busy, or feel so badly about yourself, that you spend little or no time doing things you enjoy—things like playing a musical instrument, doing a craft project, flying a kite, or going fishing. Make a list of things you enjoy doing. Then do something from that list every day. Add to the list anything new that you discover you enjoy doing.

Get something done that you have been putting off. Clean out that closet. Do that homework. Write that letter. Begin doing those things that you know will make you feel better about yourself—like going on a diet, beginning an exercise program, or keeping your living space clean.

✔ Quick Tip

Test Your Self-Confidence

If you have high self-confidence, you will agree with the following statements:

- I am eager to learn new things.
- I take pride in doing a good job and being a nice person.
- I can handle criticism without being too emotional.
- I know what things I am good at, and those that I'm not.
- It is okay if I win or if I lose.
- Before I do something, I usually think "I can do it."
- I like to try to do things without help, but I don't mind asking for help if I really need it.
- I like myself.

If you have low self-confidence, you might agree with the following statements:

- I do not like to try new things.
- I can't do anything right.
- If my friends criticize me, or if my teacher corrects a lot on my homework, I get very upset.
- I don't know what I am good at.
- I have a hard time meeting new people or making friends.
- I am embarrassed to ask a question or speak up in class.
- Before I do something, I may think "I can't do it."
- I don't like to try new things unless someone shows me how to do it first.
- I don't like myself.

Source: Excerpted from "Your Emotions," U.S. Department of Health and Human Services (www.girlshealth.gov), June 11, 2008.

Do things that make use of your own special talents and abilities. For instance, if you are good with your hands, then make things for yourself, family, and friends. If you like animals, consider having a pet or at least playing with friends' pets.

✤ It's A Fact!!
Body Image And Eating Disorders

Have you ever thought that there was something wrong with the way you look? Do you think that you are too short or too tall, too heavy or too skinny?

If you have had thoughts like these, you are not alone. These feelings about how you look are called body image. Body image and self-esteem are tied together since body image can affect how you feel about your whole self. When you put yourself down about how you look, it can lead to negative feelings about yourself in general. Poor self-esteem can also lead to eating disorders that can put your health in danger.

If you start to have negative thoughts about your body and the way you look, think about all of the traits that make you special and unique. Look at your whole self—body and mind—in a positive way and write down what you see. Need a hand getting started? Focus on the good things in your life by using the girlshealth.gov Just 4Me log (www.girlshealth.gov/emotions/feelinggood/just4me.cfm.)

Or before you go to bed at night, name three things you did that day that made you happy. By focusing on the positive aspects of your life you can feel more positive about yourself! Don't forget to give yourself compliments too! Say it out loud when the day is done! Like, "Today I played my best in our soccer game," or "My family loved the dessert I made tonight!" or "My friends really liked the jokes I told them."

If you are struggling with an eating disorder or just can't seem to feel better, talk to an adult you trust right away.

Remember: You are beautiful! You are one of a kind! Real beauty comes from inside!

Source: Excerpted from "Your Emotions: Body Image and Eating Disorders," U.S. Department of Health and Human Services (www.girlshealth.gov), March 28, 2008.

Dress in clothes that make you feel good about yourself. If you have little money to spend on new clothes, check out thrift stores in your area.

Give yourself rewards—you are a great person. Listen to a CD or tape. Make it a point to treat yourself well every day. Before you go to bed each night, write about how you treated yourself well during the day.

Spend time with people who make you feel good about yourself—people who treat you well. Avoid people who treat you badly. Do something nice for another person. Smile at someone who looks sad. Say a few kind words to the check-out cashier. Help your sibling or friend with an unpleasant chore. Send a card to an acquaintance. Volunteer for a worthy organization.

Make your living space a place that honors the person you are. If you share your room with others, see if you can work out a way to have some space that is just for you—a place where you can keep your things and know that they will not be disturbed and that you can decorate any way you choose. Display items that you find attractive or that remind you of your achievements or of special times or people in your life. If cost is a factor, use your creativity to think of inexpensive or free ways that you can add to the comfort and enjoyment of your space.

Make your meals a special time. Talk to your family about turning off the television, radio, and stereo. Encourage discussion of pleasant topics. Avoid discussing difficult issues at meals. Set the table, even if you are eating alone. Light a candle or put some flowers or an attractive object in the center of the table. Arrange your food in an attractive way on your plate.

Take advantage of opportunities to learn something new or improve your skills. Take a class or go to a seminar. For programs that are costly, ask about a possible scholarship or fee reduction.

Changing Negative Thoughts About Yourself To Positive Ones

You may be giving yourself negative messages about yourself. Many people do. These are messages that you learned when you were younger. You learned from many different sources including other children, your teachers, family members, caregivers, even from the media, and from prejudice and stigma in our society.

Some examples of common negative messages that people repeat over and over to themselves include: "I am a jerk," "I am a loser," "I never do anything right," "No one would ever like me," I am a klutz." Most people believe these messages, no matter how untrue or unreal they are. They come up immediately in the right circumstance, for instance if you get a wrong answer you think "I am so stupid." They may include words like should, ought, or must. The messages tend to imagine the worst in everything, especially you, and they are hard to turn off or unlearn.

Develop positive statements you can say to yourself to replace negative thoughts whenever you notice yourself thinking them. You can't think two thoughts at the same time. When you are thinking a positive thought about yourself, you can't be thinking a negative one. In developing these thoughts, use positive words like happy, peaceful, loving, enthusiastic, warm.

Avoid using negative words such as worried, frightened, upset, tired, bored, not, never, and can't. Don't make a statement like "I am not going to worry any more." Instead say "I focus on the positive" or whatever feels right to you. Substitute "it would be nice if" for "should." Always use the present tense, for example, "I am healthy, I am well, I am happy" as if the condition already exists. Use I, me, or your own name.

You can do this by folding a piece of paper in half the long way to make two columns. In one column write your negative thought and in the other column write a positive thought that contradicts the negative thought as shown on the next page. See the examples in Table 4.1.

You can work on changing your negative thoughts to positive ones with these tips:

- Replace the negative thought with the positive one every time you realize you are thinking the negative thought.
- Repeat your positive thought over and over to yourself, out loud whenever you get a chance and even sharing them with another person if possible.

Table 4.1. Examples Of Negative And Positive Thoughts

Negative Thought	Positive Thought
I am not worth anything.	I am a valuable person.
I have never accomplished anything.	I have accomplished many things.
I always make mistakes.	I do many things well.
I am a jerk.	I am a great person.
I don't deserve a good life.	I deserve to be happy and healthy.
I am stupid.	I am smart.

✔ Quick Tip
Celebrate Your Identity

Celebrate your uniqueness and share it with others. Make understanding your identity part of your efforts to build self-esteem and self-confidence. Don't be afraid to show your differences, and explain them to friends, classmates, teachers, and others. At the same time, be open to the differences of others. Acceptance of others is an important part of the great diversity we enjoy in the United States.

Source: Excerpted from "Your Emotions," U.S. Department of Health and Human Services (www.girlshealth.gov), June 11, 2008.

- Write your positive thoughts over and over.
- Make signs that say the positive thought. Hang them in places where you will see them often—like on the refrigerator door or on the mirror in your bathroom—and repeat the thought to yourself several times when you see it.

As you work on building your self-esteem you will notice that you feel better more and more often, that you are enjoying your life more than you did before, and that you are doing more of the things you have always wanted to do.

Chapter 5

Coping With Stress

Questions And Answers About Stress

What is stress?

Stress is what you feel when you react to pressure from others or from yourself. Pressure can come from anywhere, including school, work, activities, friends, and family members. You can also feel stress from the pressure of wanting to get good grades or wanting to feel like you belong. Stress comes in many forms and everyone feels stress.

How does my body handle stress?

Your body has a built-in response to handle stress. When something stressful happens, you may experience sweaty palms, dry mouth, or knots in your stomach. This is totally normal and means that your body is working exactly as it should. Other signs of stress include emotional signs such as feeling sad or worried, behavioral (your actions) signs such as not feeling up to doing things, and mental (your mind) signs such as not being able to concentrate or focus.

About This Chapter: This chapter begins with "Questions And Answers About Stress," excerpted from "Your Emotions: Handling Stress," U.S. Department of Health and Human Services (www.girlshealth.gov), June 11, 2008. Text under the heading "Stress-Busting Tips" is from "Feelin' Frazzled...?" BAM! Body and Mind, Centers for Disease Control and Prevention, 2003. Reviewed for currency by David A. Cooke, MD, FACP, October 2009.

What causes stress?

Just being a teen can be stressful—there is so much going on and so many changes that are happening all at once! Some specific things that might cause stress include the following:

- School work
- Not feeling good about yourself
- Changes in your body or weight
- Body shape or size
- Problems with friends, boyfriends, or other kids at school
- Living in a dangerous neighborhood

What's It Mean?

What Is Short-Term Stress?

Have you ever started a new school, argued with your best friend, or moved? Do you have to deal with the ups and downs of daily life—like homework or your parents' expectations? Then you already know about stress. In fact, everyone experiences stress. Your body is pre-wired to deal with it—whether it is expected or not. This response is known as the stress response, or fight or flight.

The fight or flight response is as old as the hills. In fact, when people used to have to fight off wild animals to survive, fight or flight is what helped them do it. Today, different things cause stress (when was the last time you had to fend off a grizzly bear?), but we still go through fight or flight. It prepares us for quick action—which is why the feeling goes away once whatever was stressing you out passes! It can also happen when something major happens—like if you change schools or have a death in your family.

Everyone has weird feelings when they are stressed. Fight or flight can cause things like sweaty palms or a dry mouth when you are nervous, or knots in your stomach after an argument with someone. This is totally normal and means that your body is working exactly like it should. There are lots of signs of stress—common types are physical (butterflies in your stomach), emotional (feeling sad or worried), behavioral (you don't feel like doing things), and mental

- Peer pressure from friends to dress or act a certain way, or smoke, drink, or use drugs
- Not fitting in or being part of a group
- Moving or friends moving away
- Separation or divorce of parents
- A family member who is ill
- Death of a loved one
- Changing schools
- Taking on too many activities at once
- Not getting along with your parents or having problems at home

(you can't concentrate). Most physical signs of stress usually don't last that long and can help you perform better, if you manage them right.

So, when you feel stress, what happens to make your body do the things it does? According to the experts, three glands "go into gear" and work together to help you cope with change or a stressful situation. Two are in your brain and are called the hypothalamus (hipe-o-thal-a-mus) and the pituitary (pi-to-i-tary) gland. The third, the adrenal (a-dree-nal) glands, are on top of your kidneys. The hypothalamus signals your pituitary gland that it is time to tell your adrenal glands to release the stress hormones called epinephrine (ep-in-efrin), norepinephrine (nor-ep-in-efrin), and cortisol (cor-ti-sol). These chemicals increase your heart rate and breathing and provide a burst of energy—which is useful if you're trying to run away from a bear! These chemicals can also control body temperature (which can make you feel hot or cold), keep you from getting hungry, and make you less sensitive to pain. Because everyone is different, everyone will have different signs. Not to worry—everyone experiences these physical signs of stress sometimes. The good news is that, once things return to normal, your body will turn off the stress response. After some rest and relaxation, you'll be good as new.

Source: From "Got Butterflies? Find Out Why," BAM! Body and Mind, Centers for Disease Control and Prevention, 2003. Reviewed for currency by David A. Cooke, MD, FACP, October 2009.

- Feeling lonely

There may be other things that cause stress for you that are not on this list. Also, it can be very tough when more than one stressful event happens at the same time or stress is ongoing.

Is stress always a bad thing?

No! A little bit of stress can work in a positive way. For instance, during a sports competition, stress might push you to perform better. Also, without the stress of deadlines, you might not be able to finish schoolwork or get to where you need to be on time.

The following items, however, can be signs that you have too much stress or are stressed out:

- Feeling down, edgy, guilty, or tired
- Having headaches or stomachaches
- Having trouble sleeping
- Laughing or crying for no reason
- Blaming others for bad things that happen to you
- Wanting to be alone all the time (withdrawal)
- Not being able to see the positive side of a situation
- Not enjoying activities that you used to enjoy
- Feeling resentful of people or things you have to do
- Feeling like you have too many things you have to do

Some of these signs can also be signs of a more serious condition called depression. For more information about depression, see the chapter titled "Depression," or talk to your health care provider.

Are you stressed about your body?

During adolescence, your body is going through many changes that are happening at a fast pace. These changes might make you feel unsure of yourself at times, or stressed. They might make you worry about your size and wanting to fit in with the rest of the crowd.

During puberty, not only will you get taller, you will also see other changes in your body because your body is starting to produce new hormones. Try not to worry! Each person changes at her own pace and all of these new changes are normal. While you are experiencing these changes keep your self-confidence up by taking good care of yourself, eating healthy foods and getting regular exercise.

What kinds of things cause stress?

Different people are stressed by different things. For example, you might get upset or stressed when you don't make good grades but your friend might not. You might be able to handle doing homework and being involved in

✎ What's It Mean?

What Is Long-Term Stress?

What happens when life continues to throw curves at you and if you have one stressful event after another? Your stress response may not be able to stop itself from running overtime, and you may not have a chance to rest, restore, and recuperate. This can add up and, suddenly, the signs of overload hit you—turning short-term stressors into long-term stress. This means that you may have even more physical signs of stress. Things like a headache, eating too much or not at all, tossing and turning all night, or feeling down and angry all the time, are all signs of long-term stress. These signs start when you just can't deal with any more.

Long-term stress can affect your health and how you feel about yourself, so it is important to learn to deal with it. No one is completely free of stress and different people respond to it in lots of different ways. The most important thing to learn about long-term stress is how to spot it. You can do that by listening to your body signals and learning healthy ways to handle it.

Source: From "Got Butterflies? Find Out Why," BAM! Body and Mind, Centers for Disease Control and Prevention, 2003. Reviewed for currency by David A. Cooke, MD, FACP, October 2009.

after-school activities but your sister or friend might feel they can't do both. Your friend might see moving to a new house as a stress but you might view it as an adventure.

How can you deal with the stress of a disaster, or a violent or tragic event?

Sometimes we are part of or have lived through a very stressful event such as a hurricane, a serious car accident, or an assault, like date rape. These kind of scary events can cause a very strong stress reaction in the victims but the reactions may be different for each person. Some become cranky or depressed; others can't sleep or have nightmares, some may keep reliving the experience, some might experience nervousness and their hearts might race, and some people put the event out of their minds. Feelings that lead to this type of stress include fear, a sense that your life is in danger, helplessness or horror.

You don't have to be hurt to experience this type of stress, You can simply be a witness to the event or be threatened with physical harm to have this type of stressful reaction.

Whether or not you were directly affected by a traumatic event, it is normal to feel nervous about your own safety and wonder how you would react in an emergency. Here are some things you can do to handle this special kind of stress:

- You may think it feels better to pretend the event did not happen, but it is best to be honest about how you are feeling. Ignoring or hiding your feelings can be worse for your health in the long run. It is okay to feel scared and uncertain.
- Try to remember that, while you might feel like a changed person and everything seems off balance right now, your life will calm down and you will find a new normal groove.
- Talk to a teacher, your parents, or a counselor about your sadness, anger, and other emotions. It can be tough to get started, but it is important to confide in someone you trust with your thoughts and feelings.
- It is common to want to strike back at people who have caused you or those you love great pain. This feeling is normal, but it is important to

understand that it is useless to respond with more violence. Nothing good can come from using hateful words or actions.

- While you will always remember and feel changed by the event, the feelings will become less painful over time. In learning to cope with tragedy, you will become stronger and better at handling stressful situations. You may also find yourself appreciating life and the people you love even more.

Can stress lead to more serious problems?

Yes! Struggling with major stress and low self-esteem issues can contribute to more serious problems such as eating disorders, hurting yourself, depression, alcohol and drug abuse, and even suicide. Continued depression and thoughts about hurting or killing yourself are signs that it is time to seek help. Talk to an adult you trust right away!

Stress-Busting Tips

Put your body in motion. Moving from the chair to the couch while watching TV is not being physically active! Physical activity is one of the most important ways to keep stress away by clearing your head and lifting your spirits. Physical activity also increases endorphin levels—the natural "feel-good" chemicals in the body which leave you with a naturally happy feeling.

Whether you like full-fledged games of football, tennis, or roller hockey, or you prefer walks with family and friends, it's important to get up, get out, and get moving!

Fuel up. Start your day off with a full tank—eating breakfast will give you the energy you need to tackle the day. Eating regular meals (this means no skipping dinner) and taking time to enjoy them (nope, eating in the car on the way to practice doesn't count) will make you feel better too.

Make sure to fuel up with fruits, vegetables, proteins (peanut butter, a chicken sandwich, or a tuna salad) and grains (wheat bread, pasta, or some crackers)—these will give you the power you need to make it through those hectic days.

Don't be fooled by the jolt of energy you get from sodas and sugary snacks—this only lasts a short time, and once it wears off, you may feel sluggish and more tired than usual. For that extra boost of energy to sail through history notes, math class, and after school activities, grab a banana, some string cheese, or a granola bar for some power-packed energy!

LOL! Some say that laughter is the best medicine—well, in many cases, it is! Did you know that it takes 15 facial muscles to laugh? Lots of laughin' can make you feel good—and, that good feeling can stay with you even after the laughter stops. So, head off stress with regular doses of laughter by watching a funny movie or cartoons, reading a joke book (you may even learn some new jokes), or even make up your own riddles… laughter can make you feel like a new person!

♣ It's A Fact!!

Discovery Of Resistance Mechanisms In Mouse Brain May Lead To Help For Stress-Related Mental Illness In Humans

Results of a new study may one day help scientists learn how to enhance a naturally occurring mechanism in the brain that promotes resilience to psychological stress. Researchers funded by the National Institutes of Health's National Institute of Mental Health (NIMH) found that, in a mouse model, the ability to adapt to stress is driven by a distinctly different molecular mechanism than is the tendency to be overwhelmed by stress. The researchers mapped out the mechanisms—components of which also are present in the human brain—that govern both kinds of responses.

In humans, stress can play a major role in the development of several mental illnesses, including post-traumatic stress disorder and depression. A key question in mental health research is: Why are some people resilient to stress, while others are not? This research indicates that resistance is not simply a passive absence of vulnerability mechanisms, as was previously thought; it is a biologically active process that results in specific adaptations in the brain's response to stress.

Results of the study were published online in *Cell*, on October 18, 2007, by Vaishnav Krishnan, Ming-Hu Han, PhD, Eric J. Nestler, MD, PhD, and colleagues from the University of Texas Southwestern Medical Center, Harvard University, and Cornell University.

Excerpted from "Stress: Brain Yields Clues About Why Some Succumb While Others Prevail," National Institute of Mental Health, press release dated October 18, 2007.

Everyone has those days when they do something really silly or stupid—instead of getting upset with yourself, laugh out loud! No one's perfect! Life should be about having fun. So, lighten up!

Have fun with friends. Being with people you like is always a good way to ditch your stress. Get a group together to go to the movies, shoot some hoops, or play a board game—or just hang out and talk. Friends can help you work through your problems and let you see the brighter side of things.

Spill to someone you trust. Instead of keeping your feelings bottled up inside, talk to someone you trust or respect about what's bothering you. It could be a friend, a parent, someone in your family, or a teacher. Talking out your problems and seeing them from a different view might help you figure out ways to deal with them. Just remember, you don't have to go it alone!

Take time to chill. Pick a comfy spot to sit and read, daydream, or even take a snooze. Listen to your favorite music. Work on a relaxing project like putting together a puzzle or making jewelry.

Stress can sometimes make you feel like a tight rubber band—stretched to the limit! If this happens, take a few deep breaths to help yourself unwind. If you're in the middle of an impossible homework problem, take a break! Finding time to relax after (and sometimes during) a hectic day or week can make all the difference.

Catch some *zzzzz*. Fatigue is a best friend to stress. When you don't get enough sleep, it's hard to deal with things—you may feel tired, cranky, or you may have trouble thinking clearly. When you're overtired, a problem may seem much bigger than it actually is. You may have a hard time doing a school assignment that usually seems easy, you don't do your best in sports or any physical activity, or you may have an argument with your friends over something really stupid.

Sleep is a big deal! Getting the right amount of sleep is especially important for kids your age. Because your body (and mind) is changing and developing, it requires more sleep to re-charge for the next day. So don't resist, hit the hay!

Keep a journal. If you're having one of those crazy days when nothing goes right, it's a good idea to write things down in a journal to get it off of your chest—like how you feel, what's going on in your life, and things you'd like to accomplish. You could even write down what you do when you're faced with a stressful situation, and then look back and think about how you handled it later. So, find a quiet spot, grab a notebook and pen, and start writing!

Get it together. Too much to do but not enough time? Forgot your homework? Feeling overwhelmed or discombobulated? Being unprepared for school, practice, or other activities can make for a very stressful day! Getting everything done can be a challenge, but all you have to do is plan a little and get organized.

Lend a hand. Get involved in an activity that helps others. It's almost impossible to feel stressed out when you're helping someone else. It's also a great way to find out about yourself and the special qualities you never knew you had! Signing up for a service project is a good idea, but helping others is as easy as saying hello, holding a door, or volunteering to keep a neighbor's pet. If you want to get involved in a more organized volunteer program, try working at a local recreation center, or helping with an after-school program. The feeling you will get from helping others is greater than you can imagine!

Most importantly, don't sweat the small stuff! Try to pick a few really important things and let the rest slide—getting worked up over every little thing will only increase your stress. So, toughen up and don't let stressful situations get to you!

Remember!!

Remember, you're not alone—everyone has stresses in their lives. It's up to you to choose how to deal with them.

Source: Centers for Disease Control and Prevention, 2003.

Chapter 6

Getting Along With Family And Friends

Healthy Relationships

What makes a relationship healthy?

Healthy relationships are fun and make you feel good about yourself. You can have a healthy relationship with anyone in your life—family, friends, and the people you date. Relationships take time and care to make them healthy. The relationships you have as a teen are a special part of your life and will teach you good lessons about who you are.

The most important part of any healthy relationship is communication. Communication means that you are able to share things about yourself and your feelings, and you listen to what the other person shares. This can happen by talking, e-mailing, writing, or even using body language. When you are talking to someone, look him or her in the eye to show you are listening.

When you have healthy communication, you both feel at ease. You can share your feelings with the other person. You know that he or she will be there to listen, support you, and keep personal things that you share private. In healthy relationships, people do not lie.

About This Chapter: This chapter includes text from "Relationships," U.S. Department of Health and Human Services (www.girlshealth.gov), June 26, 2008.

✔ Quick Tip

Arguments happen in healthy relationships, but you stay calm and talk about how you feel. Talking calmly helps you see the real reason you are not getting along. This makes it easier to figure out how to fix the problem. In healthy relationships, working through problems often makes the relationship stronger. People feel good about one another when they work through tough times rather than give up too easily.

Source: U.S. Department of Health and Human Services (www.girlshealth.gov), June 26, 2008.

How do I know that I have a healthy relationship with someone?

- You feel good about yourself when you are with that person.
- You think that both people work hard to treat the other person well.
- You feel safe around the other person.
- You like being with the other person.
- You feel that you can trust him or her with your secrets.

Keep in mind, it takes time and effort to build the trust and respect you need for a healthy relationship.

Friendships

Friendships can be tough sometimes. You may be making new friends while still trying to keep old friends. It can also be hard to know what to do when you don't agree with a friend.

How can I handle a fight with a friend?

In a healthy friendship, you should not be afraid of losing a friend because you say "no." Good friends should respect your right to say no and not give you a hard time. You should show your friends the same respect when they say no to you.

If you and your friend fight about something, it does not mean that you have an unhealthy relationship. You will not always agree with what your friend has to say. But you should always respect one another's ideas. As long as you and your friend listen to what the other has to say, you should be able to work through a fight.

The relationships you have will help you learn a lot about yourself. You will learn about the kind of friends you want to have and the kind of friend you want to be.

How can I help a friend who has a problem?

Are you worried about a friend who isn't eating? A friend who is smoking or drinking? Or maybe a friend who is having trouble at home? You can listen and give advice, but your friend's problems may be more than you can handle alone. Don't be afraid to tell a trusted adult, such as a parent/guardian, teacher, or school nurse. Even though your friend may get mad at you for telling an adult, it is the only way to protect your friend's health.

- If you think a friend may have an eating disorder, read "How to Help a Friend," available online at http://www.womenshealth.gov/bodyimage/kids/bodywise/bp/friend.pdf.
- If you have a friend who smokes, help him or her quit. Send your friend to the web site TeenQuit, online at http://www.teenquit.com.
- If you think a friend may have an alcohol or drug problem, one resource that can help you find out how you can help is the National Clearinghouse for Alcohol and Drug Information. Their "Guide for Teens" is available at http://ncadi.samhsa.gov/govpubs/phd688.
- If a friend is being abused at home, give him or her the number for the 24-hour Childhelp National Child Abuse Hotline: 800-4-A-CHILD (422-4453).
- If a friend is being hurt by someone he or she is dating, give your friend the number for the 24-hour National Domestic Violence Hotline: 800-799-SAFE (7233) or 800-787-3224 (TDD).
- If a friend is talking about suicide, you must tell a trusted adult right away. You can also give your friend the number for the National Suicide Prevention Hotline: 800-273-TALK (8255).

- If a friend is talking about hurting someone else, you must tell a trusted adult right away.
- If a friend is in trouble in other ways, the Youth Crisis Hotline at 800-HIT-HOME (448-4663) can help.

How can I handle peer pressure?

Peer pressure is when people try to pressure you to do something you usually wouldn't do, or stop doing something that you normally would do. People give in to peer pressure for many reasons. They may worry about what their friends will think, not know how to say no, or fear being left out. Some friends may pressure you to do something because "everyone else does it," such as making fun of someone, using alcohol or drugs, or smoking.

The best thing to do is say, "No, thanks" or "I don't want to." Keep in mind, you are always in charge of what you do and don't do. And it can help to talk with your parents/guardians about how to handle pressures that may come up.

How do I know if my friends really care about me?

- They want you to be happy.
- They listen and care about what you have to say.
- They are happy for you when you do well.
- They say they are sorry when they make a mistake.
- They don't expect you to be perfect.
- They give you advice in a caring way.
- They keep personal things between the two of you.

✔ Quick Tip

There are lots of things that you and your friends may do to fit in. It may be having the right clothes or being friends with the cool kids. It is normal to want to be liked by others, but it is more important to focus on what matters to YOU. Having lots of friends and dressing like everyone else may seem important right now, but try to focus on being yourself and having real friends who care about you.

Source: U.S. Department of Health and Human Services (www.girlshealth.gov), June 26, 2008.

What about cliques?

A clique is a small group of friends that is very picky about who can and cannot join the group. While it's nice to have a close group of friends, cliques often leave out others on purpose. Cliques may bully others who are not "cool enough." If you are being picked on, try to make friends with new people who care about YOU. Keep in mind, it is the quality or value of the friendship that counts, not how many friends you have. And, if you are leaving someone else out, think about how you would feel if you were the one being left out.

There can be a lot of peer pressure in cliques. You may feel like you need to do things like drink or do drugs to be part of the gang. Keep in mind, you always have the right to say no! Real friends will respect that. You also have the right to make new friends.

How can I make new friends?

It can be really tough when you are meeting a whole bunch of new people at once if you are new at school. You may feel shy or embarrassed. You may feel like you don't have anything to say. But, the other person likely feels the same way. Half the battle is feeling strong enough to talk to new people. And, it will help to just be yourself!

It can also be tough to start hanging around new people at your same school. You may need to do this if you have friends who have been getting into trouble for things like ditching school or doing drugs. Even though you may care about these friends, you have to look out for yourself and make smart choices for YOU. If you have a hard time breaking away from old friends who may be bad news, talk to a trusted adult for help on how to do your own thing.

Sometimes, you may just want to branch out and meet new people. This is totally okay and you can still keep your old friends. It's easy to hang out with people you've known a long time or have a lot in common with. But, it can also be fun to spend time with new people.

Why don't my parents/guardians like my friend(s)?

It can be common for parents/guardians and teens to run into conflict about friendships. Parents/guardians sometimes worry that their teen is hanging out with the wrong crowd. Parents/guardians may be concerned about things like drugs, alcohol, sex, skipping school, missing curfew, body piercings, or tattoos. Some parents/guardians may think body piercings and tattoos are signs of other behaviors, like drinking or smoking.

If your parents/guardians don't like your friends, the things you can do depend on the type of relationship you have with your parents/guardians. Some parents/guardians and teens can talk to each other and work through problems. Both parties trust each other and they know that they can work through things. In this case, the teen can sit down and talk with her parents/guardians and try to work things out. Sometimes, the relationship is already strained. In this case, it can be helpful to bring in an outside person to help resolve things or mediate. This could be a school counselor, school social worker, clergy member, family doctor, therapist, mentor, coach, or favorite aunt.

✤ It's A Fact!!

Getting Along With Parents, Grandparents, And Guardians

Your relationship with your parents/guardians may be confusing right now. As you get older, you can do more things on your own. You also have more freedom to spend time with other people, like friends or crushes. You may feel you are ready to choose where you go and what you do. But, you need to follow your parents'/guardians' rules. They make rules because they care about you and want you to be safe. Their rules may make you angry, though, and you may find that you're fighting with your parents/guardians more than you used to.

Each family is unique and special. No matter what type of family you have, sometimes there will be tough times as you grow up. Keep in mind, your parents/guardians make rules because they love you and want to keep you safe. It's important to listen to your parents/guardians and follow their rules.

Source: Excerpted from "Relationships," Girlshealth.gov, U.S. Department of Health and Human Services, September 3, 2008.

Dealing With Conflict

When you were younger, an adult would often step in if you had a problem with someone else, like if someone's feelings got hurt or someone took something from you without asking. Now that you're getting older, you need to learn how to deal with conflict on your own. That's because conflict is part of everyone's life—it will show up at school, at work, at home, in your community, and in relationships.

For small problems, a simple "I'm sorry" is often all it takes to feel better and move on. But not all conflicts are easily worked out. Some issues are not clear-cut, like if you and a friend are not getting along so well and you're not sure why. Other conflicts are felt by only you, like if you don't want to do what the rest of the crowd is doing, or if you are being bullied.

Avoiding a conflict can sometimes be good, but sometimes it can make things worse. In most cases, when you are angry, it's best to tell the other person what you are feeling. If you don't talk about it, your anger will most likely come out in another way, like in the tone of your voice or in your body language. This can make the problem even worse. By avoiding conflict or trying to run from the problem, you might lose a good friend, be treated unfairly at work or school, not get something you want or need, or feel like you can never make things better.

How do people react to conflict?

It's okay to feel angry, upset, annoyed, let down, or sad when you have a problem with somebody else. These feelings are normal. Still, some people deal with these feelings in unhealthy ways. You most likely know people—maybe even some adults—who yell, shout, swear, or call people names when they're upset. Maybe they try to "get back at" the person they're mad at. Or, maybe they hit others or get into fights. These types of things make it harder to work things out. Let yourself feel your emotions, but don't let them get out of hand and lead you to do these things.

How can I handle conflict in a better way?

To dealing with conflict, take it step by step.

Step 1. Cool off! Being out of control will keep you from solving the problem.

- Count down backwards from 10.

✔ Quick Tip

Cool Rules

Ever notice how quickly people get angry? It seems like people can go from totally happy to totally ticked off in no time at all. In fact, the feeling of anger is actually a series of reactions that happen in just 1/30th of a second.

The amazing thing about anger is that it's not a basic emotion like, say, happiness. It is actually a secondary emotion and it is supposed to help keep you safe and protect you from danger—the ole' fight or flight thing. But if it gets out of hand or if you try to ignore it, it can lead to some serious issues.

Here are some suggestions for dealing with anger:

Stop it at the first spark. Lots of things can trigger anger, like losing a soccer game, having to deal with your bossy little sister, or your computer crashing when you're in the middle of IM'ing your pals or writing a school paper. The important thing is to figure out what is really making you angry. Is it the same thing every time or do different things bring you to the boiling point? If it is always the same situation, person, or thing, try to avoid it. And if you can't avoid it, think of different ways you can keep from getting angry. Instead of hurling the computer out the window, think about how you avoid having it crash to begin with, like not having your e-mail and a game going at the same time. If losing the soccer game has got your goat, use your anger as motivation to improve your skills.

Consider different points of view. If your little sister is driving you nuts, maybe you need to try to look at things from her point of view—you're older and she wants to hang with you because she thinks you're cool. With that in mind, it's easier to keep your cool. Spend some time just with her so that she won't need to stalk you when all your friends are over. You might even find out that she's not half bad. By changing the way you deal with her and understanding her point of view, you can break the anger chain before you even notice you're mad.

- Close your eyes and take deep breaths.
- Think of a peaceful place or something that makes you happy.
- Slowly say over and over to yourself, "Take it easy."

Stay in control. You've tried to change your reactions to the things that you know make you crazy, you're busy looking at everything from everyone else's point of view, but you can still feel your temperature is rising. That's your body responding to your feelings. You get hot and your muscles might start to tighten and you start breathing harder. Don't let it get the best of you. Take some deep breaths, focus on relaxing your muscles, and s-l-o-w down.

Think before you speak. You catch yourself thinking or saying something in reaction to what's happening. We've all done it—we think things like, "He's so stupid." Or we say to a friend, "You're always so mean!" The words come out before we can stop ourselves. If you catch yourself doing this, take a minute to think. Try to remember that you're dealing with a person who may not know how you feel. Stay calm. Lashing back won't get you anywhere. So try to talk to your friend, let him know he hurt your feelings, and then try to move on.

Understand your feelings. The way you feel in a situation depends on your background—you may be used to people keeping their feelings in and not talking about them, or you may be used to people exploding and yelling when they are angry. Neither of these reactions is necessarily good. People who bottle up their feelings can end up exploding later or they may become depressed. People who vent and yell just tend to keep the anger cycle in motion. The trick is to deal with your anger so that you can learn how to not get riled up in the first place. Try these suggestions to help you stay calm, cool, and collected.

- Go for a walk.
- Write down your feelings on a piece of paper, then tear it up and throw it away.
- Face the mirror and practice talking to the person that you are mad at.

Source: Excerpted from "BAM! Guide to Getting Along," BAM! Body and Mind, Centers for Disease Control and Prevention, 2004.

Step 2. Keep it real! Figure out what's really bothering you.

- Do you not agree?
- Did someone say or do something that made you mad or hurt your feelings?
- Are you feeling the way you do now because of something else that upset you in the past?

✔ Quick Tip

Iron Out Your Issues

No plan will magically solve every problem or situation. There's no formula for getting along with other people, but following these tips can help.

Take a moment. Stepping back from the whole mess gives everyone a chance to cool down and think. When you're having a problem with someone, first take some time to understand your own thoughts and feelings. What's really the issue? For example, do you feel like you're not getting enough respect? What do you want? Why?

Next, find a time to work out the problem with the other person. Pick a quiet place where it's easy to talk. Make sure to give yourself enough time. (Out by the school buses 15 minutes before soccer practice probably isn't a good choice.)

Set the tone. The "tone" is the mood of the talk. When you wake up in a bad mood, it can spoil the whole day, right? You want to make sure that your talk at least starts off with a good mood. Just saying "Let's work this out" can make a huge difference.

Agree on the problem. Take turns telling your sides of the story. You can't solve a problem if you don't really understand everything that's going on.

When it's your turn, see how calm you can be. Speak softly, slowly, and firmly. No threats (like "If you don't shut up, I'll...), because they can raise the problem to a whole new level—a bad one. No need to get all excited or mad.

Try giving your point of view this way: "I feel ____(angry, sad, or upset) when you____ (take my stuff without permission, call me a name, or leave me out) because___ (you should ask first, it hurts my feelings, or makes me feel lonely)." This really works to get people to listen, because they don't feel like you're judging them. Check out the difference. You could say "You're always late to pick me up!" or "I feel

- Is this a one-time problem or one that keeps happening?

Step 3. Talk! Deal with the issue.

- Find a time when you can talk in private.
- Keep your voice calm and your body relaxed. Make eye contact to show you are serious.

embarrassed when you pick me up late because all of my friends leave right on time and it seems like no one remembered me." You can also try just stating the facts. Instead of saying "You're a thief!" try "Maybe you picked up my shirt by mistake."

When it's the other person's turn, let them explain. Listen. Don't interrupt. Try to understand where they're coming from. Show that you hear them. When people aren't getting along, each person is part of the problem—but most of us tend to blame the other person. When you've done something wrong, be ready to say you're sorry.

The goal is to decide together what the real issues are. Do not pass "Go" until you do that. It's huge!

Think of solutions. Take turns coming up with ways to solve the problem. Get creative. Usually, there are lots possible solutions. Next, talk about the good and bad points of each one.

Make a deal. Then, choose a solution that you both can agree on. Pick an idea that you both think will work. Get into the specifics—talk about exactly who will do what and when you'll do it. Everyone should give something.

Stick like glue. Keep your word and stick to what you agreed to. Give your compromise a chance. See if it sent your problem up in smoke or if the fires are still burning.

Know when to get help. Sometimes a problem gets really serious. If you aren't talking and you don't trust each other, you might need another person to step in. If it looks like the problem might turn into a fight, it's definitely time to get help. Someone like a teacher, parent, or religious advisor can help calm things down so you can safely talk out the problem with the other person.

Source: Excerpted from "BAM! Guide to Getting Along," BAM! Body and Mind, Centers for Disease Control and Prevention, 2004.

- Say exactly what is bothering you. Share how you feel by using sentences that start with "I." Don't blame or accuse the other person.

Check out the following examples and then practice changing "you" statements to "I" statements.

- Instead of: "You never want to hang out with me anymore." Try: "I feel left out when you hang out with Tracy's friends."
- Instead of: "You always pick on me in class." Try: "I feel singled out when you call on me more than other students."
- Instead of: "You're so bossy." Try: "I feel upset when you don't listen to what I think."

Keep the conflict between you and only the others involved. Don't ask friends to take sides.

Step 4. Listen! The other person might see the problem in a different way. You may each have a different point of view, but neither of you is wrong. Make sure to listen to his or her side of the story.

- Make eye contact. This shows you are interested in what the other person is saying and willing to solve the problem.
- Listen for what is behind the words—like feelings and ideas.
- Keep emotions in check. Don't interrupt, get angry, judge, or be defensive.
- Try putting yourself in the other person's shoes to see where he or she is coming from.

Step 5. Work it out! Talk about ways to settle the conflict that will meet both of your needs. Be willing to change and keep an open mind. Be willing to say you're sorry, forgive, and move on.

What if I can't work it out on my own?

Mediation means bringing in an outside person(s) to help end a fight. Parents/guardians, teachers, school nurses, coaches, counselors, and other trusted adults can help you deal with conflicts. Some schools have mediation programs that help teens figure out the real issue, talk through things, and find ways to fix their problems. Don't be shy about asking for help.

You can't always find a way to solve a conflict. If the other person doesn't want to work it out—or if the conflict gets physical—give it a rest and walk away. Keeping safe is always the smart way to go!

Sisters And Brothers

It can be really annoying to fight with sisters or brothers because they are in your house and you may feel like you can't get away from them. You may get angry if they take something that is yours, go into your room, hit you, or bother you when you have friends over. Your older sisters or brothers may try to tell you what to do. Your younger sisters or brothers may borrow your things or want to be around you all the time.

If you are having a hard time with your sisters and brothers, make rules and talk things out. Really listen to what your sister or brother has to say.

Good relationships are not just about avoiding fighting. Do fun things together like go for a bike ride or watch a movie. This will give you a chance to get to know each other as friends and have fun together.

Sometimes, your fights or worries may seem more serious if you think your family is "different." You may have step or half sisters or brothers, parents or a sister or brother who has an illness or disability, or sisters or brothers who are adopted or foster members of your family. You may have to take special care of brothers or sisters while your parents/guardians are working. But what really makes your family unique is your own rules, your own special traditions, and your own fights. Each family is different and that's what all families have in common.

Your Community

Just like you have relationships with family and friends that take work, it is also important to work on your relationship with your community. "Community" means the people around you. You have a community at your school and in your town. You can be a good member of your community by being a good person. You can be a good person by showing the good parts of your character. "Character" is a set of values that helps build your thoughts, actions, and feelings. This is a very important part of who we are.

Here are some traits of people with strong character:

- Show compassion, which is caring about other people's feelings and needs
- Always tell the truth
- Treat other people as they would like to be treated
- Show self-discipline, which is doing things like getting homework done on time without being told to
- Make good judgments, which are choices about what is right and wrong
- Show respect to others by being nice, treating others fairly, and letting other people have beliefs that may be different from their own
- Stand up for their beliefs
- Have a strong sense of responsibility, which means they take tasks such as schoolwork or taking care of a pet very seriously and work hard to do a good job
- Have self-respect, which means liking who you are and taking good care of yourself

✔ Quick Tip

Young Caregivers

There are more than one million young people in the United States who take care of someone in their family. So, if you are taking care of someone in your family, you are not alone! You might need to watch your brothers or sisters so your parents or guardians can work. Or you might take care of a family member with an illness or disability.

Caring for someone else can be tough for an adult. It can be even tougher for a young person. You may have less time for schoolwork or you may feel like you don't have any time to just be a kid. Your friends may not understand what you're going through. Sometimes it feels good to take care of someone else and sometimes you may feel sad or worried. These feelings are normal. You need to take care of yourself, too.

- If you are angry, sad, or worried, talk to a trusted adult, like your school counselor.
- Write in your diary or draw a picture about how you're feeling.
- Make some time each day for fun.
- Keep in mind, it's okay to say no sometimes and it's okay to want things for yourself.
- Ask for help. Is there someone in your family, a family friend, or a neighbor who can help you?

To learn more, visit the American Association for Caregiving Youth website at http://www.aacy.org.

Source: From "Relationships," Girlshealth.gov, U.S. Department of Health and Human Services, June 26, 2008.

Chapter 7

Love, Romance, And Heartbreak

Love And Romance

We've all experienced love. We've loved (and been loved by) parents, brothers, sisters, friends, even pets. But romantic love is different. It's an intense, new feeling unlike any of these other ways of loving.

Why Do We Fall In Love?

Loving and being loved adds richness to our lives. When people feel close to others they are happier and even healthier. Love helps us feel important, understood, and secure.

But each kind of love has its own distinctive feel. The kind of love we feel for a parent is different from our love for a baby brother or best friend. And the kind of love we feel in romantic relationships is its own unique type of love.

Our ability to feel romantic love develops during adolescence. Teens all over the world notice passionate feelings of attraction. Even in cultures where people are not allowed to act on or express these feelings, they're still there. It's

About This Chapter: This chapter includes "Love and Romance," February 2007, and "Getting Over a Break-Up," November 2007, reprinted with permission from www.kidshealth.org. This information was provided by KidsHealth, one of the largest resources online for medically reviewed health information written for parents, kids, and teens. For more articles like these, visit www.KidsHealth.org or www.TeensHealth.org.

a natural part of growing up to develop romantic feelings and sexual attractions to others. These new feelings can be exciting—or even confusing at first.

The Magical Ingredients Of Love Relationships

Love is such a powerful human emotion that experts are constantly studying it. They've discovered that love has three main qualities:

1. Attraction is the "chemistry" part of love. It's all about the physical—even sexual—interest that two people have in each other. Attraction is responsible for the desire we feel to kiss and hold the object of our affection. Attraction is also what's behind the flushed, nervous-but-excited way we feel when that person is near.

2. Closeness is the bond that develops when we share thoughts and feelings that we don't share with anyone else. When you have this feeling of closeness with your boyfriend or girlfriend, you feel supported, cared for, understood, and accepted for who you are. Trust is a big part of this.

3. Commitment is the promise or decision to stick by the other person through the ups and downs of the relationship.

> **✤ It's A Fact!!**
>
> **Programmed To Love?**
>
> The tendency to love might very well be programmed into us. After all, human survival depends on parents falling in love with their newborn babies. And, as everyone who's ever seen a lost kid in a supermarket knows, little children instinctively feel a strong attachment to their parents.
>
> Source: Copyright © 2007 The Nemours Foundation.

These three qualities of love can be combined in different ways to make different kinds of relationships. For example, closeness without attraction is the kind of love we feel for best friends. We share secrets and personal stuff with them, we support them, and they stand by us. But we are not romantically interested in them.

Attraction without closeness is more like a crush or infatuation. You're attracted to someone physically but don't know the person well enough yet to feel the closeness that comes from sharing personal experiences and feelings.

Romantic love is when attraction and closeness are combined. Lots of relationships grow out of an initial attraction (a crush or "love at first sight") and develop into closeness. It's also possible for a friendship to move from closeness into attraction as two people realize their relationship is more than "just like" and they have become interested in one another in a romantic way.

For people falling in love for the first time, it can be hard to tell the difference between the intense, new feelings of physical attraction and the deeper closeness that goes with being in love.

Lasting Love Or Fun Fling?

The third ingredient in a love relationship, commitment, is about wanting and deciding to stay together as a couple in the future—despite any changes and challenges that life brings.

Sometimes couples who fall in love in high school develop committed relationships that last. Many relationships don't last, though. But it's not because teens aren't capable of deep loving.

We typically have shorter relationships as teens because adolescence is a time when we instinctively seek lots of different experiences and try out different things. It's all part of discovering who we are, what we value, and what we want out of life.

Another reason we tend to have shorter relationships in our teens is because the things we want to get out of a romantic relationship change as we get a little older. In our teens—especially for guys—relationships are mainly about physical attraction. But

✤ It's A Fact!!

When do teens start dating?

There is no best age for teens to start dating. Every person will be ready for a dating relationship at a different time. Different families may have their own rules about dating, too. When you decide to start a dating relationship, it should be because you care about someone and not because other people are dating. A dating relationship is a special chance to get to know someone, and it should happen only when you are really ready and your parents/guardians are okay with it.

Source: Excerpted from "Relationships," U.S. Department of Health and Human Services (www.girlshealth.gov), June 26, 2008.

by the time guys reach 20 or so, they rate a person's inner qualities as most important. Teen girls emphasize closeness as most important—although they don't mind if a potential love interest is cute too!

In our teens, relationships are mostly about having fun. Dating can seem like a great way to have someone to go places with and do things with. Dating can also be a way to fit in. If our friends are all dating someone, we might put pressure on ourselves to find a boyfriend or girlfriend too.

For some people dating is even a status thing. It can almost seem like another version of cliques: The pressure to go out with the "right" person in the "right" group can make dating a lot less fun than it should be—and not so much about love!

In our late teens, though, relationships are less about going out to have fun and fitting in. Closeness, sharing, and confiding become more important to both guys and girls. By the time they reach their twenties, most girls and guys value support, closeness, and communication, as well as passion. This is the time when people start thinking about finding someone they can commit to in the long run—a love that will last.

What Makes A Good Relationship?

When people first experience falling in love, it often starts as attraction. Sexual feelings can also be a part of this attraction. People at this stage might

✤ It's A Fact!!

Do opposites attract?

It's possible to be attracted to someone who is your opposite. But when beliefs and values are extremely different, it's not likely to grow into love. People usually choose romantic partners similar to themselves—or people who have qualities that might be different from their own but are qualities that they would like to have.

Source: Copyright © 2007 The Nemours Foundation.

daydream about a crush or a new BF or GF. They may doodle the person's name or think of their special someone while a particular song is playing.

It sure feels like love. But it's not love yet. It hasn't had time to grow into emotional closeness that's needed for love. Because feelings of attraction and sexual interest are new, and they're directed at a person we want a relationship with, it's not surprising we confuse attraction with love. It's all so intense, exciting, and hard to sort out.

The crazy intensity of the passion and attraction phase fades a bit after a while. Like putting all our energy into winning a race, this kind of passion is exhilarating but far too extreme to keep going forever. If a relationship is destined to last, this is where closeness enters the picture. The early passionate intensity may fade, but a deep affectionate attachment takes its place.

Some of the ways people grow close are:

- Learning to give and receive. A healthy relationship is about both people, not how much one person can get from (or give to) the other.
- Revealing feelings. A supportive, caring relationship allows people to reveal detail about themselves—their likes and dislikes, dreams and worries, proud moments, disappointments, fears, and weaknesses.
- Listening and supporting. When two people care, they offer support when the other person is feeling vulnerable or afraid. They don't put down or insult their partner, even when they disagree.

Giving, receiving, revealing, and supporting is a back-and-forth process: One person shares a detail, then the other person shares something, then the first person feels safe enough to share a little more. In this way, the relationship gradually builds into a place of openness, trust, and support where each partner knows that the other will be there when times are tough. Both feel liked and accepted for who they are.

The passion and attraction the couple felt early on in the relationship isn't lost. It's just different. In healthy, long-term relationships, couples often find that intense passion comes and goes at different times. But the closeness is always there.

Sometimes, though, a couple loses the closeness. For adults, relationships can sometimes turn into what experts call "empty love." This means that the closeness and attraction they once felt is gone, and they stay together only out of commitment. This is not usually a problem for teens, but there are other reasons why relationships end.

Why Do Relationships End?

Love is delicate. It needs to be cared for and nurtured if it is to last through time. Just like friendships, relationships can fail if they are not given enough time and attention. This is one reason why some couples might not last—perhaps someone is so busy with school, extracurriculars, and work that he or she has less time for a relationship. Or maybe a relationship ends when people graduate and go to separate colleges or take different career paths.

For some teens, a couple may grow apart because the things that are important to them change as they mature. Or maybe each person wants different things out of the relationship. Sometimes both people realize the relationship has reached its end; sometimes one person feels this way when the other does not.

✔ Quick Tip

Communication, trust, and respect are key to healthy relationships. Healthy relationships make you feel good about who YOU are and SAFE with the other person. Feel good about yourself and get to know what makes you happy. The more you love yourself, the easier it will be to find healthy relationships.

Here are some tips for having healthy and safe relationships:

- Get to know a person by talking on the phone or at school before you go out for the first time.
- Go out with a group of friends to a public place the first few times you go out.
- Plan fun activities like going to the movies or the mall, on a picnic or for a walk.
- Tell the other person what you feel okay doing. Also, tell the person what time your parents/guardians want you to be home.
- Tell at least one friend and your parents/guardians who you are going out with and where you are going. Also tell them how to reach you.

Source: Excerpted from "Relationships," U.S. Department of Health and Human Services (www.girlshealth.gov), June 26, 2008.

Moving On

Losing love can be painful for anyone. But if it's your first real love and the relationship ends before you want it to, feelings of loss can seem overwhelming. Like the feelings of passion early in the relationship, the newness and rawness of grief and loss can be intense—and devastating. There's a reason why they call it a broken heart.

When a relationship ends, people really need support. Losing a first love isn't something we've been emotionally prepared to cope with. It can help to have close friends and family members to lean on. Unfortunately, lots of people—often adults—expect younger people to bounce back and "just get over it." If your heart is broken, find someone you can talk to who really understands the pain you're going through.

It seems hard to believe when you're brokenhearted that you can ever feel better. But gradually these feelings grow less intense. Eventually, people move on to other relationships and experiences.

Relationships—whether they last two weeks, two months, two years, or a lifetime—are all opportunities to experience love on its many different levels. We learn both how to love and how to be loved in return.

Romance provides us with a chance to discover our own selves as we share with someone new. We learn the things we love about ourselves, the things we'd like to change, and the qualities and values we look for in a partner.

Loving relationships teach us self-respect as well as respect for others. Love is one of the most fulfilling things we can have in our lives. If romance hasn't found you yet, don't worry—there's plenty of time. And the right person is worth the wait.

Getting Over A Break-Up

If you've just had a break-up and are feeling down, you're not alone. Just about everyone experiences a break-up at sometime, and many then have to deal with heartbreak—a wave of grief, anger, confusion, low self-esteem, and maybe even jealousy all at once. Millions of poems and songs have been written about having a broken heart and wars have even been fought because of heartbreak.

✤ It's A Fact!!

What is a healthy dating relationship?

Healthy dating relationships should start with the same things that healthy friendships start with: good communication, honesty, and respect. Dating relationships are a little different because they may include physical ways of showing you care, like hugging, kissing, or holding hands. You may find yourself wanting to spend all of your time with your crush, but it is important to spend some time apart, too. This will let you have a healthy relationship with your crush and with your friends and family at the same time.

Source: Excerpted from "Relationships," U.S. Department of Health and Human Services (www.girlshealth.gov), June 26, 2008.

What Exactly Is Heartbreak?

Lots of things can cause heartbreak. Some people might have had a romantic relationship that ended before they were ready. Others might have strong feelings for someone who doesn't feel the same way. Or maybe a person feels sad or angry when a close friend ends or abandons the friendship.

Although the causes may be different, the feeling of loss is the same—whether it's the loss of something real or the loss of something you only hoped for. People describe heartbreak as a feeling of heaviness, emptiness, and sadness.

How Can I Deal With How I Feel?

Most people will tell you you'll get over it or you'll meet someone else, but when it's happening to you, it can feel like no one else in the world has ever felt the same way. If you're experiencing these feelings, there are things you can do to lessen the pain.

Here are some tips that might help:

- Share your feelings. Some people find that sharing their feelings with someone they trust—someone who recognizes what they're going through—helps them feel better. That could mean talking over all the things you feel, even having a good cry on the shoulder of a comforting friend or family member. Others find they heal better if they hang out and do the things they normally enjoy, like seeing a movie or going to a concert, to take their minds off the hurt. If you feel like someone can't relate to what you're going through or is dismissive of your feelings, find someone more sympathetic to talk to. (OK, we know that sharing feelings can be tough for guys, but you don't necessarily have to tell the football team or your wrestling coach what you're going through. Talk with a friend or family member, a teacher, or counselor. It might make you more comfortable if you find a female family member or friend, like an older sister or a neighbor, to talk to.)
- Remember what's good about you. This one is really important. Sometimes people with broken hearts start to blame themselves for what's happened. They may be really down on themselves, exaggerating their faults as though they did something to deserve the unhappiness they're experiencing. If you find this happening to you, nip it in the bud! Remind yourself of your good qualities, and if you can't think of them because your broken heart is clouding your view, get your friends to remind you.
- Take good care of yourself. A broken heart can be very stressful so don't let the rest of your body get broken too. Get lots of sleep, eat healthy foods, and exercise regularly to minimize stress and depression and give your self-esteem a boost.
- Don't be afraid to cry. Going through a break-up can be really tough, and getting some of those raw emotions out can be a big help. We know this is another tough one for guys, but there's no shame in crying now and then. No one has to see you do it—you don't have to start blubbering in class or at soccer practice or anything. Just a find a place where you can be alone, like crying into your pillow at night or in the shower when you're getting ready for the day.

- Do the things you normally enjoy. Whether it's seeing a movie or going to a concert, do something fun to take your mind off the negative feelings for a while.
- Keep yourself busy. Sometimes this is difficult when you're coping with sadness and grief, but it really helps. This is a great time to redecorate your room or try a new hobby. That doesn't mean you shouldn't think about what happened—working things through in our minds is all part of the healing process—it just means you should focus on other things too.
- Give yourself time. It takes time for sadness to go away. Almost everyone thinks they won't feel normal again, but the human spirit is amazing—and the heartbreak almost always heals after a while. But how long will that take? That depends on what caused your heartbreak, how you deal with loss, and how quickly you tend to bounce back from things. Getting over a break-up can take a couple of days to many weeks—and sometimes even months.

Some people feel that nothing will make them happy again and resort to alcohol or drugs. Others feel angry and want to hurt themselves or someone else. People who drink, do drugs, or cut themselves to escape from the reality of a loss may think they are numbing their pain, but the feeling is only temporary. They're not really dealing with the pain, only masking it, which makes all their feelings build up inside and prolongs the sadness.

Sometimes the sadness is so deep—or lasts so long—that a person may need some extra support. For someone who isn't starting to feel better after a few weeks or who continues to feel depressed, talking to a counselor or therapist can be very helpful.

So be patient with yourself, and let the healing begin.

Chapter 8

Dealing With Your Parents' Divorce

For many people, their parents' divorce marks a turning point in their lives, whether the divorce happened many years ago or is taking place right now.

About half the marriages in the United States today end in divorce, so children of divorce are certainly not alone. But when it happens to you, you can feel very alone and unsure of what it all means. It may seem hard, but it is possible to cope with divorce—and have a good family life in spite of some changes divorce may bring.

Why Are My Parents Divorcing?

Parents divorce for many reasons. Usually divorce happens when couples feel they can no longer live together due to fighting and anger, or because the love they had when they married has changed. Divorce can also be because one parent falls in love with someone else, and sometimes it is due to a serious problem like drinking, abuse, or gambling.

About This Chapter: Text in this chapter is from "Dealing With Divorce," August 2007, reprinted with permission from www.kidshealth.org. Copyright © 2007 The Nemours Foundation. This information was provided by KidsHealth, one of the largest resources online for medically reviewed health information written for parents, kids, and teens. For more articles like this one, visit www.KidsHealth.org, or www.TeensHealth.org.

It's common for teens to think that their parents' divorce is somehow their fault, but nothing could be further from the truth. Some teens may wonder if they could have helped to prevent the split. Others may wish they had prevented arguments by cooperating more within the family, doing better with their behavior, or getting better grades. But separation and divorce are a result of a couple's problems with each other, not with their kids. The decisions adults make about divorce are their own.

If your parents are divorcing, you may experience a lots of feelings. Your emotions may change frequently, too. You may feel angry, frustrated, upset, or sad. You might feel protective of one parent or blame one for the situation. You may feel abandoned, afraid, worried, or guilty. You may also feel relieved, especially if there has been a lot of tension at home. These feelings are normal and talking about them with a friend, family member or trusted adult can really help.

How Will Divorce Change My Life?

Depending on what happens in your family, you may have to adjust to many changes. These could include things like moving, changing schools, spending time with both parents separately, and perhaps dealing with parents' unpleasant feelings toward one another.

Your parents may go to court to determine custody arrangements. You may end up living with one parent most of the time and visiting the other, or your parents may split their time with you evenly.

Some teens have to travel between parents, and that may create challenges both socially and practically. But with time you can create a new routine that works. Often, it takes a while for custody arrangements to be finalized. This can give people time to adapt to these big changes and let families figure out what works best.

Money matters may change for your parents, too. A parent who didn't work during the marriage may need to find a job to pay for rent or a mortgage. This might be something a parent is excited about, but he or she may also feel nervous or pressured about finances. There are also expenses associated with divorce, from lawyers' fees to the cost of moving to a new place to live.

Your family may not be able to afford all the things you were used to before the divorce. This is one of the difficult changes often associated with divorce. There can be good changes too—but how you cope with the stressful changes depends on your situation, your personality, and your support network.

What Parents And Teens Can Do To Make Divorce Easier

Keep the peace. Dealing with divorce is easiest when parents get along. Teens find it especially hard when their parents fight and argue or act with bitterness toward each other. You can't do much to influence how your parents behave during a divorce, but you can ask them to do their best to call a truce to any bickering or unkind things they might be saying about each other. No matter what problems a couple may face, as parents they need to handle visiting arrangements peacefully to minimize the stress their kids may feel.

Be fair. Most teens say it's important that parents don't try to get them to "take sides." You need to feel free to relate to one parent without the other parent acting jealous, hurt, or mad. It's unfair for anyone to feel that relating to one parent is being disloyal to the other or that the burden of one parent's happiness is on your shoulders.

When parents find it hard to let go of bitterness or anger, or if they are depressed about the changes brought on by divorce, they can find help from a counselor or therapist. This can help parents get past the pain divorce may have created, to find personal happiness, and to lift any burdens from their kids. Kids and teens can also benefit from seeing a family therapist or someone who specializes in helping them get through the stress of a family breakup.

Keep in touch. Going back and forth between two homes can be tough, especially if parents live far apart. It can be a good idea to keep in touch with a parent you see less often because of distance. Even a quick email saying "I'm thinking of you" helps ease the feelings of missing each other. Making an effort to stay in touch when you're apart can keep both of you up to date on everyday activities and ideas.

Work it out. You may want both parents to come to special events, like games, meets, plays, or recitals. But sometimes a parent may find it awkward to attend if the other is present. It helps if parents can figure out a way to make this work, especially because you may need to feel the support and presence of both parents even more during divorce. You might be able to come up with an idea for a compromise or solution to this problem and suggest it to both parents.

Figure out your strengths. How do you deal with stress? Do you get angry and take it out on siblings, friends, or yourself? Or are you someone who is a more of a pleaser who puts others first? Do you tend to avoid conflict altogether and just hope that problems will magically disappear? A life-changing event like a divorce can put people through some tough times, but it can also help them learn about their strengths, and put in place some new coping skills. For example, how can you cope if one parent bad-mouths another? Sometimes staying quiet until the anger has subsided and then discussing it calmly with your mom or dad can help. You may want to tell them you have a right to love both your parents, no matter what they are doing to each other.

✔ Quick Tip
Talk About The Future

Lots of teens whose parents divorce worry that their own plans for the future could be affected. Some are concerned that the costs of divorce (like legal fees and expenses of two households) might mean there will be less money for college or other things.

Pick a good time to tell your parents about your concerns—when there's enough time to sit down with one or both parents to discuss how the divorce will affect you. Don't worry about putting added stress on your parents. It's better to bring your concerns into the open than to keep them to yourself and let worries or resentment build. There are solutions for most problems and counselors who can help teens and their parents find those solutions.

If you need help figuring out your strengths or how to cope—like from a favorite aunt or from your school counselor—ask for it. And if you find it hard to confront your parents, try writing them a letter. Figure out what works for you.

Live your life. Sometimes during a divorce, parents may be so caught up in their own changes it can feel like your own life is on hold. In addition to staying focused on your own plans and dreams, make sure you participate in as many of your normal activities as possible. When things are changing at home, it can really help to keep some things, such as school activities and friends, the same. If things get too hard at home, see if you can stay with a friend or relative until things calm down. Take care of yourself by eating right and getting regular exercise—two great stress busters.

Let others support you. Talk about your feelings and reactions to the divorce with someone you trust. If you're feeling down or upset, let your friends and family members support you. These feelings usually pass. If they don't, and if you're feeling depressed or stressed out, or if it's hard to concentrate on your normal activities, let a counselor or therapist help you. Your parents, school counselor, or a doctor or other health professional can help you find one. Many communities and schools have support groups for kids and teens whose parents have divorced. It can really help to talk with other people your age who are going through similar experiences.

Bringing Out The Positive

There will be ups and downs in the process, but teens can cope successfully with their parents' divorce and the changes it brings. You may even discover some unexpected positives. Many teens find their parents are actually happier after the divorce or they may develop new and better ways of relating to both parents when they have separate time with each one.

Some teens learn compassion and caring skills when a younger brother or sister needs their support and care. Siblings who are closer in age may form tighter bonds, learning to count on each other more because they're facing the challenges of their parents' divorce together. Coping well with divorce also can bring out strength and maturity. Some become more responsible, better problem solvers, better listeners, or better friends. Looking back on the experience, lots of people say that they learned coping skills they never knew they had and feel stronger and more resilient as a result of what they went through.

Many movies have been made about divorce and stepfamilies—some with happy endings, some not. That's how it is in real life too. But most teens who go through a divorce learn (sometimes to their surprise) that they can make it through this difficult situation successfully. Giving it time, letting others support you along the way, and keeping an eye on the good things in your life can make all the difference.

Chapter 9

The Moving Blues

Caroline didn't want to move. It had been hard enough to make the transition from junior high to high school, especially when many of her friends went to different schools. Now she liked her friends, she liked her school, and she liked her routine. She didn't want to leave the big city for a small town and felt angry with her parents and out of step with everyone else.

It isn't easy for anyone to pack up and leave everything that is familiar and try to fit into a new environment. But it's especially hard during a time in your life when there are already so many physical and emotional changes taking place.

Why Do I Feel Upset About Moving?

Experts consider moving to be one of the major stresses in life. Leaving behind friends, familiar places, and activities creates anxiety for everyone involved—parents included. And it's hard work to pack and prepare for a move and then settle into a new home.

About This Chapter: Text in this chapter is from "The Moving Blues," July 2008, reprinted with permission from www.kidshealth.org. This information was provided by KidsHealth, one of the largest resources online for medically reviewed health information written for parents, kids, and teens. For more articles like this one, visit www.KidsHealth.org, or www.TeensHealth.org.

The reasons behind a move can sometimes be upsetting, and that can add to the stress. A parent may be forced to take a job in a new town because of company layoffs or staff reorganizations. Sometimes a death or divorce in the family can lead to a move, or your family may have to move to take care of a sick family member, such as a grandparent.

During the busy, stressful time of planning, preparing, and packing for a move, your mom and dad may be too preoccupied to realize how the change is affecting you. They may not even realize you are unhappy if you don't discuss it with them. Be open with your parents and try to talk reasonably about the move and how it is affecting you. Your parents or siblings may have the same concerns or fears.

A move can lead some people to become depressed. If you find that you can't shake feelings of sadness or anxiety, talk to an adult. Don't worry that your parents are too focused on organizing their own lives and don't worry that you'll be bothering them. Most parents appreciate knowing how you feel. Or you can talk to your brother or sister or a school counselor. Not dealing with feelings now may lead to problems later.

It can help to remember that the problems involved in moving are always temporary. People usually feel better once they've had time to settle in.

What To Expect

Even when the reasons for a move are good (such as a promotion or better job for a parent) and you're excited about it, it's still a good idea to be prepared for unexpected changes. It's easy to get caught up in the excitement and expect everything to be perfect.

Ali remembers her move to Germany. Like many military families, she'd moved many times before so it seemed like no big deal. In fact, Ali was so excited at the prospect of living abroad that she didn't think about the challenges involved in living in a place where she didn't speak the language. She was also surprised by some of the cultural differences—things she hadn't anticipated because she'd assumed that Germany would be pretty much like the United States. Today she says she makes a list of positives and negatives before she moves to help keep her expectations realistic.

One unexpected difference may be school. It's easy to assume that one school is pretty much like another, but your new school may not use the same textbooks or procedures. Some of your classes may be different, or the teacher may have already covered topics you haven't learned about yet. It can be particularly hard if you're moving in the middle of a school year, but your teachers will understand and work with you to be sure you feel comfortable.

It's common for people who move to feel like they're starting all over again. You have to learn new streets, new faces, and new ways of doing things. People may dress or speak differently. The slang and accents may sound different in your new community, depending on how far you move. It's natural for people to feel out of place in a new situation where they don't know the customs and rules.

Making The Best Of It

Although there is no way to eliminate the anxiety of moving, there are many ways to make the move easier. Before you even begin packing, you can start to get to know your new home. The internet and library may contain lots of good information about your new community. Make a list of your interests and hobbies, and then find the locations and phone numbers of places where those activities take place. When you're visiting your new school, find out if there are deadlines for activities you're interested in and see if you can still join.

A new place seems more familiar, and it's easier to make friends, when you can participate in a common interest with people who do the things you enjoy.

Look for opportunities to try new activities as well. If you have a job, ask your current boss to write a reference letter for you. If you work for a food chain or a chain of stores, you might be able to arrange a transfer and have a job waiting for you.

See if you can get a city map and highlight where you will be living, where your new school is, and the location of places of worship, movie theaters, skate parks, and other places you like to go. Ask if your realtor can videotape your new house if you haven't been able to see it yet (most realtors post indoor and outdoor pictures of properties online).

It can help to learn about what makes your new city or town unique. Share the information with your friends and make them feel part of your moving experience. Soon you will feel like you already know your new community.

Packing It Up

You can pick up a copy of the "United States Postal Service Mover's Guide" in any post office or online; it will give you and your parents some tips. The guide includes change of address forms, a checklist of things to do, and suggestions for a survival kit that will contain items you may need to have at hand and might otherwise be packed out of reach during the move.

You can help—and feel more in control—by making a list of things that need to be done before the move. Offer to help your parents with some of their items. The more you participate and keep busy, the more it will feel like your own experience rather than something that is being done to you. For example, organize a yard sale to sell the stuff you don't want to take with you. You may find that friends and neighbors are interested in participating in a yard sale, too.

✔ Quick Tip

As soon as you know you are moving, start preparing by:

- sorting out clothes and giving away items that you aren't going to take;
- packing away items you are going to take, but won't need until after you've moved;
- spreading out the chores you have to do so you won't be overwhelmed during the last few days;
- cleaning up your room or any other areas you are responsible for to make packing easier;
- labeling your boxes so you can easily identify where things are when you get to your new home.

Keeping In Touch

One of the fears of moving is losing old friends. Remember your friends when you get to your new destination by putting pictures up around your new room. Print out copies of pictures for your friends to keep, too.

Saying goodbye is never easy, but it doesn't mean it's forever. Luckily, today it's easier than ever to stay in touch with social networking sites and IM. Share pictures and videos. Let your friends know about the differences, both good and bad, between your old home and your new place. You might be able to plan summer visits to see old friends or for a friend to visit you.

Moving is hard, but you may discover that it has taught you some valuable skills: how to make new friends, be flexible, and find your way around strange places. Although learning these lessons can feel tough at the time, once you've settled in, you may find you like the new place better. And be sure to say "hi" to the next new kid in town—you can relate.

Chapter 10

Dealing With Grief

Death And Grief

People React Emotionally And Physically

When coping with a death, you may go through all kinds of emotions. You may be sad, worried, or scared. You might be shocked, unprepared, or confused. You might be feeling angry, cheated, relieved, guilty, exhausted, or just plain empty. Your emotions might be stronger or deeper than usual or mixed together in ways you've never experienced before.

Some people find they have trouble concentrating, studying, sleeping, or eating when they're coping with a death. Others lose interest in activities they used to enjoy. Some people lose themselves in playing computer games or eat or drink to excess. And some people feel numb, as if nothing has happened.

All of these are normal ways to react to a death.

About This Chapter: Text in this chapter is from "Death and Grief," April 2007, and "My Pet Died. How Can I Feel Better?" October 2007, reprinted with permission from www.kidshealth.org. This information was provided by KidsHealth, one of the largest resources online for medically reviewed health information written for parents, kids, and teens. For more articles like these, visit www.KidsHealth.org or www.TeensHealth.org.

What Is Grief?

When we have emotional, physical, and spiritual reactions in response to a death or loss, it's known as grief or grieving. People who are grieving might:

- Feel strong emotions, such as sadness and anger;
- Have physical reactions, such as not sleeping or even waves of nausea;
- Have spiritual reactions to a death—for example, some people find themselves questioning their beliefs and feeling disappointed in their religion while others find that they feel more strongly than ever about their faith.

The grieving process takes time and healing usually happens gradually. The intensity of grief may be related to how sudden or predictable the loss was and how you felt about the person who died.

Some people write about grief happening in stages, but usually it feels more like "waves" or cycles of grief that come and go depending on what you are doing and if there are triggers for remembering the person who has died.

Different Ways Of Grieving

If you've lost someone in your immediate family, such as a parent, brother, or sister, you may feel cheated out of time you wanted to have with that person. It can also feel hard to express your own grief when other family members are grieving, too.

✎ What's It Mean?

Grief: Grief is the normal response of sorrow, emotion, and confusion that comes from losing someone or something important to you. It is a natural part of life. Grief is a typical reaction to death, divorce, job loss, a move away from friends and family, or loss of good health due to illness.

Source: Excerpted from "How to Deal with Grief," National Mental Health Information Center, Substance Abuse and Mental Health Services Administration (http://mentalhealth.samhsa.gov).

✤ It's A Fact!!

There are many different types of loss, and not all of them are related to death. A person can also grieve over the breakup of an intimate relationship or after a parent, sibling, or friend moves away.

Source: Copyright © April 2007 The Nemours Foundation.

Some people may hold back their own grief or avoid talking about the person who died because they worry that it may make a parent or other family member sad. It's also natural to feel some guilt over a past argument or a difficult relationship with the person who died.

We don't always grieve over the death of another person. The death of a beloved pet can trigger strong feelings of grief. People may be surprised by how painful this loss can be. But the loving bonds we share with pets are real, and so are the feelings of loss and grief when they die.

All of these feelings and reactions are OK—but what can people do to get through them? How long does grief last? Will things ever get back to normal? And how will you go on without the person who has died?

Coping With Grief

Just as people feel grief in many different ways, they handle it differently, too.

Some people reach out for support from others and find comfort in good memories. Others become very busy to take their minds off the loss. Some people become depressed and withdraw from their peers or go out of the way to avoid the places or situations that remind them of the person who has died.

For some people, it can help to talk about the loss with others. Some do this naturally and easily with friends and family, while others talk to a professional therapist.

Some people may not feel like talking about it much at all because it's hard to find the words to express such deep and personal emotion or they wonder whether talking will make them feel the hurt more. This is fine, as long you find other ways to deal with your pain.

People sometimes deal with their sorrow by engaging in dangerous or self-destructive activities. Doing things like drinking, drugs, or cutting yourself to escape from the reality of a loss may seem to numb the pain, but the feeling is only temporary. This isn't really dealing with the pain, only masking it, which makes all those feelings build up inside and only prolongs the grief.

If your pain just seems to get worse, or if you feel like hurting yourself or have suicidal thoughts, tell someone you trust about how you feel.

✤ It's A Fact!!
Coping With Suicide

Losing someone to suicide can be especially difficult to deal with. People who lose friends or family members to suicide may feel intense despair and sadness because they feel unable to understand what could have led to such an extreme action. They may feel angry at the person—a completely normal emotion. Or they could feel guilty and wonder if there was something they might have done to prevent the suicide. Sometimes, after a traumatic loss, a person can become depressed and may need extra help to heal.

Source: Copyright © April 2007 The Nemours Foundation.

What To Expect

It may feel like it might be impossible to recover after losing someone you love. But grief does get gradually better and become less intense as time goes by. To help get through the pain, it can help to know some of the things you might expect during the grieving process.

The first few days after someone dies can be intense, with people expressing strong emotions, perhaps crying, comforting each other, and gathering to express their support and condolences to the ones most affected by the loss. It is common to feel as if you are "going crazy" and feel extremes of anxiety, panic, sadness, and helplessness. Some people describe feeling "unreal," as if they're looking at the world from a faraway place. Others feel moody, irritable, and resentful.

Family and friends often participate in rituals that may be part of their religious, cultural, community, or family traditions, such as memorial services, wakes, or funerals. These activities can help people get through the first days after a death and honor the person who died. People might spend time together talking and sharing memories about their loved one. This may continue for days or weeks following the loss as friends and family bring food, send cards, or stop by to visit.

Many times, people show their emotions during this time. But sometimes a person can be so shocked or overwhelmed by the death that he or she doesn't show any emotion right away—even though the loss is very hard. And it's not uncommon to see people smiling and talking with others at a funeral, as if something sad had not happened. But being among other mourners can be a comfort, reminding us that some things will stay the same.

Sometimes, when the rituals associated with grieving end, people might feel like they should be "over it" because everything seems to have gone back to normal. When those who are grieving first go back to their normal activities, it might be hard to put their hearts into everyday things. Many people go back to doing regular things after a few days or a week. But although they may not talk about their loss as much, the grieving process continues.

It's natural to continue to have feelings and questions for a while after someone dies. It's also natural to begin to feel somewhat better. A lot depends on how your loss affects your life. It's OK to feel grief for days, weeks, or even longer, depending on how close you were to the person who died.

No matter how you choose to grieve, there's no one right way to do it. The grieving process is a gradual one that lasts longer for some people than others. There may be times when you worry that you'll never enjoy life the same way again, but this is a natural reaction after a loss.

Caring For Yourself

The loss of someone close to you can be stressful. It can help you to cope if you take care of yourself in certain small but important ways. Here are some that might help:

- **Remember that grief is a normal emotion.** Know that you can (and will) heal over time.
- **Participate in rituals.** Memorial services, funerals, and other traditions help people get through the first few days and honor the person who died.
- **Be with others.** Even informal gatherings of family and friends bring a sense of support and help people not to feel so isolated in the first days and weeks of their grief.
- **Talk about it when you can.** Some people find it helpful to tell the story of their loss or talk about their feelings. Sometimes a person doesn't feel like talking, and that's OK, too. No one should feel pressured to talk.
- **Express yourself.** Even if you don't feel like talking, find ways to express your emotions and thoughts. Start writing in a journal about the memories you have of the person you lost and how you're feeling since the loss. Or write a song, poem, or tribute about your loved one. You can do this privately or share it with others.
- **Exercise.** Exercise can help your mood. It may be hard to get motivated, so modify your usual routine if you need to.
- **Eat right.** You may feel like skipping meals or you may not feel hungry, but your body still needs nutritious foods.
- **Join a support group.** If you think you may be interested in attending a support group, ask an adult or school counselor about how to become involved. The thing to remember is that you don't have to be alone with your feelings or your pain.
- **Let your emotions be expressed and released.** Don't stop yourself from having a good cry if you feel one coming on. Don't worry if listening to particular songs or doing other activities is painful because it brings back memories of the person that you lost; this is common. After a while, it becomes less painful.
- **Create a memorial or tribute.** Plant a tree or garden, or memorialize the person in some fitting way, such as running in a charity run or walk (a breast cancer race, for example) in honor of the lost loved one.

Getting Help For Intense Grief

If your grief isn't letting up for a while after the death of your loved one, you may want to reach out for help. If grief has turned into depression, it's very important to tell someone.

How do you know if your grief has been going on too long? Here are some signs:

- You've been grieving for four months or more and you aren't feeling any better.
- You feel depressed.
- Your grief is so intense that you feel you can't go on with your normal activities.
- Your grief is affecting your ability to concentrate, sleep, eat, or socialize as you normally do.
- You feel you can't go on living after the loss or you think about suicide, dying, or hurting yourself.

It's natural for loss to cause people to think about death to some degree. But if a loss has caused you to think about suicide or hurting yourself in some way, or if you feel that you can't go on living, it's important that you tell someone right away.

Counseling with a professional therapist can help because it allows you to talk about your loss and express strong feelings. Many counselors specialize in working with teens who are struggling with loss and depression. If you'd like to talk to a therapist and you're not sure where to begin, ask an adult or school counselor. Your doctor may also be able to recommend someone.

Will I Ever Get Over This?

Well-meaning friends and family might tell a grieving person they need to "move on" after a loss. Unfortunately, that type of advice can sometimes make people hesitate to talk about their loss, or make people think they're grieving wrong or too long, or that they're not normal. It can help to remember that the grieving process is very personal and individual—there's no right or wrong way to grieve. We all take our own time to heal.

It's important for grieving people to not drop out of life, though. If you don't like the idea of moving on, maybe the idea of "keeping on" seems like a better fit. Sometimes it helps to remind yourself to just keep on doing the best you can for now. If you feel sad, let yourself have your feelings and try not to run away from your emotions. But also keep on doing things you normally would such as being with friends, caring for your pet, working out, or doing your schoolwork.

Going forward and healing from grief doesn't mean forgetting about the person you lost. Getting back to enjoying your life doesn't mean you no longer miss the person. And how long it takes until you start to feel better isn't a measure of how much you loved the person. With time, the loving support of family and friends, and your own positive actions, you can find ways to cope with even the deepest loss.

✤ It's A Fact!!

How does grief differ from depression?

Depression is more than a feeling of grief after losing someone or something you love. Clinical depression is a whole body disorder. It can take over the way you think and feel. Symptoms of depression include the following:

- A sad, anxious, or "empty" mood that won't go away
- Loss of interest in what you used to enjoy
- Low energy, fatigue, feeling "slowed down"
- Changes in sleep patterns
- Loss of appetite, weight loss, or weight gain
- Trouble concentrating, remembering, or making decisions
- Feeling hopeless or gloomy
- Feeling guilty, worthless, or helpless
- Thoughts of death or suicide or a suicide attempt
- Recurring aches and pains that don't respond to treatment

If you recently experienced a death or other loss, these feelings may be part of a normal grief reaction. But if these feelings persist with no lifting mood, ask for help.

Source: Excerpted from "How to Deal with Grief," National Mental Health Information Center, Substance Abuse and Mental Health Services Administration (http://mentalhealth.samhsa.gov).

✔ Quick Tip

How will I know when I'm done grieving?

Every person who experiences a death or other loss must complete a four-step grieving process:

1. Accept the loss.
2. Work through and feel the physical and emotional pain of grief.
3. Adjust to living in a world without the person or item lost.
4. Move on with life.

The grieving process is over only when a person completes the four steps.

Source: Excerpted from "How to Deal with Grief," National Mental Health Information Center, Substance Abuse and Mental Health Services Administration (http://mentalhealth.samhsa.gov).

My Pet Died: How Can I Feel Better?

A pet can be a great friend. Even if you're having a bad day, if you don't feel popular, or if you're having trouble at school, your pet loves you. No strings attached. Millions of families throughout the world own pets, which means that every day someone goes through the heartbreak of losing an animal friend.

Whether it's old age, illness, or because of an accident, animals—like people—will die sometime. Veterinarians can do wonderful things for pets. But sometimes all the medical skill in the world can't save an animal. And if a pet is in a lot of pain and will never get better, the vet may have to put it to sleep. This is known as euthanasia (pronounced: yoo-thuh-nay-zhuh). The vet will give the animal an injection (shot) that first puts it to sleep and then stops the heart from beating. Euthanasia allows pets to die peacefully without any pain or fear. But deciding to help a pet die is still a hard thing to do.

Coping With The Death Of A Pet

Emotions can get pretty complicated when a pet dies. You probably expect to feel sad, but you may have other emotions, too. For example, you may feel angry if your friends don't seem to realize how much losing your pet means to you. Or perhaps you feel guilty that you didn't spend more time with your pet before he or she died. It's natural to feel a range of emotions when a pet dies.

If you're like a lot of people, you may have had someone say to you, "Sorry, but it was only an animal." So is it normal to get upset over the death of a pet? Absolutely. After all, by the time we reach our teenage years, many of us have grown up with our pets, and they're part of the family. Just like losing a family member, when a pet dies people can go through a period of grieving.

Grief can show up in many ways. Some people cry a lot. For others, the death may take a while to sink in. Some people temporarily lose interest in the things they enjoy doing or want to spend some quiet time alone. Others will want to keep busy to take their minds off the loss. It's also natural to feel like avoiding situations that involved your pet—such as the park where you used to walk your dog or the trail where you rode your horse.

✤ It's A Fact!!

Some people feel ready to get another pet right away. Other people need more time. Sometimes, members of a family have different timetables for getting through their grief and loss—one person may feel ready for a new pet, but someone else may not. It's important to take the time you need to grieve and to respect the time that others need as well.

Source: Copyright © October 2007 The Nemours Foundation.

For many people, losing a pet can be their first experience with death. Recognizing and sorting out feelings can be a big help. Talking about a loss is one of the best ways to cope, which is why people get together after a funeral and share memories or stories about the person who has died. Acknowledging your grief by talking about it with friends and family members can help you begin to feel better.

There are also additional ways to express your feelings and thoughts. Recording them in a journal is helpful to many people, as is keeping a scrapbook. You can also write about your pet in a story or poem, draw a picture, or compose music. Or plan a funeral or memorial service for your pet. Some people choose to make a donation in a pet's memory to an animal shelter or even volunteer there. All of these ideas can help you hold on to the good and happy memories.

Everyone has to deal with grief sometime, and most people work through it given time. But if you're under stress or trying to deal with other serious problems at the same time, grief can feel overwhelming. If your sadness is intense or you think you're upset about more than the death of your pet, it can be a good idea to talk with a professional counselor or therapist to help sort everything out. It's normal for a death to raise questions about our own lives, but you may also want to talk to someone if you find yourself focusing on death a lot.

You'll never forget your pet. But in time the painful feelings will ease. And when the time comes, you may even find yourself ready to open your home to a new pet in need of a loving family.

Part Two

Mood And Anxiety Disorders

Chapter 11

Depression

When the Blues Don't Go Away

Everyone occasionally feels blue or sad, but these feelings usually pass within a couple of days. When a person has depression, it interferes with his or her daily life and routine, such as going to work or school, taking care of children, and relationships with family and friends. Depression causes pain for the person who has it and for those who care about him or her.

Depression can be very different in different people or in the same person over time. It is a common but serious illness. Treatment can help those with even the most severe depression get better.

What are the symptoms of depression?

- Ongoing sad, anxious, or empty feelings
- Feelings of hopelessness
- Feelings of guilt, worthlessness, or helplessness
- Feeling irritable or restless
- Loss of interest in activities or hobbies that were once enjoyable
- Feeling tired all the time

About This Chapter: Text in this chapter is from "Depression (Easy to Read)," National Institute of Mental Health (www.nimh.nih.gov), 2007.

- Difficulty concentrating, remembering details, or difficulty making decisions
- Not able to go to sleep or stay asleep (insomnia); may wake in the middle of the night, or sleep all the time
- Overeating or loss of appetite
- Thoughts of suicide or making suicide attempts
- Ongoing aches and pains, headaches, cramps or digestive problems that do not go away

Not everyone diagnosed with depression will have all of these symptoms. The signs and symptoms may be different in men, women, younger children, and older adults.

Can a person have depression and another illness at the same time?

Often, people have other illnesses along with depression. Sometimes other illnesses come first, but other times the depression comes first. Each person and situation is different, but it is important not to ignore these illnesses and to get treatment for them and the depression. Some illnesses or disorders that may occur along with depression include the following:

- Anxiety disorders, including post-traumatic stress disorder (PTSD), obsessive-compulsive disorder (OCD), panic disorder, social phobia, and generalized anxiety disorder (GAD)
- Alcohol and other substance abuse or dependence
- Heart disease, stroke, cancer, HIV/AIDS, diabetes, and Parkinson's disease

Studies have found that treating depression can help in treating these other illnesses.

When does depression start?

Young children and teens can get depression but it can occur at other ages also. Depression is more common in women than in men, but men do get depression too. Loss of a loved one, stress and hormonal changes, or traumatic events may trigger depression at any age.

✎ What's It Mean?

There are several forms of depressive disorders. The most common are major depressive disorder and dysthymic disorder.

- **Major Depressive Disorder:** Also called major depression. Is characterized by a combination of symptoms that interfere with a person's ability to work, sleep, study, eat, and enjoy once-pleasurable activities. Major depression is disabling and prevents a person from functioning normally. An episode of major depression may occur only once in a person's lifetime, but more often, it recurs throughout a person's life.
- **Dysthymic Disorder:** Also called dysthymia. Is characterized by long-term (two years or longer) but less severe symptoms that may not disable a person but can prevent one from functioning normally or feeling well. People with dysthymia may also experience one or more episodes of major depression during their lifetimes.

Some forms of depressive disorder exhibit slightly different characteristics than those described above, or they may develop under unique circumstances. However, not all scientists agree on how to characterize and define these forms of depression. They include the following:

- **Psychotic Depression:** Occurs when a severe depressive illness is accompanied by some form of psychosis, such as a break with reality, hallucinations, and delusions.
- **Postpartum Depression:** Diagnosed if a new mother develops a major depressive episode within one month after delivery. It is estimated that 10 to 15 percent of women experience postpartum depression after giving birth.
- **Seasonal Affective Disorder (SAD):** Characterized by the onset of a depressive illness during the winter months, when there is less natural sunlight. The depression generally lifts during spring and summer. SAD may be effectively treated with light therapy, but nearly half of those with SAD do not respond to light therapy alone. Antidepressant medication and psychotherapy can reduce SAD symptoms, either alone or in combination with light therapy.
- **Bipolar Disorder:** Also called manic-depressive illness. Not as common as major depression or dysthymia. Bipolar disorder is characterized by cycling mood changes—from extreme highs (mania) to extreme lows (depression).

Source: Excerpted from "Depression," National Institute of Mental Health, March 20, 2009.

Is there help?

There is help for someone who has depression. Even in severe cases, depression is highly treatable. The first step is to visit a doctor. Your family doctor or a health clinic is a good place to start. A doctor can make sure that the symptoms of depression are not being caused by another medical condition. A doctor may refer you to a mental health professional.

The most common treatments of depression are psychotherapy and medication.

✔ Quick Tip

As a teenager, there are so many changes taking place in your body and with your emotions that it can be very overwhelming. You might feel like you are in a great mood one minute and a bad one the next. This roller coaster of emotions is normal. It's OK to have the blues sometimes and there are things you can do to feel better. Try these tips to improve your mood:

- Know that what you are going through is very common.
- Find a way to relax, such as sitting down and taking a deep breath or taking a shower.
- Talk to your friends, parents/guardians, teachers, counselors, or doctors about what you are feeling. They can help you sort through your emotions.
- Get some exercise. When you exercise, your body makes more special chemicals called endorphins. Endorphins can help improve your mood.
- Make sure that you get enough rest. Being tired can make you feel more stressed.

There is a big difference between having the blues and having depression. Depression is a serious illness that affects many young people. The good news is that depression can be treated. Make sure to talk to your doctor or school counselor about any worries you have about depression.

Source: Excerpted from "Your Emotions: Depression Or Feeling 'Blue'," Girlshealth.gov, U.S. Department of Health and Human Services, March 28, 2008.

Psychotherapy: Several types of psychotherapy—or "talk therapy"—can help people with depression. There are two main types of psychotherapy commonly used to treat depression: cognitive-behavioral therapy (CBT) and interpersonal therapy (IPT). CBT teaches people to change negative styles of thinking and behaving that may contribute to their depression. IPT helps people understand and work through troubled personal relationships that may cause their depression or make it worse.

For mild to moderate depression, psychotherapy may be the best treatment option. However, for major depression or for certain people, psychotherapy may not be enough. For teens, a combination of medication and psychotherapy may work the best to treat major depression and help keep the depression from happening again. Also, a study about treating depression in older adults found that those who got better with medication and IPT were less likely to have depression again if they continued their combination treatment for at least two years.

Medications: Medications help balance chemicals in the brain called neurotransmitters. Although scientists are not sure exactly how these chemicals work, they do know they affect a person's mood. The following are types of antidepressant medications that help keep the neurotransmitters at the correct levels:

- SSRIs (selective serotonin reuptake inhibitors)
- SNRIs (serotonin and norepinephrine reuptake inhibitors)
- MAOIs (monoamine oxidase inhibitors)
- Tricyclics

These different types of medications affect different chemicals in the brain.

Medications affect everyone differently. Sometimes several different types have to be tried before finding the one that works. If you start taking medication, tell your doctor about any side effects right away. Depending on which type of medication, these are some possible side effects:

- Headache
- Nausea

- Insomnia and nervousness
- Agitation or feeling jittery
- Sexual problems
- Dry mouth
- Constipation
- Bladder problems
- Blurred vision
- Drowsiness during the day

Despite the fact that SSRIs and other antidepressants are generally safe and reliable, some studies have shown that they may have unintentional effects on some people, especially young people. In 2004, the U.S. Food and Drug Administration (FDA) reviewed data from studies of antidepressants that involved nearly 4,400 children and teenagers being treated for depression. The review showed that 4% of those who took antidepressants thought about or attempted suicide (although no suicides occurred), compared to 2% of those who took sugar pills (placebo).

This information prompted the FDA, in 2005, to adopt a "black box" warning label on all antidepressant medications to alert the public about the potential increased risk of suicidal thinking or attempts in children and teenagers taking antidepressants. In 2007, the FDA proposed that makers of all antidepressant medications extend the black box warning on their labels to include young patients up through age 24 who are taking these medications for depression treatment. A "black box" warning is the most serious type of warning on prescription drug labeling.

The warning also emphasizes that children, teenagers and young adults taking antidepressants should be closely monitored, especially during the initial weeks of treatment, for any worsening depression or suicidal thinking or behavior. These include any unusual changes in behavior such as sleeplessness, agitation, or withdrawal from normal social situations.

Results of a review of pediatric trials between 1988 and 2006 suggested that the benefits of antidepressant medications likely outweigh their risks to children and adolescents with major depression and anxiety disorders. The study was funded in part by the National Institute of Mental Health.

St. John's Wort: The extract from St. John's wort (*Hypericum perforatum*), a bushy, wild-growing plant with yellow flowers, has been used for centuries in many folk and herbal remedies. The National Institutes of Health conducted a clinical trial to determine the effectiveness of the herb in treating adults who have major depression. Involving 340 patients diagnosed with major depression, the trial found that St. John's wort was no more effective than a "sugar pill" (placebo) in treating major depression. Another study is looking at whether St. John's wort is effective for treating mild or minor depression.

Other research has shown that St. John's wort may interfere with other medications, including those used to control HIV infection. On February 10, 2000, the FDA issued a Public Health Advisory letter stating that the herb may interfere with certain medications used to treat heart disease, depression, seizures, certain cancers, and organ transplant rejection. The herb also may interfere with the effectiveness of oral contraceptives. Because of these potential interactions, patients should always consult with their doctors before taking any herbal supplement.

Electroconvulsive Therapy: For cases in which medication and/or psychotherapy does not help treat depression, electroconvulsive therapy (ECT) may be useful. ECT, once known as "shock therapy," formerly had a bad reputation. But in recent years, it has greatly improved and can provide relief for people with severe depression who have not been able to feel better with other treatments.

ECT may cause short-term side effects, including confusion, disorientation, and memory loss. But these side effects typically clear soon after treatment. Research has indicated that after one year of ECT treatments, patients show no adverse cognitive effects.

How can I find treatment and who pays?

Most insurance plans cover treatment for depression. Check with your own insurance company to find out what type of treatment is covered. If you don't have insurance, local city or county governments may offer treatment at a clinic or health center, where the cost is based on income. Medicaid plans also may pay for depression treatment.

If you are unsure where to go for help, ask your family doctor. Others who can help include the following:

- Psychiatrists, psychologists, licensed social workers, or licensed mental health counselors
- Health maintenance organizations
- Community mental health centers
- Hospital psychiatry departments and outpatient clinics
- Mental health programs at universities or medical schools
- State hospital outpatient clinics
- Family services, social agencies or clergy
- Peer support groups
- Private clinics and facilities
- Employee assistance programs
- Local medical and/or psychiatric societies

You can also check the phone book under "mental health," "health," "social services," "hotlines," or "physicians" for phone numbers and addresses. An emergency room doctor also can provide temporary help and can tell you where and how to get further help.

Why do people get depression?

There is no single cause of depression. Depression happens because of a combination of things including the following:

Genes: Some types of depression tend to run in families. Genes are the "blueprints" for who we are, and we inherit them from our parents. Scientists are looking for the specific genes that may be involved in depression.

Brain Chemistry And Structure: When chemicals in the brain are not at the right levels, depression can occur. These chemicals, called neurotransmitters, help cells in the brain communicate with each other. By looking at

✤ It's A Fact!!

Certain circumstances may predict suicidal thinking or behavior among teens with treatment-resistant major depression who are undergoing second-step treatment, according to an analysis of data from a study funded by the National Institute of Mental Health (NIMH). The study was published online ahead of print February 17, 2009, in the *American Journal of Psychiatry*.

In the Treatment of SSRI-resistant Depression in Adolescents (TORDIA) study, 334 teens who did not get well after taking a type of antidepressant called a selective serotonin reuptake inhibitor (SSRI) before the trial were randomly assigned to one of four treatments for 12 weeks:

- Switch to another SSRI
- Switch to venlafaxine (Effexor), a different type of antidepressant
- Switch to another SSRI and add cognitive behavioral therapy (CBT), a type of psychotherapy
- Switch to venlafaxine and add CBT

Results of the trial were previously reported in February 2008. They showed that teens who received combination therapy, with either type of antidepressant, were more likely to get well than those on medication alone.

Using data from spontaneous reports by the participants and from systematic assessment by clinicians, David Brent, M.D., of the Western Psychiatric Institute and Clinic, and colleagues aimed to identify characteristics or circumstances that may predict whether a teen is likely to have suicidal thoughts or behavior during treatment. Nearly 60 percent of TORDIA participants had suicidal thinking or behavior at the beginning of the trial.

Fifty-eight suicidal events—which include serious suicidal thinking or a recent suicide attempt—occurred in 48 participants during the trial, most of which happened early in the trial. The researchers found that teens who had higher levels of suicidal thinking, higher levels of parent-child conflict, and who used drugs or alcohol at the trial's beginning were more likely to experience a suicidal event during treatment and less likely to respond to treatment. They were also less likely to have completed treatment.

Source: Excerpted from "Suicidal Thinking May Be Predicted Among Certain Teens With Depression," a Science Update from the National Institute of Mental Health, February 17, 2009.

pictures of the brain, scientists can also see that the structure of the brain in people who have depression looks different than in people who do not have depression. Scientists are working to figure out why these differences occur.

Environmental And Psychological Factors: Trauma, loss of a loved one, a difficult relationship, and other stressors can trigger depression. Scientists are working to figure out why depression occurs in some people but not in others with the same or similar experiences. They are also studying why some people recover quickly from depression and others do not.

What if I or someone I know is in crisis?

If you are thinking about harming yourself, or know someone who is, tell someone who can help immediately.

- Call your doctor.
- Call 911 or go to a hospital emergency room to get immediate help or ask a friend or family member to help you do these things.
- Call the toll-free, 24-hour hotline of the National Suicide Prevention Lifeline at 800-273-TALK (800-273-8255); TTY: 800-799-4TTY (4889) to talk to a trained counselor.
- Make sure you or the suicidal person is not left alone.

Chapter 12

Premenstrual Syndrome

Risk Factors

Premenstrual syndrome (PMS) is reported in women in many cultures worldwide. About 80% of women in their reproductive years have some emotional and physical symptoms before their periods that impair daily activities. Between 3–8% of women report very severe symptoms, notably premenstrual dysphoric disorder (PMDD). A number of factors may put a woman at higher risk for PMS.

Age: The risk for severe PMS is higher in younger women, and onset usually begins around the mid-twenties. Some evidence suggests that PMS symptoms diminish after age 35. Naturally, PMS and any manifestation of it end at menopause.

Psychologic Factors: Women with a history of or susceptibility to depression may be at increased risk for PMS and premenstrual dysphoric disorder (PMDD). Cultural factors may also affect the perception and severity of PMS symptoms.

Other Factors Associated With PMS: Studies have found some factors associated with a higher risk for PMS or more severe symptoms, (although the evidence behind these claims is not very strong):

- Having a mother who had PMS
- Being sedentary
- Stress
- High-sugar diet
- Consumption of large amounts of caffeine
- Alcohol abuse
- Women with more children may experience more severe symptoms than those with fewer children

Complications

PMS, and in particular premenstrual dysphoric disorder (PMDD), can have an adverse effect on women's relationships with co-workers, partners, and children.

Risk For Major Depression: Depression and PMS often coincide, and may in some cases be due to common factors. Some studies suggest that PMDD may lead to or predict perimenopausal depression in some women.

Substance Abuse: Women who abuse alcohol or have close relatives who are alcoholics, have a much higher risk for drinking during the premenstrual period. Alcohol worsens PMS symptoms and may increase the risk for prolonged cramping (dysmenorrhea) during menstruation. Studies also have found a higher incidence of smoking in women with premenstrual dysphoric disorder than in women without PMDD.

Magnification Of Other Medical Conditions

A number of conditions worsen during the premenstrual or menstrual phase of the cycle, a phenomenon sometimes referred to as menstrual magnification.

Migraines: About half of women with migraines report an association with menstruation, usually in the first days before or after menstruation begins. Compared to migraines that occur at other times of the month, menstrual migraines tend to be more severe, last longer, and not have auras.

Asthma: Asthma attacks often increase or worsen during the premenstrual period.

Other Disorders: Many other chronic medical conditions may be exacerbated during the premenstrual phase, including epilepsy and other seizure disorders, multiple sclerosis, systemic lupus erythematosus, inflammatory bowel disease, and irritable bowel syndrome.

Symptoms

Nearly every woman at some point has some symptoms as menstruation approaches. For about half of these women, symptoms are mild and do not affect normal daily life. The other half report symptoms severe enough to impair daily life and relationships. Between 3–5% of women report extremely severe symptoms.

In general, premenstrual syndrome (PMS) is a set of physical, emotional, and behavioral symptoms that occur during the last week of the luteal phase (1–2 weeks before menstruation) in most cycles. The symptoms typically go away within four days after bleeding starts and do not start again until at least day 13 in the cycle. Women may begin to experience premenstrual syndrome symptoms at any time during their reproductive years. Once established, the symptoms tend to remain fairly constant until menopause, although they can vary from cycle to cycle.

✤ It's A Fact!!

Researchers are still uncertain about the causes of premenstrual syndrome. Fluctuations in gonadal hormones (progesterone or estrogen) and brain chemicals may play a role although their exact significance is unclear. Hormonal levels seem to be the same in women whether or not they have premenstrual syndrome. It is possible that women with premenstrual syndrome are somehow more responsive to these changing levels of hormones.

Physical Symptoms

- Breast engorgement and tenderness
- Abdominal bloating
- Constipation or diarrhea
- Headache and migraine (migraine may increase severity of PMS symptoms)
- Swelling of the hands or feet
- Weight gain
- Clumsiness
- Nausea and vomiting
- Muscle and joint aches or pains

Emotional And Behavioral Symptoms

- Depression (severe depression before menstruation, called premenstrual dysphoric disorder, occurs in about 5% of women with PMS)
- Anxiety and panic attacks
- Insomnia
- Change in sexual interest and desire (although some women lose interest, others have a heightened drive)
- Irritability
- Hostility and outbursts of anger (in severe cases, violence toward self and others)
- Increased appetite often with specific food cravings (especially salt and sugar)
- Mood swings (although angry outburst or negative emotions are common, some women experience very positive bursts of creative energy before a period)
- Inability to concentrate and some memory loss (although women often report these symptoms, studies have indicate no actual differences in mental and thinking tasks between women with PMS

✎ What's It Mean?

Premenstrual Dysphoric Disorder: Premenstrual dysphoric disorder (PMDD) is a specific psychiatric condition marked by severe depression, irritability, and tension before menstruation. For a doctor to confirm a diagnosis of PMDD, the patient must have symptoms during the last week of the premenstrual phase and that resolve within a few days after menstruation starts. Five or more of the following symptoms must occur:

- Feeling of sadness or hopelessness, possible suicidal thoughts
- Feelings of tension or anxiety (panic attacks, in fact, may be much more common in patients with PMDD than in the general population)
- Mood swings marked by periods of teariness
- Persistent irritability or anger that affects other people
- Disinterest in daily activities and relationships
- Trouble concentrating
- Fatigue or low energy
- Food cravings or bingeing
- Sleep disturbances
- Feeling out of control
- Physical symptoms, such as bloating, breast tenderness, headaches, and joint or muscle pain

or premenstrual dysphoric disorder and women without these syndromes)
- Withdrawal from other people
- Confusion
- Being accident prone
- Lethargy and fatigue

Treatment

Lifestyle Changes: A healthy lifestyle, including regular exercise and a healthy diet, is the first step towards managing premenstrual syndrome. For many women with mild symptoms, lifestyle approaches are sufficient to control symptoms.

Dietary Factors: Women should follow the general guidelines for a healthy diet. These guidelines include eating plenty of whole grains and fresh fruits and vegetables and avoiding saturated fats and commercial junk foods. Making dietary adjustments starting about 14 days before a period may help some women control premenstrual symptoms.

Drinking plenty of fluids (water or juice, not soft drinks or caffeine) may help reduce bloating, fluid retention, and other symptoms.

Increasing complex carbohydrate intake may be helpful. Carbohydrates increase blood levels of tryptophan, an amino acid that converts to serotonin, the brain chemical important for feelings of well-being. Meals should be high in complex carbohydrates, which are found in whole grains and vegetables. (Complex carbohydrates should always be preferred over simple carbohydrates found in sugar and starch-heavy foods, such as pastas, baked goods, white-flour products, and white potatoes.)

It is best to eat frequent small meals, with no more than three hours between snacks, and avoid overeating. Unfortunately many women not only overeat during the premenstrual stage but also tend to eat sugar-rich foods or high-fat salty snack foods—the worst choices for PMS. Overeating such foods may worsen some PMS symptoms, including water retention and negative mood.

Limiting salt intake can help bloating. Reducing caffeine, sugar, and alcohol intake may be beneficial.

Exercise And Stress Reduction: Exercise, especially aerobic exercise, increases natural opioids in the brain (endorphins) and improves mood. Exercise is also very important for maintaining good physical health. Even taking a 30-minute walk every day is beneficial. Although not an aerobic exercise, yoga releases muscle tension, regulates breathing, and reduces stress. Relaxation techniques, including meditation, can also help reduce stress.

Vitamins And Minerals: Some evidence indicates that calcium with vitamin D, and vitamin B6 supplements, may help with PMS symptoms.

Improved Sleep: Many women with PMS suffer from sleep problems, either sleeping too much or too little. Achieving better sleep habits may help relieve symptoms.

Herbs And Supplements: Generally, manufacturers of herbal remedies and dietary supplements do not need U.S. Food and Drug Administration (FDA) approval to sell their products. Just like a drug, herbs and supplements can affect the body's chemistry, and therefore have the potential to produce side effects that may be harmful. There have been a number of reported cases of serious and even lethal side effects from herbal products. Always check with your doctor before using any herbal remedies or dietary supplements.

✤ It's A Fact!!

The effects of magnesium are not as well established as with calcium, but some evidence suggests that it may be helpful in reducing fluid retention in women with mild PMS. A number of factors can cause magnesium deficiencies, including intake of too much alcohol, salt, soda, coffee, as well as profuse sweating, intense stress, and excessive menstruation. Magnesium can be toxic in high amounts and can interact with certain drugs. Women should discuss supplements with their doctor.

A number of herbal remedies are used for PMS symptoms. With a few exceptions, studies have not found any herbal or dietary supplement remedy to be any more effective than placebo for relieving PMS symptoms.

Some women have reported that taking evening primrose oil helped PMS. However, studies vary as to its effectiveness for PMS symptoms and two rigorous studies reported no benefit. It may be helpful for relieving breast symptoms.

Ginger tea is safe and may help soothe mild nausea and other minor symptoms of PMS.

The following are special concerns for people taking natural remedies for PMS:

- St. John's wort (*Hypericum perforatum*) is an herbal remedy that may help some patients with mild-to-moderate depression. It can increase the risk for bleeding when used with blood-thinning drugs. It can also reduce the effectiveness of certain drugs, including cancer and HIV treatments. St. John's wort can increase sensitivity to sunlight.
- Dong quai is a Chinese herb used to treat menstrual symptoms. Dong quai can lengthen the time it takes for blood to clot. People with bleeding disorders should not use dong quai. Dong quai should not be taken with drugs that prevent blood clotting, such as warfarin or aspirin.
- L-tryptophan supplements have caused eosinophilia-myalgia syndrome (EMS) in some people. EMS is a disorder that elevates certain white blood cells and can be fatal.

Medications: Nonsteroidal anti-inflammatory drugs (NSAIDs) block prostaglandins, substances that dilate blood vessels and cause inflammation. NSAIDs are usually among the first drugs recommended for almost any kind of minor pain. The most common ones used for PMS are nonprescription ibuprofen (Advil, Motrin, Midol) and naproxen (Aleve) or prescription mefenamic acid (Postel). Studies indicate that NSAIDs are most helpful when started seven days before menstruation and continued for four days into the cycle. Long-term daily use of any NSAID can increase the risk for gastrointestinal bleeding and ulcers. Long-term NSAID use can also increase the risk for heart attack and stroke.

Acetaminophen (Tylenol) is a good alternative to NSAIDs, especially when stomach problems, ulcers, or allergic reactions prohibit their use. Products that combine acetaminophen with other drugs that reduce PMS symptoms may be helpful. Brands include Pamprin and Premsyn. Such drugs typically also include a diuretic to reduce fluid and an antihistamine. Little evidence exists to indicate whether they are more or less effective than NSAIDs or other mild pain relievers.

Selective serotonin-reuptake inhibitors (SSRIs) are drugs that keep higher levels of serotonin available in the brain. They have become the most effective treatments for premenstrual dysphoric disorder (PMDD) and for severe PMS symptoms. SSRIs currently approved by the FDA for the treatment of PMDD symptoms include fluoxetine (Prozac, Sarafem), sertraline (Zoloft), paroxetine (Paxil), citalopram (Celexa), [and] ecitalopram (Lexapro).

Non-SSRI antidepressants sometimes prescribed for PMDD include the serotonin-noradrenaline reuptake inhibitor venlafaxine (Effexor) and the tricyclic antidepressant clomipramine (Anafranil). Patients should not take tricyclics with either SSRIs or other antidepressants known as monoamine oxidase inhibitors (MAOIs).

Antianxiety drugs (called anxiolytics) may be helpful for women with severe premenstrual anxiety that is not relieved by SSRIs or other treatments.

Hormone Therapies: Hormone therapies are used to interrupt the hormonal cycle that triggers premenstrual syndrome symptoms. One method to accomplish this is through birth control pills.

Oral contraceptives (OCs), commonly called "the Pill" collectively, contain combinations of an estrogen (usually estradiol) and a progestin (either a natural progesterone or the synthetic form called progestin). Some women may experience worsening of symptoms with oral contraceptives.

One birth control pill, Yaz, is approved specifically for treatment of premenstrual dysmorphic disorder (PMSS). Yaz is a low-dose birth control pill that combines the estrogen estradiol with a newer type of progestin called drospirenone. This type of progestin is related to spironolactone,

✤ It's A Fact!!

In May 2007, the FDA proposed that all antidepressant medications should carry a warning about increased risks for suicidal thinking and behavior in young adults ages 18–24. This risk for "suicidality" generally occurs during the first few months of treatment.

a diuretic. Yaz uses a 24-day dosing regimen (24 days active pills, four days placebo pills).

Newer "continuous-dosing" (also called "continuous-use") oral contraceptives aim to reduce—or even eliminate—monthly periods and thereby prevent the pain and discomfort that often accompanies menstruation. These OCs contain a combination of estradiol and the progesterone levonorgestrel, but use extending dosing of active pills.

Gonadotropin-releasing hormone (GnRH) agonists (also called analogs) are powerful hormonal drugs that suppress ovulation and, thereby, the hormonal fluctuations that produce PMS. They are sometimes used for very severe PMS symptoms and to improve breast tenderness, fatigue, and irritability. GnRH analogs, however, appear to have little effect on depression.

Danazol (Danocrine) is a synthetic substance that resembles male hormones and should be used only if other therapies fail. It suppresses estrogen and menstruation and is used in low doses for severe PMS and premenstrual migraines. Taking it only during the luteal phase relieves cyclical mastalgia (severe breast pain) and avoids major side effects, but this intermittent regimen has no effect on other PMS symptoms. Side effects from continuous use of Danazol can be severe.

Diuretics are drugs that increase urination and help eliminate water and salt from the body. They reduce bloating in women with PMS and may also have a beneficial effect on mood, breast tenderness, and food craving. Diuretics can have considerable side effects and should not be used for mild or moderate PMS symptoms.

Chapter 13

Seasonal Affective Disorder

Maggie started off her junior year of high school with great energy. She had no trouble keeping up with her schoolwork and was involved in several after-school activities. But after the Thanksgiving break, she began to have difficulty getting through her assigned reading and had to work harder to apply herself. She couldn't concentrate in class, and after school all she wanted to do was sleep.

Maggie's grades began to drop and she rarely felt like socializing. Even though Maggie was always punctual before, she began to have trouble getting up on time and was absent or late from school many days during the winter.

At first, Maggie's parents thought she was slacking off. They were upset with her, but figured it was just a phase—especially since her energy finally seemed to return in the spring. But when the same thing happened the following November, they took Maggie to the doctor, who diagnosed her with a type of depression called seasonal affective disorder.

About This Chapter: Text in this chapter is from "Seasonal Affective Disorder," January 2007, reprinted with permission from www.kidshealth.org. Copyright © 2007 The Nemours Foundation. This information was provided by KidsHealth, one of the largest resources online for medically reviewed health information written for parents, kids, and teens. For more articles like this one, visit www.KidsHealth.org, or www.TeensHealth.org.

What Is Seasonal Affective Disorder?

Seasonal affective disorder (SAD) is a form of depression that appears at the same time each year. With SAD, a person typically has symptoms of depression and unexplained fatigue as winter approaches and daylight hours become shorter. When spring returns and days become longer again, people with SAD experience relief from their symptoms, returning to their usual mood and energy level.

What Causes SAD?

Experts believe that, with SAD, depression is somehow triggered by the brain's response to decreased daylight exposure. No one really understands how and why this happens. Current theories about what causes SAD focus on the role that sunlight might play in the brain's production of key hormones.

Experts think that two specific chemicals in the brain, melatonin and serotonin may be involved in SAD. These two hormones help regulate a person's sleep-wake cycles, energy, and mood. Shorter days and longer hours of darkness in fall and winter may cause increased levels of melatonin and decreased levels of serotonin, creating the biological conditions for depression.

Melatonin is linked to sleep. The body produces this hormone in greater quantities when it's dark or when days are shorter. This increased production of melatonin can cause a person to feel sleepy and lethargic.

With serotonin, it's the reverse—serotonin production goes up when a person is exposed to sunlight, so it's likely that a person will have lower levels of serotonin during the winter when the days are shorter. Low levels of serotonin are associated with depression, whereas increasing the availability of serotonin helps to combat depression.

What Are the Symptoms Of SAD?

Someone with SAD will show several particular changes from the way he or she normally feels and acts. These changes occur in a predictable seasonal pattern. The symptoms of SAD are the same as symptoms of depression, and a person with SAD may notice several or all of these symptoms:

- **Changes In Mood:** A person may feel sad or be in an irritable mood most of the time for at least 2 weeks during a specific time of year. During that time, a guy or girl may feel a sense of hopelessness or worthlessness. As part of the mood change that goes with SAD, people can be self-critical; they may also be more sensitive than usual to criticism and cry or get upset more often or more easily.
- **Lack Of Enjoyment:** Someone with SAD may lose interest in things he or she normally likes to do and may seem unable to enjoy things as before. People with SAD can also feel like they no longer do certain tasks as well as they used to, and they may have feelings of dissatisfaction or guilt. A person with SAD may seem to lose interest in friends and may stop participating in social activities.
- **Low Energy:** Unusual tiredness or unexplained fatigue is also part of SAD and can cause people to feel low on energy.
- **Changes In Sleep:** A person may sleep much more than usual. Excessive sleeping can make it impossible for a student to get up and get ready for school in the morning.
- **Changes In Eating:** Changes in eating and appetite related to SAD may include cravings for simple carbohydrates (think comfort foods and sugary foods) and the tendency to overeat. Because of this change in eating, SAD can result in weight gain during the winter months.
- **Difficulty Concentrating:** SAD can affect concentration, too, interfering with a person's school performance and grades. A student may have more trouble than usual completing assignments on time or seem to lack his or her usual motivation. Someone with SAD may notice that his or her grades may drop, and teachers may comment that the student seems less motivated or is making less effort in school.
- **Less Time Socializing:** People with SAD may spend less time with friends, in social activities, or in extracurricular activities.

The problems caused by SAD, such as lower-than-usual grades or less energy for socializing with friends, can affect self-esteem and leave a person feeling disappointed, isolated, and lonely—especially if he or she doesn't realize what's causing the changes in energy, mood, and motivation.

Who Gets SAD?

SAD can affect adults, teens, and children. It's estimated that about six in every 100 people (6%) experience SAD.

The number of people with SAD varies from region to region. One study of SAD in the United States found the rates of SAD were seven times higher among people in New Hampshire than in Florida, suggesting that the farther people live from the equator, the more likely they are to develop SAD.

✤ It's A Fact!!

Like other forms of depression, the symptoms of SAD can be mild, severe, or anywhere in between. Milder symptoms interfere less with someone's ability to participate in everyday activities, but stronger symptoms can interfere much more. It's the seasonal pattern of SAD—the fact that symptoms occur only for a few months each winter (for at least two years in a row) but not during other seasons—that distinguishes SAD from other forms of depression.

Most people don't get seasonal depression (SAD), even if they live in areas where days are shorter during winter months. Experts don't fully understand why certain people are more likely to experience SAD than others. It may be that some people are more sensitive than others to variations in light, and therefore may experience more dramatic shifts in hormone production, depending on their exposure to light.

Like other forms of depression, females are about four times more likely than males to develop SAD. People with relatives who have experienced depression are also more likely to develop it. Individual biology, brain chemistry, family history, environment, and life experiences may also make certain individuals more prone to SAD and other forms of depression.

✤ It's A Fact!!

Interestingly, when people who get SAD travel to areas far south of the equator that have longer daylight hours during winter months, they do not get their seasonal symptoms. This supports the theory that SAD is related to light exposure.

Researchers are continuing to investigate what leads to SAD, as well as why some people are more likely than others to experience it.

How Is SAD Diagnosed And Treated?

Doctors and mental health professionals make a diagnosis of SAD after a careful evaluation. A medical checkup is also important to make sure that symptoms aren't due to a medical condition that needs treatment. Tiredness, fatigue, and low energy could be a sign of another medical condition such as hypothyroidism, hypoglycemia, or mononucleosis. Other medical conditions can cause appetite changes, sleep changes, or extreme fatigue.

Once a person's been diagnosed with SAD, doctors may recommend one of several treatments:

Increased Light Exposure: Because the symptoms of SAD are triggered by lack of exposure to light, and they tend to go away on their own when available light increases, treatment for SAD often involves increased exposure to light during winter months. For someone with mild symptoms, it may be enough to spend more time outside during the daylight hours, perhaps by exercising outdoors or taking a daily walk. Full spectrum (daylight) light bulbs that fit in regular lamps can help bring a bit more daylight into your home in winter months and might help with mild symptoms.

Light Therapy: Stronger symptoms of SAD may be treated with light therapy (also called phototherapy). Light therapy involves the use of a special light that simulates daylight. A special light box or panel is placed on a tabletop or desk, and the person sits in front of the light for a short period of time every day (45 minutes a day or so, usually in the morning). The person should occasionally glance at the light (the light has to be absorbed through the retinas in order to work), but not stare into it for long periods. Symptoms tend to improve within a few days in some cases or within a few weeks in others. Generally, doctors recommend the use of light therapy until enough sunlight is available outdoors.

Like any medical treatment, light treatment should only be used under the supervision of a doctor. People who have another type of depressive disorder, skin that's sensitive to light, or medical conditions that may make the eyes vulnerable to light damage should use light therapy with caution. The lights that are used for SAD phototherapy must filter out harmful UV rays. Tanning beds or booths should not be used to alleviate symptoms of SAD. Some mild side effects of phototherapy might include headache or eyestrain.

Talk Therapy: Talk therapy (psychotherapy) is also used to treat people with SAD. Talk therapy focuses on revising the negative thoughts and feelings associated with depression and helps ease the sense of isolation or loneliness that people with depression often feel. The support and guidance of a professional therapist can be helpful for someone experiencing SAD. Talk therapy can also help someone to learn about and understand their condition as well as learn what to do to prevent or minimize future bouts of seasonal depression.

Medication: Doctors may also prescribe medications for teens with SAD. Antidepressant medications help to regulate the balance of serotonin and other neurotransmitters in the brain that affect mood and energy. Medications need to be prescribed and monitored by a doctor. If your doctor prescribes medication for SAD or another form of depression, be sure to let him or her know about any other medications or remedies you may be taking, including over-the-counter or herbal medicines. These can interfere with prescription medications.

Dealing With SAD

When symptoms of SAD first develop, it can be confusing, both for the person with SAD and family and friends. Some parents or teachers may mistakenly think that teens with SAD are slacking off or not trying their best. If you think you're experiencing some of the symptoms of SAD, talk to a parent, guidance counselor, or other trusted adult about what you're feeling.

If you've been diagnosed with SAD, there are a few things you can do to help:

- Follow your doctor's recommendations for treatment.
- Learn all you can about SAD and explain the condition to others so they can work with you.
- Get plenty of exercise, especially outdoors. Exercise can be a mood lifter.

- Spend time with friends and loved ones who understand what you're going through — they can help provide you with personal contact and a sense of connection.
- Be patient. Don't expect your symptoms to go away immediately.
- Ask for help with homework and other assignments if you need it. If you feel you can't concentrate on things, remember that it's part of the disorder and that things will get better again. Talk to your teachers and work out a plan to get your assignments done.
- Eat right. It may be hard, but avoiding simple carbohydrates and sugary snacks and concentrating on plenty of whole grains, vegetables, and fruits can help you feel better in the long term.
- Develop a sleep routine. Regular bedtimes can help you reap the mental health benefits of daytime light.
- Depression in any form can be serious. If you think you have symptoms of any type of depression, talk to someone who can help you get treatment.

Chapter 14

Bipolar Disorder

What is bipolar disorder?

Bipolar disorder is a serious brain illness. It is also called manic-depressive illness. Children with bipolar disorder go through unusual mood changes. Sometimes they feel very happy or "up," and are much more active than usual. This is called mania. And sometimes children with bipolar disorder feel very sad and "down" and are much less active than usual. This is called depression.

Bipolar disorder is not the same as the normal ups and downs every kid goes through. Bipolar symptoms are more powerful than that. The illness can make it hard for a child to do well in school or get along with friends and family members. The illness can also be dangerous. Some young people with bipolar disorder try to hurt themselves or attempt suicide.

Children and teens with bipolar disorder should get treatment. With help, they can manage their symptoms and lead successful lives.

Who develops bipolar disorder?

Anyone can develop bipolar disorder, including children and teens. However, most people with bipolar disorder develop it in their late teen or early adult years. The illness usually lasts a lifetime.

About This Chapter: Text in this chapter is from "Bipolar Disorder in Children and Teens (Easy to Read)," National Institute of Mental Health (www.nimh.nih.gov), February 27, 2009.

✤ It's A Fact!!

Do other illnesses co-occur with bipolar disorder?

Alcohol and drug abuse are very common among people with bipolar disorder. Research findings suggest that many factors may contribute to these substance abuse problems, including self-medication of symptoms, mood symptoms either brought on or perpetuated by substance abuse, and risk factors that may influence the occurrence of both bipolar disorder and substance use disorders. Treatment for co-occurring substance abuse, when present, is an important part of the overall treatment plan.

Anxiety disorders, such as post-traumatic stress disorder and obsessive-compulsive disorder, also may be common in people with bipolar disorder. Co-occurring anxiety disorders may respond to the treatments used for bipolar disorder, or they may require separate treatment.

Source: Excerpted from "Bipolar Disorder," National Institute of Mental Illness (www.nimh.nih.gov), January 22, 2009.

How is bipolar disorder different in children and teens than it is in adults?

When children develop the illness, it is called early-onset bipolar disorder. This type can be more severe than bipolar disorder in older teens and adults. Also, young people with bipolar disorder may have symptoms more often and switch moods more frequently than adults with the illness.

What causes bipolar disorder?

Several factors may contribute to bipolar disorder, including the following:

- Genes, because the illness runs in families. Children with a parent or sibling with bipolar disorder are more likely to get the illness than other children.

- Abnormal brain structure and brain function.
- Anxiety disorders. Children with anxiety disorders are more likely to develop bipolar disorder.

The causes of bipolar disorder aren't always clear. Scientists are studying it to find out more about possible causes and risk factors. This research may help doctors predict whether a person will get bipolar disorder. One day, it may also help doctors prevent the illness in some people.

✤ It's A Fact!!

Symptoms Persist As Bipolar Children Grow Up

Bipolar disorder identified in childhood often persisted into adulthood in the first large follow-up study of its kind. Forty-four percent of children diagnosed with bipolar disorder continued to have manic episodes as adults, in the study by National Institute of Mental Health (NIMH) grantee Barbara Geller, M.D., and colleagues at Washington University in St. Louis. They report on their findings in the October 2008 issue of the *Archives of General Psychiatry.*

"Serious mental illnesses do not emerge de novo (anew) when individuals reach adulthood, but rather reflect early developmental processes," explained NIMH's Ellen Leibenluft, M.D., in an accompanying editorial titled "Pediatric Bipolar Disorder Comes of Age."

The study adds to mounting evidence for the legitimacy of the diagnosis of bipolar in children, and reflects the "field's continuing efforts to nurture developmental conceptualizations of psychiatric illnesses," notes Leibenluft. The results are consistent with a 2006 study by Geller and colleagues, which found that child and adult forms of bipolar disorder occurred within the same families. In taking stock of what has been learned about pediatric bipolar disorder over the past couple of decades, Leibenluft points to a growing consensus that "unequivocal," classic bipolar disorder occurs in youth—albeit with continuing debate about whether children with persistent, severe irritability, but without distinct episodes of mania, should be assigned the bipolar disorder diagnosis. There is also consensus that children with bipolar disorder are severely impaired, with frequent relapses and other apparent psychopathology.

Source: Excerpted from "Symptoms Persist as Bipolar Children Grow Up," a Science Update from the National Institute of Mental Health, October 27, 2008.

What are the symptoms of bipolar disorder?

Bipolar mood changes are called "mood episodes." A child may have manic episodes, depressive episodes, or "mixed" episodes. A mixed episode has both manic and depressive symptoms. Children and teens with bipolar disorder may have more mixed episodes than adults with the illness.

Mood episodes last a week or two—sometimes longer. During an episode, the symptoms last every day for most of the day.

Mood episodes are intense. The feelings are strong and happen along with extreme changes in behavior and energy levels.

✤ It's A Fact!!

Largest Study Of Its Kind Implicates Gene Abnormalities In Bipolar Disorder

The largest genetic analysis of its kind to date for bipolar disorder has implicated machinery involved in the balance of sodium and calcium in brain cells. Researchers supported in part by the National Institute of Mental Health, part of the National Institutes of Health, found an association between the disorder and variation in two genes that make components of channels that manage the flow of the elements into and out of cells, including neurons.

"A neuron's excitability—whether it will fire—hinges on this delicate equilibrium," explained Pamela Sklar, M.D., Ph.D., of Massachusetts General Hospital (MGH) and the Stanley Center for Psychiatric Research at the Broad Institute of MIT and Harvard, who led the research. "Finding statistically robust associations linked to two proteins that may be involved in regulating such ion channels—and that are also thought to be targets of drugs used to clinically to treat bipolar disorder—is astonishing."

Although it's not yet known if or how the suspect genetic variation might affect the balance machinery, the results point to the possibility that bipolar disorder might stem, at least in part, from malfunction of ion channels.

Source: Excerpted from "Largest Study of Its Kind Implicates Gene Abnormalities in Bipolar Disorder," a National Institute of Mental Health press release dated August 18, 2008.

Children and teens having a manic episode may have symptoms such as the following:

- Feel very happy or act silly in a way that's unusual
- Have a very short temper
- Talk really fast about a lot of different things
- Have trouble sleeping but not feel tired
- Have trouble staying focused
- Talk and think about sex more often
- Do risky things

Children and teens having a depressive episode may have symptoms such as the following:

- Feel very sad
- Complain about pain a lot, like stomachaches and headaches
- Sleep too little or too much
- Feel guilty and worthless
- Eat too little or too much
- Have little energy and no interest in fun activities
- Think about death or suicide

Do children and teens with bipolar disorder have other problems?

Bipolar disorder in young people can co-exist with several problems.

- **Substance Abuse:** Both adults and kids with bipolar disorder are at risk of drinking or taking drugs.
- **Attention Deficit/Hyperactivity Disorder (ADHD):** Children with bipolar disorder and ADHD may have trouble staying focused.
- **Anxiety Disorders** (like separation anxiety): Children with both types of disorders may need to go to the hospital more often than other people with bipolar disorder.

- **Other Mental Illnesses** (like depression): Some mental illnesses cause symptoms that look like bipolar disorder. Tell a doctor about any manic or depressive symptoms you have had.

Sometimes behavior problems go along with mood episodes. Young people may take a lot of risks, like drive too fast or spend too much money. Some young people with bipolar disorder think about suicide. Watch out for any sign of suicidal thinking. Take these signs seriously and call your doctor.

How is bipolar disorder diagnosed?

An experienced doctor will carefully examine you. There are no blood tests or brain scans that can diagnose bipolar disorder. Instead, the doctor will ask questions about your mood and sleeping patterns. The doctor will also ask about your energy and behavior. Sometimes doctors need to know about medical problems in your family, such as depression or alcoholism. The doctor may use tests to see if an illness other than bipolar disorder is causing your symptoms.

How is bipolar disorder treated?

Right now, there is no cure for bipolar disorder. Doctors often treat children who have the illness in a similar way they treat adults. Treatment can help control symptoms. Treatment works best when it is ongoing, instead of on and off.

Medication: Different types of medication can help. Children respond to medications in different ways, so the type of medication depends on the child. Some children may need more than one type of medication because their symptoms are so complex. Sometimes they need to try different types of medicine to see which are best for them.

Children should take the fewest number and smallest amounts of medications as possible to help their symptoms. A good way to remember this is "start low, go slow". Always tell your doctor about any problems with side effects. Do not stop taking your medication without a doctor's help. Stopping medication suddenly can be dangerous, and it can make bipolar symptoms worse.

Therapy: Different kinds of psychotherapy, or "talk" therapy, can help children with bipolar disorder. Therapy can help children change their behavior and manage their routines. It can also help young people get along better with family and friends. Sometimes therapy includes family members.

What can children and teens expect from treatment?

With treatment, children and teens with bipolar disorder can get better over time. It helps when doctors, parents, and young people work together.

Sometimes a child's bipolar disorder changes. When this happens, treatment needs to change too. For example, you may need to try a different medication. The doctor may also recommend other treatment changes. Symptoms

✤ It's A Fact!!
Family-Focused Therapy Effective In Treating Depressive Episodes Of Bipolar Youth

Adolescents with bipolar disorder who received a nine-month course of family-focused therapy (FFT) recovered more quickly from depressive episodes and stayed free of depression for longer periods than a control group, according to a study funded by the National Institute of Mental Health (NIMH) published September 2008 in the *Archives of General Psychiatry*.

In FFT, the patient and his or her family are heavily involved in psychosocial treatment sessions. They learn to identify the symptoms of bipolar disorder, its course, and how to spot impending episodes or relapses. Patients and families also learn communication and problem-solving skills, and illness management strategies. For this trial, David Miklowitz, Ph.D., of the University of Colorado, and colleagues adapted the therapy to the needs of adolescents and their families.

Source: Excerpted from "Family-Focused Therapy Effective in Treating Depressive Episodes of Bipolar Youth," a Science Update from the National Institute of Mental Health, September 1, 2008.

may come back after a while, and more adjustments may be needed. Treatment can take time, but sticking with it helps many children and teens have fewer bipolar symptoms.

You can help treatment be more effective. Try keeping a chart of your moods, behaviors, and sleep patterns. This is called a "daily life chart" or "mood chart." It can help you understand and track the illness. A chart can also help the doctor see whether treatment is working.

Where do I go for help?

If you're not sure where to get help, call your family doctor. You can also check the phone book for mental health professionals. Hospital doctors can help in an emergency.

I know someone who is in crisis. What do I do?

If you're thinking about hurting yourself, or if you know someone who might, get help quickly.

- Do not leave the person alone.
- Call your doctor.
- Call 911 or go to the emergency room.
- Call a toll-free suicide hotline: 800-273-TALK (8255) for the National Suicide Prevention Lifeline. The TTY number is 800-799-4TTY (4889).

Chapter 15

Generalized Anxiety Disorder

All of us worry about things like health, money, or family problems at one time or another. But people with generalized anxiety disorders (GAD) are extremely worried about these and many other things, even when there is little or no reason to worry about them. They may be very anxious about just getting through the day. They think things will always go badly. At times, worrying keeps people with GAD from doing everyday tasks.

This is a list of common symptoms that people with GAD may experience:

- Worry very much about everyday things for at least six months, even if there is little or no reason to worry about them
- Can't control their constant worries
- Know that they worry much more than they should
- Can't relax
- Have a hard time concentrating
- Are easily startled
- Have trouble falling asleep or staying asleep

About This Chapter: Text in this chapter is from "Generalized Anxiety Disorder," National Institute of Mental Health (www.nimh.nih.gov), February 11, 2009.

People with GAD may also experience common body symptoms including the following:

- Feeling tired for no reason
- Headaches
- Muscle tension and aches
- Having a hard time swallowing
- Trembling or twitching
- Being irritable
- Sweating
- Nausea
- Feeling lightheaded
- Feeling out of breath
- Having to go to the bathroom a lot
- Hot flashes

✤ It's A Fact!!

Anxiety Disorders

People with anxiety disorders feel extremely fearful and unsure. Most people feel anxious about something for a short time now and again, but people with anxiety disorders feel this way most of the time. Their fears and worries make it hard for them to do everyday tasks. About 18% of American adults have anxiety disorders. Children also may have them.

Treatment is available for people with anxiety disorders. Researchers are also looking for new treatments that will help relieve symptoms.

When does GAD start?

GAD develops slowly. It often starts during the time between childhood and middle age. Symptoms may get better or worse at different times, and often are worse during times of stress.

People with GAD may visit a doctor many times before they find out they have this disorder. They ask their doctors to help them with the signs of GAD, such as headaches or trouble falling asleep, but don't always get the help they need right away. It may take doctors some time to be sure that a person has GAD instead of something else.

Is there help?

There is help for people with GAD. The first step is to go to a doctor or health clinic to talk about symptoms. People who think they have GAD may want to bring this information to the doctor to help them talk about the symptoms in it. The doctor will do an exam to make sure that another physical problem isn't causing the symptoms. The doctor may make a referral to a mental health specialist.

Doctors may prescribe medication to help relieve GAD. It's important to know that some of these medicines may take a few weeks to start working. In most states only a medical doctor (a family doctor or psychiatrist) can prescribe medications.

The kinds of medicines used to treat GAD are listed below. Some are used to treat other problems, such as depression, but also are helpful for GAD:

- Antidepressants
- Anti-anxiety medicines
- Beta blockers

Doctors also may ask people with GAD to go to therapy with a licensed social worker, psychologist, or psychiatrist. This treatment can help people with GAD feel less anxious and fearful.

There is no cure for GAD yet, but treatments can give relief to people who have it and help them live a more normal life. If you know someone with signs of GAD, talk to him or her about seeing a doctor. Offer to go along for support. To find out more about GAD, call the National Institute of Mental Health at 866-615-NIMH (866-615-6464) to have free information mailed to you.

Who pays for treatment?

Most insurance plans cover treatment for anxiety disorders. People who are going to have treatment should check with their own insurance companies to find out about coverage. For people who don't have insurance, local city or county governments may offer treatment at a clinic or health center, where the cost is based on income. Medicaid plans also may pay for GAD treatment.

Chapter 16

Panic Disorder

Anxiety Disorders

Most people feel anxious about something for a short time now and again, but people with anxiety disorders feel this way most of the time. Their fears and worries make it hard for them to do everyday tasks. About 18% of American adults have anxiety disorders. Children also may have them. This chapter is about one kind of anxiety disorder called panic disorder.

Panic Disorder

People with panic disorder have sudden and repeated attacks of fear that last for several minutes, but sometimes symptoms may last longer. These are called panic attacks. Panic attacks are characterized by a fear of certain disaster or a fear of losing control. A person may also have a strong physical reaction. It may feel like having a heart attack. Panic attacks can occur at any time, and many people worry about and dread the possibility of having another attack.

A person with panic disorder may become discouraged and feel ashamed because he or she cannot carry out normal routines like going to the grocery store, or driving. Having panic disorder can also interfere with school or work.

About This Chapter: This chapter includes excerpts from "When Fear Overwhelms: Panic Disorder," National Institute of Mental Health (www.nimh.nih.gov), 2008.

What are the symptoms of panic disorder?

People with panic disorder have these symptoms:

- Sudden and repeated attacks of fear
- A feeling of being out of control during a panic attack
- A feeling that things are not real
- An intense worry about when the next attack will happen
- A fear or avoidance of places where panic attacks have occurred in the past
- Physical symptoms including pounding heart; sweating; weakness, faintness, or dizziness; feeling a hot flush or a cold chill; tingly or numb hands; chest pain; or feeling nauseous or stomach pain

✤ It's A Fact!!

Panic attacks are characterized by a fear of certain disaster or a fear of losing control.

Source: National Institute of Mental Health, 2008.

If you or someone you know develops these symptoms, talk to a doctor or health care provider. There is help available.

When does panic disorder start?

Panic disorder often begins in the late teens or early adulthood. More women than men have panic disorder. But not everyone who experiences panic attacks will develop panic disorder.

Is there help?

There is help for people with panic disorder. In fact, it is one of the most treatable anxiety disorders. First, a person should visit a doctor or health care provider to discuss the symptoms or feelings he or she is having. The list of symptoms in this chapter can be a useful guide when talking with the doctor. The doctor will do an examination to make sure that another physical problem is not causing the symptoms. The doctor may make a referral to a specialist such as a psychiatrist, psychologist, or licensed social worker.

Medications can help reduce the severity and frequency of panic attacks, but they may take several weeks to start working. A doctor can prescribe medications. Different types of medications are used to treat panic disorder. They are antidepressants, anti-anxiety drugs, and beta blockers. These same medications are used to treat other types of disorders as well.

Psychotherapy, or "talk therapy" with a specialist can help people learn to control the symptoms of a panic attack. Therapy can be with a licensed social worker, counselor, psychologist, or psychiatrist. There is no cure for panic disorder, but most people can live a normal life when they receive treatment with medicine and/or therapy.

Who pays for treatment?

Most insurance plans cover treatment for anxiety disorders. Check with your insurance company to find out. If you do not have insurance, the health or human services agency of your city or county government may offer care at a clinic or health center where payment is usually based on a person's income. If you receive Medicaid, the plan you are in may pay for treatment.

Why do people get panic disorder?

Panic disorder sometimes runs in families, but no one knows for sure why some people have it, while others don't. When chemicals in the brain are not at a certain level it can cause a person to have panic disorder. That is why medications often help with symptoms because they help the brain chemicals stay at the correct levels.

✔ Quick Tip

Panic disorder is one of the most treatable anxiety disorders. If you know someone with symptoms of panic disorder, talk to him or her about seeing a doctor. Offer to go with your friend to the doctor's appointment for support. To find out more about panic disorder, call the National Institute of Mental Health, 866-615-NIMH (866-615-6464).

Source: National Institute of Mental Health, 2008.

To improve treatment, scientists are studying how well different medicines and therapies work. In one kind of research, people with panic disorder choose to take part in a clinical trial to help doctors find out what treatments work best for most people, or what works best for different symptoms. Usually, the treatment is free. Scientists are learning more about how the brain works so that they can discover new treatments.

✤ It's A Fact!!

Three brain areas of panic disorder patients are lacking in a key component of a chemical messenger system that regulates emotion, researchers at the National Institute of Mental Health (NIMH) have discovered. Brain scans revealed that a type of serotonin receptor is reduced by nearly a third in three structures straddling the center of the brain. The finding is the first in living humans to show that the receptor, which is pivotal to the action of widely prescribed anti-anxiety medications, may be abnormal in the disorder, and may help to explain how genes might influence vulnerability. Drs. Alexander Neumeister and Wayne Drevets, NIMH Mood and Anxiety Disorders Program, and colleagues, reported on their findings in the January 21, 2004 *Journal of Neuroscience*.

Source: Excerpted from "Emotion-Regulating Protein Lacking in Panic Disorder," a National Institute of Mental Health press release dated January 20, 2004.

Chapter 17

Post-Traumatic Stress Disorder

What is post-traumatic stress disorder, or PTSD?

PTSD is an anxiety disorder that some people get after seeing or living through a dangerous event.

When in danger, it's natural to feel afraid. This fear triggers many split-second changes in the body to prepare to defend against the danger or to avoid it. This "fight-or-flight" response is a healthy reaction meant to protect a person from harm. But in PTSD, this reaction is changed or damaged. People who have PTSD may feel stressed or frightened even when they're no longer in danger.

Who gets PTSD?

Anyone can get PTSD at any age. This includes war veterans and survivors of physical and sexual assault, abuse, accidents, disasters, and many other serious events.

Not everyone with PTSD has been through a dangerous event. Some people get PTSD after a friend or family member experiences danger or is harmed. The sudden, unexpected death of a loved one can also cause PTSD.

About This Chapter: Text in this chapter is excerpted from "Post-Traumatic Stress Disorder," National Institute of Mental Health (www.nimh.nih.gov), February 14, 2009.

✔ Quick Tip

Tips For Kids And Teens

After a traumatic or violent event it is normal to feel anxious about your safety and security. Even if you were not directly involved, you may worry about whether this type of event may someday affect you. How can you deal with these fears? Start by looking at the tips below for some ideas.

Talk to an adult who you can trust: This might be your parent, another relative, a friend, neighbor, teacher, coach, school nurse, counselor, family doctor, or member of your church or temple. If you've seen or experienced violence of any kind, not talking about it can make feelings build up inside and cause problems. If you are not sure where to turn, call your local crisis intervention center or a national hotline.

Stay active: Go for a walk, volunteer with a community group, play sports, write a play or poem, play a musical instrument, or join an after-school program. Trying any of these can be a positive way to handle your emotions.

Be a leader in making your school or community safer: Join an existing group that is promoting non-violence in your school or community, or launch your own effort.

Stay in touch with family: If possible, stay in touch with trusted family, friends, and neighbors to talk things out and help deal with any stress or worry.

Take care of yourself: Losing sleep, not eating, and worrying too much can make you sick. As much as possible, try to get enough sleep, eat right, exercise, and keep a normal routine. It may be hard to do, but it can keep you healthy and better able to handle a tough time.

Source: Excerpted from "Tips for Coping with Stress," Centers for Disease Control and Prevention, April 20, 2009.

What are the symptoms of PTSD?

PTSD can cause many symptoms. These symptoms can be grouped into three categories:

1. Re-Experiencing Symptoms

- Flashbacks—reliving the trauma over and over, including physical symptoms like a racing heart or sweating
- Bad dreams
- Frightening thoughts

Re-experiencing symptoms may cause problems in a person's everyday routine. They can start from the person's own thoughts and feelings. Words, objects, or situations that are reminders of the event can also trigger re-experiencing.

2. Avoidance Symptoms

- Staying away from places, events, or objects that are reminders of the experience
- Feeling emotionally numb
- Feeling strong guilt, depression, or worry
- Losing interest in activities that were enjoyable in the past
- Having trouble remembering the dangerous event

Things that remind a person of the traumatic event can trigger avoidance symptoms. These symptoms may cause a person to change his or her personal routine. For example, after a bad car accident, a person who usually drives may avoid driving or riding in a car.

3. Hyperarousal Symptoms

- Being easily startled
- Feeling tense or "on edge"
- Having difficulty sleeping, and/or having angry outbursts

Hyperarousal symptoms are usually constant, instead of being triggered by things that remind one of the traumatic event. They can make the person feel stressed and angry. These symptoms may make it hard to do daily tasks, such as sleeping, eating, or concentrating.

It's natural to have some of these symptoms after a dangerous event. Sometimes people have very serious symptoms that go away after a few weeks. This is called acute stress disorder, or ASD. When the symptoms last more than a few weeks and become an ongoing problem, they might be PTSD. Some people with PTSD don't show any symptoms for weeks or months.

Do children react differently than adults?

Children and teens can have extreme reactions to trauma, but their symptoms may not be the same as adults. In very young children, these symptoms can include the following:

- Bedwetting, when they'd learned how to use the toilet before
- Forgetting how or being unable to talk
- Acting out the scary event during playtime
- Being unusually clingy with a parent or other adult

Older children and teens usually show symptoms more like those seen in adults. They may also develop disruptive, disrespectful, or destructive behaviors. Older children and teens may feel guilty for not preventing injury or deaths. They may also have thoughts of revenge.

☞ Remember!!

Risk factors for PTSD include the following:

- Living through dangerous events and traumas
- Having a history of mental illness
- Getting hurt
- Seeing people hurt or killed
- Feeling horror, helplessness, or extreme fear
- Having little or no social support after the event
- Dealing with extra stress after the event, such as loss of a loved one, pain and injury, or loss of a job or home.

Resilience factors that may reduce the risk of PTSD include the following:

- Seeking out support from other people, such as friends and family
- Finding a support group after a traumatic event
- Feeling good about one's own actions in the face of danger
- Having a coping strategy, or a way of getting through the bad event and learning from it
- Being able to act and respond effectively despite feeling fear.

Source: NIMH, 2009.

How is PTSD detected?

A doctor who has experience helping people with mental illnesses, such as a psychiatrist or psychologist, can diagnose PTSD. The diagnosis is made after the doctor talks with the person who has symptoms of PTSD.

To be diagnosed with PTSD, a person must have all of the following for at least one month:

- At least one re-experiencing symptom
- At least three avoidance symptoms
- At least two hyperarousal symptoms

Symptoms that make it hard to go about daily life, go to school or work, be with friends, and take care of important tasks.

Why do some people get PTSD and other people do not?

It is important to remember that not everyone who lives through a dangerous event gets PTSD. In fact, most will not get the disorder.

Many factors play a part in whether a person will get PTSD. Some of these are risk factors that make a person more likely to get PTSD. Other factors, called resilience factors, can help reduce the risk of the disorder. Some of these risk and resilience factors are present before the trauma and others become important during and after a traumatic event.

Researchers are studying the importance of various risk and resilience factors. With more study, it may be possible someday to predict who is likely to get PTSD and prevent it.

How is PTSD treated?

The main treatments for people with PTSD are psychotherapy ("talk" therapy), medications, or both. Everyone is different, so a treatment that works for one person may not work for another. It is important for anyone with PTSD to be treated by a mental health care provider who is experienced with PTSD. Some people with PTSD need to try different treatments to find what works for their symptoms.

If someone with PTSD is going through an ongoing trauma, such as being in an abusive relationship, both of the problems need to be treated. Other ongoing problems can include panic disorder, depression, substance abuse, and feeling suicidal.

Psychotherapy: Psychotherapy is "talk" therapy. It involves talking with a mental health professional to treat a mental illness. Psychotherapy can occur one-on-one or in a group. Talk therapy treatment for PTSD usually lasts six to 12 weeks, but can take more time. Research shows that support from family and friends can be an important part of therapy.

Many types of psychotherapy can help people with PTSD. Some types target the symptoms of PTSD directly. Other therapies focus on social, family, or job-related problems. The doctor or therapist may combine different therapies depending on each person's needs.

One helpful therapy is called cognitive behavioral therapy, or CBT. There are several parts to CBT, including the following:

- *Exposure Therapy:* This therapy helps people face and control their fear. It exposes them to the trauma they experienced in a safe way. It uses mental imagery, writing, or visits to the place where the event happened. The therapist uses these tools to help people with PTSD cope with their feelings.

✤ It's A Fact!! How Talk Therapies Help People Overcome PTSD

Talk therapies teach people helpful ways to react to frightening events that trigger their PTSD symptoms. Based on this general goal, different types of therapy may:

- Teach about trauma and its effects.
- Use relaxation and anger control skills.
- Provide tips for better sleep, diet, and exercise habits.
- Help people identify and deal with guilt, shame, and other feelings about the event.
- Focus on changing how people react to their PTSD symptoms. For example, therapy helps people visit places and people that are reminders of the trauma.

Source: NIMH, 2009.

- *Cognitive Restructuring:* This therapy helps people make sense of the bad memories. Sometimes people remember the event differently than how it happened. They may feel guilt or shame about what is not their fault. The therapist helps people with PTSD look at what happened in a realistic way.
- *Stress Inoculation Training:* This therapy tries to reduce PTSD symptoms by teaching a person how to reduce anxiety. Like cognitive restructuring, this treatment helps people look at their memories in a healthy way.

Other types of treatment can also help people with PTSD. People with PTSD should talk about all treatment options with their therapist.

Medications: The U.S. Food and Drug Administration (FDA) has approved two medications for treating adults with PTSD:

- Sertraline (Zoloft)
- Paroxetine (Paxil)

Both of these medications are antidepressants, which are also used to treat depression. They may help control PTSD symptoms such as sadness, worry, anger, and feeling numb inside. Taking these medications may make it easier to go through psychotherapy.

Sometimes people taking these medications have side effects. The effects can be annoying, but they usually go away. However, medications affect everyone differently. Any side effects or unusual reactions should be reported to a doctor immediately.

The most common side effects of antidepressants like sertraline and paroxetine are the following:

- Headache, which usually goes away within a few days
- Nausea (feeling sick to your stomach), which usually goes away within a few days
- Sleeplessness or drowsiness, which may occur during the first few weeks but then goes away
- Sometimes the medication dose needs to be reduced or the time of day it is taken needs to be adjusted to help lessen these side effects

- Agitation (feeling jittery)
- Sexual problems, which can affect both men and women, including reduced sex drive, and problems having and enjoying sex

FDA Warning On Antidepressants: Despite the relative safety and popularity of selective serotonin reuptake inhibitors (SSRIs) and other antidepressants, some studies have suggested that they may have unintentional effects on some people, especially adolescents and young adults. In 2004, the Food and Drug Administration (FDA) conducted a thorough review of published and unpublished controlled clinical trials of antidepressants that involved nearly 4,400 children and adolescents. The review revealed that four percent of those taking antidepressants thought about or attempted suicide (although no suicides occurred), compared to two percent of those receiving placebos.

This information prompted the FDA, in 2005, to adopt a "black box" warning label on all antidepressant medications to alert the public about the potential increased risk of suicidal thinking or attempts in children and adolescents taking antidepressants. In 2007, the FDA proposed that makers of all antidepressant medications extend the warning to include young adults up through age 24. A "black box" warning is the most serious type of warning on prescription drug labeling.

The warning emphasizes that patients of all ages taking antidepressants should be closely monitored, especially during the initial weeks of treatment. Possible side effects to look for are worsening depression, suicidal thinking or behavior, or any unusual changes in behavior such as sleeplessness, agitation, or withdrawal from normal social situations. The warning adds that families and caregivers should also be told of the need for close monitoring and report any changes to the physician. The latest information can be found on the FDA Web site.

Results of a comprehensive review of pediatric trials conducted between 1988 and 2006 suggested that the benefits of antidepressant medications likely outweigh their risks to children and adolescents with major depression and anxiety disorders. The study was funded in part by the National Institute of Mental Health.

Other Medications: Doctors may also prescribe other types of medications, such as the ones listed below. There is little information on how well these work for people with PTSD.

- *Benzodiazepines:* These medications may be given to help people relax and sleep. People who take benzodiazepines may have memory problems or become dependent on the medication.
- *Antipsychotics:* These medications are usually given to people with other mental disorders, like schizophrenia. People who take antipsychotics may gain weight and have a higher chance of getting heart disease and diabetes.
- *Other Antidepressants:* Like sertraline and paroxetine, the antidepressants fluoxetine (Prozac) and citalopram (Celexa) can help people with PTSD feel less tense or sad. For people with PTSD who also have other anxiety disorders or depression, antidepressants may be useful in reducing symptoms of these co-occurring illnesses.

How can PTSD be treated after mass trauma?

Sometimes large numbers of people are affected by the same event. For example, a lot of people needed help after Hurricane Katrina in 2005 and the terrorist attacks of September 11, 2001. Most people will have some PTSD symptoms in the first few weeks after events like these. This is a normal and expected response to serious trauma, and for most people, symptoms generally lessen with time.

But some people do not get better on their own. A study of Hurricane Katrina survivors found that, over time, more people were having problems with PTSD, depression, and related mental disorders. This pattern is unlike the recovery from other natural disasters, where the number of people who have mental health problems gradually lessens. As communities try to rebuild after a mass trauma, people may experience ongoing stress from loss of jobs and schools, and trouble paying bills, finding housing, and getting health care. This delay in community recovery may in turn delay recovery from PTSD.

In the first couple weeks after a mass trauma, brief versions of CBT may be helpful to some people who are having severe distress.

Mass Trauma Affects Hospitals And Other Providers: Hospitals, health care systems, and health care providers are also affected by a mass trauma. The number of people who need immediate physical and psychological help may be too much for health systems to handle. Some patients may not find help when they need it because hospitals do not have enough staff or supplies. In some cases, health care providers themselves may be struggling to recover as well.

✔ Quick Tip

After mass trauma, most people can be helped with basic support, including the following:

- Getting to a safe place
- Seeing a doctor if injured
- Getting food and water
- Contacting loved ones or friends
- Learning what is being done to help

Source: NIMH, 2009.

What efforts are under way to improve the detection and treatment of PTSD?

Researchers have learned a lot in the last decade about fear, stress, and PTSD. Scientists are also learning about how people form memories. This is important because creating very powerful fear-related memories seems to be a major part of PTSD. Researchers are also exploring how people can create "safety" memories to replace the bad memories that form after a trauma. The National Institute of Mental Health (NIMH)'s goal in supporting this research is to improve treatment and find ways to prevent the disorder.

PTSD research also includes the following examples:

- Using powerful new research methods, such as brain imaging and the study of genes, to find out more about what leads to PTSD, when it happens, and who is most at risk.
- Trying to understand why some people get PTSD and others do not. Knowing this can help health care professionals predict who might get PTSD and provide early treatment.
- Focusing on ways to examine pre-trauma, trauma, and post-trauma risk and resilience factors all at once.

- Looking for treatments that reduce the impact traumatic memories have on our emotions.
- Improving the way people are screened for PTSD, given early treatment, and tracked after a mass trauma.
- Developing new approaches in self-testing and screening to help people know when it's time to call a doctor.
- Testing ways to help family doctors detect and treat PTSD or refer people with PTSD to mental health specialists.

How can I help a friend or relative who has PTSD?

If you know someone who has PTSD, it affects you too. The first and most important thing you can do to help a friend or relative is to help him or her get the right diagnosis and treatment. You may need to make an appointment for your friend or relative and go with him or her to see the doctor. Encourage him or her to stay in treatment, or to seek different treatment if his or her symptoms don't get better after 6 to 8 weeks.

To help a friend or relative, you can take these steps:

- Offer emotional support, understanding, patience, and encouragement.
- Learn about PTSD so you can understand what your friend or relative is experiencing.
- Talk to your friend or relative, and listen carefully.
- Listen to feelings your friend or relative expresses and be understanding of situations that may trigger PTSD symptoms.
- Invite your friend or relative out for positive distractions such as walks, outings, and other activities.
- Remind your friend or relative that, with time and treatment, he or she can get better.
- Never ignore comments about your friend or relative harming him or herself, and report such comments to your friend's or relative's therapist or doctor.

How can I help myself?

It may be very hard to take that first step to help yourself. It is important to realize that although it may take some time, with treatment, you can get better.

To help yourself, try these steps:

- Talk to your doctor about treatment options.
- Engage in mild activity or exercise to help reduce stress.
- Set realistic goals for yourself.
- Break up large tasks into small ones, set some priorities, and do what you can as you can.
- Try to spend time with other people and confide in a trusted friend or relative. Tell others about things that may trigger symptoms.
- Expect your symptoms to improve gradually, not immediately.
- Identify and seek out comforting situations, places, and people.

✔ Quick Tip

If you or someone you know needs immediate help please contact the one of the following crisis hotlines:

- National Suicide Prevention Lifeline: 800-273-TALK (888-628-9454 for Spanish-speaking callers)
- Youth Mental Health Line: 888-568-1112
- Child-Help USA: 800-422-4453 (24 hour toll free)

Source: Excerpted from "Tips for Coping with Stress," Centers for Disease Control and Prevention, April 20, 2009.

Chapter 18

Obsessive-Compulsive Disorder

What are anxiety disorders?

People with anxiety disorders feel extremely fearful and unsure. Most people feel anxious about something for a short time now and again, but people with anxiety disorders feel this way most of the time. Their fears and worries make it hard for them to do everyday tasks. About 18% of American adults have anxiety disorders. Children also may have them.

Treatment is available for people with anxiety disorders. Researchers are also looking for new treatments that will help relieve symptoms.

This chapter is about one kind of anxiety disorder called obsessive-compulsive disorder, or OCD.

What is obsessive-compulsive disorder?

Everyone double-checks things sometimes—for example, checking the stove before leaving the house, to make sure it's turned off. But people with OCD feel the need to check things over and over, or have certain thoughts or perform routines and rituals over and over. The thoughts and rituals of OCD cause distress and get in the way of daily life.

About This Chapter: Text in this chapter is from "When Unwanted Thoughts Take Over: Obsessive-Compulsive Disorder," National Institute of Mental Health (www.nimh.nih.gov), April 9, 2009.

The repeated, upsetting thoughts of OCD are called obsessions. To try to control them, people with OCD repeat rituals or behaviors, which are called compulsions. People with OCD can't control these thoughts and rituals.

Examples of obsessions are fear of germs, of being hurt or of hurting others, and troubling religious or sexual thoughts. Examples of compulsions are repeatedly counting things, cleaning things, washing the body or parts of it, or putting things in a certain order, when these actions are not needed, and checking things over and over.

People with OCD have these thoughts and do these rituals for at least an hour on most days, often longer. The reason OCD gets in the way of their lives is that they can't stop the thoughts or rituals, so they sometimes miss school, work, or meetings with friends, for example.

What are the symptoms of OCD?

People with OCD can have the following symptoms:

- Having repeated thoughts or images about many different things:
    - fears such as germs, dirt, and intruders
    - violence
    - hurting loved ones
    - sexual acts
    - conflicts with religious beliefs
    - being overly neat
- Doing the same rituals over and over such as washing hands, locking and unlocking doors, counting, keeping unneeded items, or repeating the same steps again and again
- Unwanted thoughts and behaviors they can't control
- Not getting pleasure from the behaviors or rituals, but get brief relief from the anxiety the thoughts cause
- Spending at least an hour a day on the thoughts and rituals, which cause distress and get in the way of daily life

When does OCD start?

For many people, OCD starts during childhood or the teen years. Most people are diagnosed at about age 19. Symptoms of OCD may come and go and be better or worse at different times.

Is there help?

There is help for people with OCD. The first step is to go to a physician or health clinic to talk about symptoms. People who think they have OCD may want to bring this booklet to the physician, to help them talk about the symptoms in it. The physician will do an exam to make sure that another physical problem isn't causing the symptoms. The physician may make a referral to a mental health specialist.

✤ It's A Fact!!

A likely mechanism by which a bacterial infection triggers obsessive compulsive disorder (OCD) in some children has been demonstrated by scientists at the National Institutes of Health's (NIH) National Institute of Mental Health (NIMH) and collaborators at California State University (CSU) and the University of Oklahoma (UO). Their research suggests that an antibody against strep throat bacteria sometimes mistakenly acts on a brain enzyme, disrupting communications between neurons and causing a form of obsessive compulsive and related tic disorder in children—pediatric autoimmune neuropsychiatric disorders associated with streptococci (PANDAS).

Source: Excerpted from "How Strep Triggers Obsessive Compulsive Disorder—New Clues," a Science Update from the National Institute of Mental Health, October 11, 2006.

Physicians may prescribe medication to help relieve OCD. It's important to know that some of these medicines may take a few weeks to start working. Only a physician (a family physician or psychiatrist) can prescribe medications. (In two states, psychologists with specific training and certification may prescribe medications for anxiety disorders.)

The kinds of medicines used to treat OCD are listed below. Some of these medicines are used to treat other problems, such as depression, but also are helpful for OCD.

- Antidepressants
- Antianxiety medicines
- Beta-blockers

Physicians also may ask people with OCD to go to therapy with a licensed social worker, psychologist, or psychiatrist. This treatment can help people with OCD feel less anxious and fearful.

There is no cure for OCD yet, but treatments can give relief to people who have it and help them live a more normal life. If you know someone with signs of OCD, talk to him or her about seeing a physician. Offer to go along for support.

✤ It's A Fact!!

OCD Risk Higher When Several Variations In Gene Occur Together

Several variations within the same gene act together to raise the risk of obsessive-compulsive disorder (OCD), new National Institute of Mental Health (NIMH) research suggests. The gene produces a protein that helps make the brain chemical serotonin available to brain cells.

Previously, the gene variations had been implicated in OCD individually, in separate studies—but other studies sometimes found that the variations had no impact on risk of OCD. The reason for the inconsistent results appears to be that the variations have an impact on OCD risk when they occur together, not individually, NIMH researchers Jens R. Wendland, Pablo R. Moya, Dennis L. Murphy, and colleagues reported in the March 1, 2008 issue of *Human Molecular Genetics*.

The gene in which the variations occur is called SLC6A4, and the protein it makes is called the serotonin transporter.

The new findings suggest not only that the serotonin transporter is involved in OCD, but also that part of the problem may be excess activity of the gene that makes the transporter. Excessive activity of this gene results in too much serotonin being shuttled out of the areas between brain cells, making less of it available for important cell functions.

Reference: Wendland JR, Moya PR, Kruse MR, Ren-Patterson RF, Jensen CL, Cromer KR, Murphy DL. A Novel, Putative Gain-of-Function Haplotype at SLC6A4 Associates with Obsessive-Compulsive Disorder. *Human Molecular Genetics*, 17(5):717-23. March 1, 2008.

Source: Excerpted from "OCD Risk Higher When Several Variations in Gene Occur Together," a Science Update from the National Institute of Mental Health, April 7, 2008.

Who pays for treatment?

Most insurance plans cover treatment for anxiety disorders. People who are going to have treatment should check with their own insurance companies to find out about coverage. For people who don't have insurance, local city or county governments may offer treatment at a clinic or health center, where the cost is based on income. Medicaid plans also may pay for OCD treatment.

Why do people get OCD?

OCD sometimes runs in families, but no one knows for sure why some people have it, while others don't. When chemicals in the brain are not at a certain level it may result in OCD. Medications can often help the brain chemicals stay at the correct levels.

To improve treatment, scientists are studying how well different medicines and therapies work. In one kind of research, people with OCD choose to take part in a clinical trial to help physicians find out what treatments work best for most people, or what works best for different symptoms. Usually, the treatment is free. Scientists are learning more about how the brain works, so that they can discover new treatments.

Chapter 19

Social Phobia

What are anxiety disorders?

People with anxiety disorders feel extremely fearful and unsure. Most people feel anxious about something for a short time now and again, but people with anxiety disorders feel this way most of the time. Their fears and worries make it hard for them to do everyday tasks. About 18% of American adults have anxiety disorders. Children also may have them.

Treatment is available for people with anxiety disorders. Researchers are also looking for new treatments that will help relieve symptoms.

This chapter is about one kind of anxiety disorder called social phobia. Some people also call it social anxiety disorder.

What is social phobia?

Social phobia is a strong fear of being judged by others and of being embarrassed. This fear can be so strong that it gets in the way of going to work or school or doing other everyday things.

People with social phobia are afraid of doing common things in front of other people; for example, they might be afraid to sign a check in front of a

About This Chapter: Text in this chapter is from "Always Embarrassed: Social Phobia (Social Anxiety Disorder)," National Institute of Mental Health (www.nimh.nih.gov), March 25, 2009.

cashier at the grocery store, or they might be afraid to eat or drink in front of other people. All of us have been a little bit nervous, at one time or another, about things like meeting new people or giving a speech. But people with social phobia worry about these and other things for weeks before they happen.

Most of the people who have social phobia know that they shouldn't be as afraid as they are, but they can't control their fear. Sometimes, they end up staying away from places or events where they think they might have to do something that will embarrass them. That can keep them from doing the everyday tasks of living and from enjoying times with family and friends.

What are common symptoms of social phobia?

People with social phobia may experience the following symptoms:

- Very anxious about being with other people
- Very self-conscious in front of other people; that is, they are very worried about how they themselves will act
- Very afraid of being embarrassed in front of other people
- Very afraid that other people will judge them
- Worry for days or weeks before an event where other people will be
- Stay away from places where there are other people
- Have a hard time making friends and keeping friends

✤ It's A Fact!!

In a study using functional brain imaging, National Institute of Mental Health (NIMH) scientists found that when people with generalized social phobia were presented with a variety of verbal comments about themselves and others ("you are ugly," or "he's a genius," for example) they had heightened brain responses only to negative comments about themselves. Knowledge of the social cues that trigger anxiety and what parts of the brain are engaged when this happens can help scientists understand and better treat this anxiety disorder.

Source: Excerpted from "Social Phobia Patients Have Heightened Reactions to Negative Comments," a Science Update from the National Institute of Mental Health, October 22, 2008.

- Those with social phobia may have body symptoms when they are with other people, such as blushing, heavy sweating, trembling, nausea, and having a hard time talking

When does social phobia start?

Social phobia usually starts during the child or teen years, usually at about age 13. A doctor can tell that a person has social phobia if the person has had symptoms for at least six months. Without treatment, social phobia can last for many years or a lifetime.

Is there help?

There is help for people with social phobia. The first step is to go to a doctor or health clinic to talk about symptoms. People who think they have social phobia may want to bring this booklet to the doctor to help them talk about the symptoms in it. The doctor will do an exam to make sure that another physical problem isn't causing the symptoms. The doctor may make a referral to a mental health specialist.

Doctors may prescribe medication to help relieve social phobia. It's important to know that some of these medicines may take a few weeks to start working. In most states only a medical doctor (a family doctor or psychiatrist) can prescribe medications.

The kinds of medicines used to treat social phobia are listed below. Some of these medicines are used to treat other problems, such as depression, but also are helpful for social phobia:

- Antidepressants
- Anti-anxiety medicines
- Beta blockers

Doctors also may ask people with social phobia to go to therapy with a licensed social worker, psychologist, or psychiatrist. This treatment can help people with social phobia feel less anxious and fearful.

There is no cure for social phobia yet, but treatments can give relief to people who have it and help them live a more normal life. If you know someone with signs of social phobia, talk to him or her about seeing a doctor. Offer to go along for support.

Who pays for treatment?

Most insurance plans cover treatment for anxiety disorders. People who are going to have treatment should check with their own insurance companies to find out about coverage. For people who don't have insurance, local city or county governments may offer treatment at a clinic or health center, where the cost is based on income. Medicaid plans also may pay for social phobia treatment.

Why do people get social phobia?

Social phobia sometimes runs in families, but no one knows for sure why some people have it, while others don't. When chemicals in the brain are not at a certain level it can cause a person to have social phobia. That is why medications often help with the symptoms because they help the brain chemicals stay at the correct levels.

To improve treatment, scientists are studying how well different medicines and therapies work. In one kind of research, people with social phobia choose to take part in a clinical trial to help doctors find out what treatments work best for most people, or what works best for different symptoms. Usually, the treatment is free. Scientists are learning more about how the brain works, so that they can discover new treatments.

Chapter 20

Specific Phobias

About Phobias

What is a phobia?

We all have things that frighten us or make us uneasy. New places, insects, driving over high bridges, or creaky elevators. And although we sometimes try to avoid things that make us uncomfortable, we generally manage to control our fears and carry on with daily activities. Some people, however, have very strong irrational, involuntary fear reactions that lead them to avoid common everyday places, situations, or objects even though they know logically there isn't any danger. The fear doesn't make any sense, but it seems nothing can stop it. When confronted with the feared situation, they may even have a panic attack, the spontaneous onset of intense fear that makes people feel as if they might stop breathing and pass out, are having a heart attack, or will lose control and die.

People who experience these seemingly out-of-control fears have a phobia. There are three types of phobias—agoraphobia, social phobia (also known as social anxiety disorder) and specific phobias. This chapter focuses on specific phobias. For information about agoraphobia and social phobia visit the Anxiety Disorders Association of America (ADAA) website at www.adaa.org.

What is a specific phobia?

People with a specific phobias have an excessive and unreasonable fear in the presence of or anticipation of a specific object, place, or situation. Common specific phobias include animals, insects, heights, thunder, driving, public transportation, flying, dental or medical procedures, and elevators. Although the person with a phobia realizes that the fear is irrational, even thinking about it can cause extreme anxiety.

About Anxiety Disorders

Anxiety is a normal part of living. It's the body's way of telling us something isn't right. It keeps us from harm's way and prepares us to act quickly in the face of danger. However, for some people, anxiety is persistent, irrational, and overwhelming. It may get in the way of day-to-day activities or even make them impossible. This may be a sign of an anxiety disorder.

The term "anxiety disorders" describes a group of conditions including generalized anxiety disorder (GAD), obsessive-compulsive disorder (OCD), panic disorder, posttraumatic stress disorder (PTSD), social anxiety disorder, and specific phobias. For more information about anxiety disorders, visit www.adaa.org.

✎ What's It Mean?

Phobias: A phobia is a type of anxiety disorder. It is a strong, irrational fear of something that poses little or no actual danger. There are many specific phobias. Acrophobia is a fear of heights. You may be able to ski the world's tallest mountains but be unable to go above the fifth floor of an office building. Agoraphobia is a fear of public places, and claustrophobia is a fear of closed-in places. If you become anxious and extremely self-conscious in everyday social situations, you could have a social phobia. Other common phobias involve tunnels, highway driving, water, flying, animals, and blood.

People with phobias try to avoid what they are afraid of. If they cannot, they may experience symptoms such as the following:

- Panic and fear
- Rapid heartbeat
- Shortness of breath
- Trembling
- A strong desire to get away

Treatment helps most people with phobias. Options include medicines, therapy, or both.

Source: Excerpted from "Phobias," MedlinePlus, National Library of Medicine (www.nlm.nih.gov), March 28, 2009.

What's the difference between normal anxiety and a phobia?

Normal Anxiety

- Feeling queasy while climbing a tall ladder
- Worrying about taking off in an airplane during a lightening storm
- Feeling anxious around your neighbor's pit bull

Phobia

- Refusing to attend your best friend's wedding because it's on the 25th floor of a hotel
- Turning down a big promotion because it involves air travel
- Avoiding visiting your neighbors for fear of seeing a dog

About Specific Phobias

How can specific phobias affect your life?

The impact of a phobia on one's life depends on how easy it is to avoid the feared object, place, or situation. Since individuals do whatever they can to avoid the uncomfortable and often terrifying feelings of phobic anxiety, phobias can disrupt daily routines, limit work efficiency, reduce self-esteem, and place a strain on relationships.

What causes specific phobias?

Specific phobias are the most common type of anxiety disorder, affecting 19 million American adults. Most phobias seem to come out of the blue, usually arising in childhood or early adulthood. Scientists believe that phobias can be traced to a combination of genetic tendencies, brain chemistry and other biological, psychological, and environmental factors.

What treatments are available?

Most individuals who seek treatment for phobias and other anxiety disorders see significant improvement and enjoy a better quality of life. A variety of treatment options exists, including cognitive-behavioral therapy (CBT), exposure therapy, anxiety management, relaxation techniques, and medications.

One or a combination of these may be recommended. Details about these treatments are available on the ADAA website at www.adaa.org.

It is important to remember that there is no single "right" treatment. What works for one person may not be the best choice for someone else. A course of treatment should be tailored to individual needs. Ask your doctor to explain why a particular type of treatment is being recommended, what other options are available, and what you need to do to fully participate in your recovery.

How can ADAA help you?

Suffering from a specific phobia or any anxiety disorder can interfere with many aspects of your life. You may feel alone, embarrassed, or frightened. ADAA can provide the resources that will help you and your loved ones better understand your condition, connect you with a community of people who know what you are experiencing, and assist you in finding local mental health professionals. Visit the ADAA website at www.adaa.org to locate mental health professionals who treat phobias and other anxiety disorders in your area, as well as local support groups. Learn about the causes, symptoms, and best treatments for anxiety disorders, review questions to ask a therapist or doctor, and find helpful materials for family and loved ones. ADAA's mission is to help you make good decisions so that you can get on with your life.

Specific Phobias Self-Test

If you think you might have a specific phobia, take the test below. Answer "yes" or "no" to the questions and discuss the results with your doctor.

Yes or No? Are you troubled by...

- Fear of places or situations where getting help or escape might be difficult, such as in a crowd or on a bridge?
- Shortness of breath or a racing heart for no apparent reason when confronting certain situations?
- Persistent and unreasonable fear of an object or situation, such as flying, heights, animals, blood, etc.?
- Being unable to travel alone?

- Fears that continue despite causing problems for you or your loved ones?
- Fear that interferes with your daily life?

Having more than one illness at the same time can make it difficult to diagnose and treat the different conditions. Conditions that sometimes complicate anxiety disorders include depression and substance abuse, among others. The following information will help your health care professional in evaluating you for a specific phobia.

Yes or No? In the last year, have you experienced...

- Changes in sleeping or eating habits?
- Feeling sad or depressed more days than not?
- A disinterest in life more days than not?
- A feeling of worthlessness or guilt more days than not?

Yes or No? During the last year, has your use of alcohol or drugs...

- Resulted in failure at work, or school, or difficulties with your family?
- Placed you in a dangerous situation, such as driving under the influence?
- Gotten you arrested?
- Continued despite causing problems for you or your loved ones?

✔ Quick Tip

Take Five And Manage Your Anxiety

Whether you have normal anxiety or an anxiety disorder, these strategies will help you cope:

- **Exercise:** Go for a walk or jog. Do yoga. Dance. Just get moving!
- **Talk To Someone:** A spouse, significant other, friend, child, or doctor.
- **Keep A Daily Journal:** Become aware of what triggers your anxiety.
- **Eat A Balanced Diet:** Don't skip meals. Avoid caffeine, which can trigger anxiety symptoms.
- **Visit The Anxiety Disorders Association Of America Website:** It's online at www.adaa.org. Let them help you help yourself.

You are not alone. Talk to someone—a friend, loved one, or doctor. Get help. Anxiety disorders are real, serious, and treatable.

Source: © 2008 Anxiety Disorders Association of America.

Part Three

Behavioral, Personality, And Psychotic Disorders

Chapter 21

Adjustment Disorders

An adjustment disorder is a debilitating reaction, usually lasting less than six months, to a stressful event or situation. The development of emotional or behavioral symptoms in response to an identifiable stressor(s) occurring within three months of the onset of the stressor(s).

These symptoms or behaviors are clinically significant as evidenced by either of the following:

- Distress that is in excess of what would be expected from exposure to the stressor
- Significant impairment in social, occupational, or educational functioning

The symptoms are not caused by bereavement.

The stress-related disturbance does not meet the criteria for another specific disorder. Once the stressor (or its consequences) has terminated, the symptoms do not persist for more than an additional six months.

Adjustment Disorders Subtypes

- With depressed mood
- With anxiety

- With mixed anxiety and depressed mood
- With disturbance of conduct
- With mixed disturbance of emotions and conduct
- Unspecified

Associated Features

- Depressed mood
- Somatic/sexual dysfunction
- Guilt/obsession

Differential Diagnosis

Some disorders display similar or sometimes even the same symptom. The clinician, therefore, in his diagnostic attempt has to differentiate against the following disorders which one needs to be ruled out to establish a precise diagnosis.

- Personality disorders
- Not otherwise specified disorders (for example, anxiety disorder not otherwise specified)
- Posttraumatic stress disorder, and acute stress disorder
- Psychological factors affecting medical condition
- Bereavement
- Nonpathological reactions to stress

Treatment

Counseling And Psychotherapy: The primary goals of treatment are to relieve symptoms and assist with achieving a level of adaptation that is comparable to the affected person's level of functioning before the stressful event.

Most mental health professionals recommend a form of psychosocial treatment for this disorder. Treatments include individual psychotherapy, family therapy, behavior therapy, and self-help groups.

✤ It's A Fact!!

Cause

Many people have difficulties adjusting to stressful events. Stressful events include starting a new job, ending an important relationship, or conflicts with work colleagues. As a result, the individual may have difficulty with his or her mood and behavior several months after the event. There are as many different responses to stressful events as there are stressful events. Some who have recently experienced a stressor may be more sad or irritable than usual and feeling somewhat hopeless. Others become more nervous and worried. And other individuals combine these two emotional patterns. The symptoms associated with adjustment difficulties usually subside within about six months after the stressful event.

Pharmacotherapy: Mental health professionals generally do not use medication to treat this disorder. When medications are used, they are usually in addition to other forms of treatment.

Expectations: Adjustment disorders are less severe than other disorders. People with behavior disorders are more likely to later develop antisocial personality disorder. People with multiple psychiatric disorders are less likely to return to a previous level of functioning.

Complications: Major depression may develop if help is not obtained.

Chapter 22

Conduct Disorder

What is conduct disorder?

Children with conduct disorder repeatedly violate the personal or property rights of others and the basic expectations of society. A diagnosis of conduct disorder is likely when symptoms continue for six months or longer. Conduct disorder is known as a "disruptive behavior disorder" because of its impact on children and their families, neighbors, and schools.

Another disruptive behavior disorder, called oppositional defiant disorder, may be a precursor of conduct disorder. A child is diagnosed with oppositional defiant disorder when he or she shows signs of being hostile and defiant for at least six months. Oppositional defiant disorder may start as early as the preschool years, while conduct disorder generally appears when children are older. Oppositional defiant disorder and conduct disorder are not co-occurring conditions.

How common is conduct disorder?

Conduct disorder affects 1 to 4 percent of 9- to 17-year-olds, depending on exactly how the disorder is defined. The disorder appears to be more common in boys than in girls and more common in cities than in rural areas.

About This Chapter: Information in this chapter is from "Children's Mental Health Facts: Children and Adolescents with Conduct Disorder," Substance Abuse and Mental Health Services Administration (SAMHSA), April 2003. Reviewed for currency by David A. Cooke, MD, FACP, October 2009.

Who is at risk for conduct disorder?

Research shows that some cases of conduct disorder begin in early childhood, often by the preschool years. In fact, some infants who are especially "fussy" appear to be at risk for developing conduct disorder. Other factors that may make a child more likely to develop conduct disorder include the following:

- Early maternal rejection
- Separation from parents, without an adequate alternative caregiver
- Early institutionalization
- Family neglect
- Abuse or violence
- Parental mental illness
- Parental marital discord
- Large family size
- Crowding
- Poverty

> ✤ **It's A Fact!!**
>
> **Symptoms Of Conduct Disorder**
>
> - Aggressive behavior that harms or threatens other people or animals
> - Destructive behavior that damages or destroys property
> - Lying or theft
> - Truancy or other serious violations of rules
> - Early tobacco, alcohol, and substance use and abuse
> - Precocious sexual activity.
>
> Children with conduct disorder or oppositional defiant disorder also may experience the following:
>
> - Higher rates of depression, suicidal thoughts, suicide attempts, and suicide
> - Academic difficulties
> - Poor relationships with peers or adults
> - Sexually transmitted diseases
> - Difficulty staying in adoptive, foster, or group homes
> - Higher rates of injuries, school expulsions, and problems with the law

What help is available for families?

Although conduct disorder is one of the most difficult behavior disorders to treat, young people often benefit from a range of services that include the following:

- Training for parents on how to handle child or adolescent behavior
- Family therapy
- Training in problem solving skills for children or adolescents
- Community-based services that focus on the young person within the context of family and community influences

☞ Remember!!

Some child and adolescent behaviors are hard to change after they have become ingrained. Therefore, the earlier the conduct disorder is identified and treated, the better the chance for success. Most children or adolescents with conduct disorder are probably reacting to events and situations in their lives. Some recent studies have focused on promising ways to prevent conduct disorder among at-risk children and adolescents. In addition, more research is needed to determine if biology is a factor in conduct disorder.

Chapter 23

Intermittent Explosive Disorder And Oppositional Defiant Disorder

Intermittent Explosive Disorder

Road rage. Domestic abuse. Angry outbursts or temper tantrums that involve throwing or breaking objects. Sometimes such erratic eruptions can be caused by a condition known as intermittent explosive disorder.

Intermittent explosive disorder (IED) is characterized by repeated episodes of aggressive, violent behavior that are grossly out of proportion to the situation. The National Institute of Mental Health funded a study done in June 2006 that showed intermittent explosive disorder is more common than once thought. Intermittent explosive disorder occurs most often in young men and may affect as many as 7.3 percent of adults in the Unites States.

Individuals with intermittent explosive disorder may attack others and their possessions, causing bodily injury and property damage. Later, they may feel remorse, regret, or embarrassment about the aggression.

About This Chapter: This chapter includes "Intermittent Explosive Disorder," and "Oppositional Defiant Disorder," *Court Flash Newsletter*, © July 2006. Reprinted with permission from the Public Health Nursing Program, Riverside County Department of Public Health [California].

Signs And Symptoms

Explosive disruptions, usually lasting 10 to 20 minutes, often result in injuries and the deliberate destruction of property. These episodes may occur in clusters or be separated by weeks or months of nonaggression.

Aggressive episodes may be preceded or accompanied by these symptoms:

- Tingling
- Tremor
- Palpitations
- Chest tightness
- Head pressure
- Hearing an echo

Causes

The cause of intermittent explosive disorder appears to be a combination of biological and environmental factors. Lives have been torn apart by this disorder, but medications can help control the aggressive impulses.

Most people with this disorder grew up in families where explosive behavior and verbal and physical abuse were common. Being exposed to this type of violence at an early age makes it more likely for these children to exhibit these same traits as they mature.

There may also be a genetic component, causing this disorder to be passed down from parents to children.

Risk Factors

People with other mental health problems—such as mood disorder, anxiety disorders and eating disorders—may be more likely to also have intermittent explosive disorder. Substance abuse is another risk factor.

Individuals with narcissistic, obsessive, paranoid or schizoid traits may be especially prone to intermittent explosive disorder. As children, they may have exhibited severe temper tantrums and other behavioral problems such as stealing and fire setting.

✤ It's A Fact!!

Evidence suggests that intermittent explosive disorder (IED) might predispose toward depression, anxiety, alcohol and drug abuse disorders by increasing stressful life experiences. Given its earlier age-of-onset, identifying IED early—perhaps in school-based violence prevention programs—and providing early treatment might prevent some of the associated pathology.

Source: Excerpted from "Intermittent Explosive Disorder Affects up to 16 Million Americans," a National Institute of Mental Health press release dated June 5, 2006.

Screening And Diagnosis

The diagnosis is based on these criteria:

- Multiple incidents in which the person failed to resist aggressive impulses that resulted in deliberate destruction of property or assault of another person.
- The degree of aggressiveness expressed during the incident is completely out of proportion to the precipitating event.
- The aggressive episodes are not accounted for by another mental disorder, and are not due to the effects of a drug or general medical condition.

Other conditions that must be ruled out before making a diagnosis of intermittent explosive disorder include delirium, dementia, oppositional defiant disorder, antisocial personality disorder, schizophrenia, panic attacks and substance withdrawal or intoxication.

People with intermittent explosive disorder may have an imbalance in the amount of serotonin and testosterone in their brains.

Complications

This disorder may result in job loss, school suspension, divorce, auto accidents, or incarceration.

Treatment

Many different types of drugs are used to help control intermittent explosive disorder, including: anticonvulsants, anti-anxiety agents in the benzodiazepine family, mood regulators and antidepressants. Group counseling and anger management sessions can also be helpful. Relaxation techniques have been found to be useful in neutralizing anger.

Oppositional Defiant Disorder

Introduction

Even the best-behaved children can be difficult and challenging at times. Teens are often moody and argumentative. But if the child or teen has a persistent pattern of tantrums, arguing, and angry or disruptive behaviors toward parents and other authority figures, he or she may have oppositional defiant disorder (ODD). Emotionally draining for the parents and distressing for the child, oppositional defiant disorder can add fuel to what may already be a stressful and turbulent family life.

Signs And Symptoms

It may be tough at times to recognize the difference between a strong-willed or emotional child and a child who has oppositional defiant disorder. It is normal for children to exhibit oppositional behaviors at certain stages of their development. However, if the child's oppositional behaviors are persistent, have lasted at least six months and are clearly disruptive to the family and home or school environment, the issue may be oppositional defiant disorder.

The following behaviors are associated with ODD:

- Negativity
- Defiance
- Disobedience
- Hostility directed towards authority figures

These behaviors might cause a child to regularly and consistently show these symptoms:

- Frequent temper tantrums
- Argumentativeness with adults
- Refusal to comply with adult requests or rules
- Blaming others for mistakes or misbehavior
- Acting touchy and easily annoyed
- Anger and resentment
- Spiteful or vindictive behavior
- Aggressiveness toward peers

Oppositional defiant disorder occurs along with other behavioral or mental health problems such as attention-deficit/hyperactivity disorder (ADHD), anxiety, or depression. The symptoms of ODD may be hard to distinguish from other behavioral or mental health problems.

Causes

There is no clear cause underpinning oppositional defiant disorder. Contributing causes may include the following:

- The child's inherent temperament
- The family's response to the child's style
- A genetic component that when coupled with environmental factors, such as lack of supervision, poor quality daycare, family instability, can increase risk of ODD
- A biochemical or neurological factor
- The child's perception that he or she is not getting enough of the parent's time or attention

Risk Factors

A number of factors play a role in the development of oppositional defiant disorder. Possible risk factors include the following:

- Having a parent with a mood or substance abuse disorder
- Being abused or neglected

- Harsh or inconsistent discipline
- Lack of supervision
- Poor relationships with one or both parents
- Family instability such as multiple moves, changing schools frequently
- Parents with a history of ADHD, ODD, or conduct disorders
- Financial problems in the family
- Peer rejection
- Exposure to violence
- Frequent changes in daycare providers
- Parents with a troubled marriage or are divorced

Screening and Diagnosis

Doctors usually diagnose oppositional defiant disorder through information provided by parents and teachers. It can be difficult for doctors to sort and exclude other associated disorders—for example, ADHD versus ODD.

Physicians rely on clinical judgment and experience, information gathered from parents and teachers who may fill out questionnaires, and possibly from interviewing the child.

Treatment

Oppositional defiant disorder is not something a child can overcome on their own, nor can it be solved with medication, herbal supplements, vitamins, or special diet. Successful treatment of oppositional defiant disorder requires commitment and follow-through by the parents and others involved in the child's care. But most important in treatment is for parents to show consistent, unconditional love, and acceptance of the child—even during difficult and disruptive situations.

Ideally treatment for oppositional defiant disorder involves the primary care physician and a mental health or child development professional. These health professionals can screen for and treat other mental health problems that may be interfering with oppositional deficit disorder, such as ADHD, anxiety, or depression. Successful treatment of the often co-existing conditions will improve the effectiveness of treatment for ODD. In some case, the symptoms of ODD disappear entirely.

A mental health professional can help the parent learn or strengthen specific skills and parenting techniques to help improve the child's behavior and strengthen the relationship between the parent and child. For example, the parent may learn how to use the following tactics:

- Give effective time-outs
- Avoid power struggles
- Remain calm and unemotional in the face of opposition
- Recognize and praise the child's good behaviors and positive characteristics
- Offer acceptable choices to the child, giving him or her certain amount of control

✔ Quick Tip
Self-Care

At home, parents can begin chipping away at problem behaviors by practicing the following:

- Recognize and praise the child's positive behaviors
- Model the behavior they want the child to have
- Picking battles
- Set limits and enforce consistent reasonable consequences
- Develop a consistent daily schedule for the child
- Work together with spouses and other members of the household to assure consistent and appropriate discipline procedures
- Assign the child a household chore that is essential and that won't get done unless the child does it

Source: © July 2006 Public Health Nursing Program, Riverside County Department of Public Health [California].

Although some parent management techniques seem like common sense, learning to use them in the face of opposition is not easy, especially if there are other stressors at home. Learning these skills may require counseling, parenting classes, or other forms of education, and consistent practice and patience. At first, the child is not likely to be cooperative or appreciate that parents have changed responses to his or her behavior. Families should expect that there will be set backs and relapses and be prepared with a plan to manage those times.

Individual counseling may help the child learn to manage his or her anger. Family counseling may help to improve communication and relationships and help family members learn how to work together. Again it is crucial to identify and treat any other disorders that may be affecting the child along with oppositional defiant disorder.

Resources

Mayo Clinic. (2006). Intermittent Explosive Disorder. Retrieved on July 5, 2006 from the World Wide Web: http://www.mayoclinic.com/health/intermitten-explosive%20-disorder/DS00730

Mayo Clinic. (2006). Oppositional Defiant Disorder. Retrieved on July 5, 2006 from the World Wide Web: http://www.mayoclinic.com/health/oppositional-defiant-disorder/DS00630

Chapter 24

Impulse Control Disorders

Pyromania (Fire Starting)

The pyromaniac sets main deliberate fires and takes enjoyment in watching what others have to do as a result of this. Therefore the pyromaniac is often one of the spectators of the fire he has generated.

- More than once, the person has deliberately and purposefully set fires.
- Before the fire-setting, the person experiences tension or excited mood.
- The person is interested in or attracted to fire and its circumstances and outcomes.
- The person experiences gratification, pleasure or relief when setting fires or experiencing their consequences.
- These fires are not set: for profit; to express a political agenda; to conceal crimes; to express anger or revenge; to improve the patient's living circumstances; in response to a delusion or hallucination; as a result of impaired judgment.
- The fire-setting is not better explained by antisocial personality disorder, conduct disorder, or manic episode.

Associated Features

- Childhood enuresis
- Learning disabilities
- Cruelty—to animals

Differential Diagnosis

Some disorders have similar or even the same symptoms. The clinician, therefore, in his/her diagnostic attempt, has to differentiate against the following disorders which need to be ruled out to establish a precise diagnosis.

- Antisocial personality disorder
- Conduct disorder
- Manic episode
- Substance abuse
- Mental retardation
- Psychosis

✤ It's A Fact!!

Cause: Pyromania is a strong need to set things on fire. It is all about the pleasure it gives to see what other people have to do to extinguish the fire and the pyromaniac may enjoy reading about the effects of his/her activities.

Treatment

- Behavioral therapy is used to direct the persons interest away from fire setting activities and have these replace with more socially acceptable forms of tension reduction.
- Counseling and psychotherapy

Kleptomania

Kleptomania involves a failure to resist impulses to steal items that are not needed or sought for personal use or monetary value. Kleptomania should be distinguished from shoplifting, in which the action is usually well-planned and motivated by need or monetary gain. Some clinicians view kleptomania as part of the obsessive-compulsive spectrum of disorders, reasoning that many individuals experience the impulse to steal as an alien, unwanted intrusion into their mental state. Other evidence suggests that kleptomania may be related to, or a variant of, mood disorders, such as depression. The main diagnostic features are:

- The person repeatedly yields to the impulse to steal objects that are needed neither for personal use nor for their monetary worth.
- Just before the theft, the patient experiences increasing tension.
- At the time of theft, the patient feels gratification, pleasure, or relief.
- These thefts are committed neither out of anger or revenge nor in response to delusions or hallucinations.
- The thefts are not better explained by antisocial personality disorder, conduct disorder, or a manic episode.

Associated Features

- Depressed or guilty (concerning the thefts)
- Major depressive disorder
- Anxiety

Differential Diagnosis

Some disorders have similar or even the same symptoms. The clinician, therefore, in his/her diagnostic attempt, has to differentiate against the following disorders which need to be ruled out to establish a precise diagnosis.

- An ordinary criminal act
- Bipolar mood disorder
- Conduct disorder
- Antisocial personality disorder
- Manic episode in response to delusions or dementia

♣ It's A Fact!!

Cause: Most person's with this disorder seem to be women; their average age is about 35 and the duration of illness is roughly 16 years. Some individuals report the onset of kleptomania as early as age five. While we do not know the causes of kleptomania, there is indirect evidence linking it with abnormalities in the brain chemical serotonin. Stressors such as major losses may also precipitate kleptomanic behavior.

Treatment

Treatment will include counseling and psychotherapeutic approaches and in some cases combined with drug therapy.

- **Counseling And Psychotherapy:** A variety of psychotherapies have been used to treat this disorder, but it is not clear which one is best. Family therapy may also be important, since this disorder can be very disruptive to families.
- **Pharmacotherapy:** Prozac, an antidepressant that boosts levels of serotonin, has been found useful in some cases of kleptomania.

Pathological Gambling

Pathological gambling is persistent and recurrent maladaptive gambling behavior that disrupts personal, family, or vocational pursuits. The individual may be preoccupied with gambling (for example, reliving past gambling experiences, planning the next gambling venture, or thinking of ways to get money with which to gamble). Most individuals with pathological gambling say that they are seeking an aroused, euphoric state that the gambling gives them which appears more exhilarating than the money. Increasingly larger bets, or greater risks, may be needed to continue to produce the desired level of excitement.

- Persistent, maladaptive gambling is expressed by five or more of the following: the patient needs to put increasing amounts of money into play to get the desired excitement; has repeatedly tried (and failed) to control or stop gambling; feels restless or irritable when trying to control gambling; uses gambling to escape from problems; often tries to recoup loses; lies to cover up the extent of gambling; has stolen to finance gambling; has jeopardized a job or important relationship; has had to rely on others for money to relieve the consequences of gambling; is preoccupied with gambling.
- A manic episode doesn't better explain this behavior.

Associated Features

- General medical conditions that are associated with stress
- Mood disorders

- Attention deficit/hyperactivity disorder
- Substance abuse or dependence
- Borderline personality disorders

Differential Diagnosis

Some disorders have similar or even the same symptoms. The clinician, therefore, in his/her diagnostic attempt, has to differentiate against the following disorders which need to be ruled out to establish a precise diagnosis.

- Social gambling
- Manic episode
- Antisocial, narcissistic personality disorders

Treatment

Treatment for the person with compulsive gambling begins with the recognition of the problem. It is often associated with denial, allowing the person to believe there is no need for treatment. Most people affected by compulsive gambling enter treatment under pressure from others, rather than a voluntary acceptance of the need for treatment. Addicts to gambling need professional help and they should get behavioral therapy. Often this happens too late and the patient has already accumulated large debts.

> ### ✤ It's A Fact!!
>
> **Cause:** Pathological gamblers were found to exhibit certain physiological traits, such as high energy levels, hyperactivity, and high tolerance of stress. The sociological view that pathological gamblers have positive rewards convincing them of the benefits of gambling was supported with evidence of a big win early in the career of the pathological gambler.
>
> Pathological gambling is very similar in definition and symptoms to substance dependence. Various studies of pathological gamblers in treatment reveal that approximately 50 percent have histories of alcohol or drug abuse. In males, the disorder typically begins in adolescence. Females typically start gambling later in life, are more apt to be depressed, and gamble as a means of escaping the depression. It is not unusual for male gamblers to have a history of 20 to 30 years when they seek treatment, compared with three years for females.

Counseling And Psychotherapy: Treatment options include individual and group psychotherapy, and self-help support groups such as Gamblers Anonymous. Abstinence principles that apply to other types of addiction, such as substance abuse and alcohol dependence, are also relevant in the treatment of compulsive gambling behavior.

Trichotillomania

Trichotillomania involves the repetitive, uncontrollable pulling of one's body hair. Most commonly, scalp hair, eyelashes, and eyebrows are pulled, although hair may be pulled from any location. Typical symptoms include:

- Recurrent pulling out of one's hair resulting in noticeable hair loss.
- An increasing sense of tension immediately before pulling out the hair or when attempting to resist the behavior.
- Pleasure, gratification, or relief when pulling out the hair.
- The disturbance causes clinically significant distress or impairment in social, occupational, or other important areas of functioning.
- The disturbance is not better accounted for by another mental disorder and is not due to a general medical condition (for example, a dermatological condition).

Associated Features

Associated features of trichotillomania include: examining the hair root; twirling it off; pulling the strand between the teeth, or trichophagia (eating hairs). Nail biting, scratching, gnawing, and excoriation may be associated with trichotillomania.

- Mood disorder
- Anxiety disorder
- Mental retardation

> ✤ **It's A Fact!!**
>
> **Cause:** Trichotillomania is found predominantly in females and tends to occur more often in children than adults. The disorder usually begins between early childhood and adolescence. In some cases, trichotillomania is related to an increased stress level at home or school, while for other children, it is simply a learned habit that has strengthened over time.

Differential Diagnosis

Some disorders have similar or even the same symptoms. The clinician, therefore, in his/her diagnostic attempt, has to differentiate against the following disorders which need to be ruled out to establish a precise diagnosis.

- Obsessive-compulsive disorder
- Tourette syndrome
- Pervasive developmental disorder (infantile autism)
- Stereotypy disorder
- Factitious disorder (Munchausen syndrome)

Treatment

The primary treatment approach for trichotillomania is habit reversal combined with stress management and behavioral contracting. Parents can help by recognizing the problem in its early stages and getting involved in its treatment.

Counseling And Psychotherapy: Treatment may involve self-monitoring of hair-pulling episodes as well as the feelings and situations that are most likely to lead to hair pulling. Youngsters are then systematically introduced to new behaviors, for example, squeezing a ball or tightening their fist, whenever they feel the urge to pull at their hair.

Relaxation training and other stress reduction techniques may also be used including reward charts that help track and monitor a child's progress with the added incentive of earning small rewards for continued progress. In addition, cognitive therapy, is found to be effective.

Skin Picking

Compulsive skin picking (CSP), also called pathological skin picking, neurotic excoriation, or dermatillomania, is defined as the habitual picking of skin lesions or the excessive scratching, picking, or squeezing of otherwise healthy skin is a poorly understood disorder.

Some researchers now believe that compulsive hair pulling, skin picking, and nail biting form a subgroup of what is becoming known as the obsessive-compulsive disorder (OCD) spectrum. OCD has been previously been regarded as only a single disorder but may in fact represent a range of related disorders, including classic OCD, body dysmorphic disorder, anorexia nervosa, bulimia, trichotillomania, onychophagia, compulsive skin picking, compulsive nail biting, and Tourette syndrome.

The characteristics of skin picking include:

- Recurrent skin picking—face, lips, scalp, hands or arms.
- Tension increase immediately before picking.
- Pleasure, gratification, tension decrease or relief when skin picking.
- The picking causes significant difficulties in life, or stress.
- Sensations such as itching, tingling, burning, or an uncontrollable urge to pick their skin.

Associated Features

- Stereotypic behaviors—body rocking, thumb sucking, knuckle cracking, cheek chewing, and head banging
- Anxiety
- Depression

Differential Diagnosis

Some disorders have similar symptoms. The clinician, therefore, in his diagnostic attempt has to differentiate against the following disorders which need to be ruled out to establish a precise diagnosis.

- Depression
- Anxiety
- Substance abuse
- Body dysmorphic disorder
- Obsessive compulsive disorder
- Trichotillomania
- Dermatological skin disorder

✤ It's A Fact!!

Cause: Most people develop this problem in their teens or 20s. An episode may be a conscious response to anxiety or depression, but is frequently done as an unconscious habit.

Treatment

The primary treatment modality for CSP depends on the level of awareness the individual has regarding the problem. If the CSP is generally an unconscious habit, the primary treatment is a form of cognitive-behavioral therapy and drug therapy.

Counseling And Psychotherapy: Cognitive behavioral therapy and habit reversal training (HRT) may be used, as it appears that skin-picking is a conditioned response to specific situations and events, and that the individual with CSP is frequently unaware of these triggers. HRT challenges the problem in a two ways. Firstly, the individual learns how to become more consciously aware of situations and events that trigger skin-picking episodes and secondly, the individual learns to utilize alternative behaviors in response to these situations and events.

Pharmacotherapy: Antidepressants—Anafranil; Prozac; Zoloft; Paxil; Luvox; Celexa; Lexapro; Serzone; Effexor.

Chapter 25

Eating Disorders

What Are Eating Disorders?

An eating disorder is marked by extremes. It is present when a person experiences severe disturbances in eating behavior, such as extreme reduction of food intake or extreme overeating, or feelings of extreme distress or concern about body weight or shape.

A person with an eating disorder may have started out just eating smaller or larger amounts of food than usual, but at some point, the urge to eat less or more spirals out of control. Eating disorders are very complex, and despite scientific research to understand them, the biological, behavioral, and social underpinnings of these illnesses remain elusive.

The two main types of eating disorders are anorexia nervosa and bulimia nervosa. A third category is "eating disorders not otherwise specified (EDNOS)," which includes several variations of eating disorders. Most of these disorders are similar to anorexia or bulimia but with slightly different characteristics. Binge-eating disorder, which has received increasing research and media attention in recent years, is one type of EDNOS.

About This Chapter: This chapter begins with "What Are Eating Disorders," excerpted from "Eating Disorders," National Institute of Mental Health, February 11, 2009. It continues with excerpts from the following publications of the National Women's Health Information Center: "Frequently Asked Questions: Anorexia Nervosa," July 1, 2006; "Frequently Asked Questions: Bulimia Nervosa," January 1, 2007; and "Frequently Asked Questions: Binge Eating Disorder," January 1, 2005.

Eating disorders frequently appear during adolescence or young adulthood, but some reports indicate that they can develop during childhood or later in adulthood. Women and girls are much more likely than males to develop an eating disorder. Men and boys account for an estimated five to 15 percent of patients with anorexia or bulimia and an estimated 35 percent of those with binge-eating disorder. Eating disorders are real, treatable medical illnesses with complex underlying psychological and biological causes. They frequently co-exist with other psychiatric disorders such as depression, substance abuse, or anxiety disorders. People with eating disorders also can suffer from numerous other physical health complications, such as heart conditions or kidney failure, which can lead to death.

✎ What's It Mean?

Anorexia Nervosa: Self-starvation. People with this disorder eat very little even though they are thin. They have an intense and overpowering fear of body fat and weight gain.

Binge Eating Disorder: Eating large amounts of food in a short period of time, usually alone, without being able to stop when full. The overeating or bingeing is often accompanied by feeling out of control and then depressed, guilty, or disgusted.

Bulimia Nervosa: Characterized by cycles of binge eating and purging, either by vomiting or taking laxatives or diuretics (water pills). People with bulimia have a fear of body fat even though their size and weight may be normal.

Disordered Eating: Troublesome eating behaviors, such as restrictive dieting, bingeing, or purging, which occur less frequently or are less severe than those required to meet the full criteria for the diagnosis of an eating disorder.

Overexercising: Exercising compulsively for long periods of time as a way to burn calories from food that has just been eaten. People with anorexia or bulimia may overexercise.

Source: Excerpted from "At Risk: All Ethnic and Cultural Groups," *BodyWise*, Office on Women's Health, U.S. Department of Health and Human Services, 2004.

Frequently Asked Questions About Anorexia Nervosa

What is anorexia nervosa?

A person with anorexia (a-neh-RECK-see-ah) nervosa, often called anorexia, has an intense fear of gaining weight. Someone with anorexia thinks about food a lot and limits the food she or he eats, even though she or he is too thin. Anorexia is more than just a problem with food. It's a way of using food or starving oneself to feel more in control of life and to ease tension, anger, and anxiety. Most people with anorexia are female. The following characteristics may describe an anorexic:

- Has a low body weight for her or his height
- Resists keeping a normal body weight
- Has an intense fear of gaining weight
- Thinks she or he is fat even when very thin
- Misses three menstrual periods in a row (for girls/women who have started having their periods)

Who becomes anorexic?

While anorexia mostly affects girls and women (90–95 percent), it can also affect boys and men. It was once thought that women of color were shielded from eating disorders by their cultures, which tend to be more accepting of different body sizes. Sadly, research shows that as African American, Latina, Asian/Pacific Islander, and American Indian and Alaska Native women are more exposed to images of thin women, they also become more likely to develop eating disorders.

What causes anorexia?

There is no single known cause of anorexia. But some things may play a part:

- **Culture:** Women in the U.S. are under constant pressure to fit a certain ideal of beauty. Seeing images of flawless, thin females everywhere makes it hard for women to feel good about their bodies. More and more, men are also feeling pressure to have a perfect body.

- **Families:** If you have a mother or sister with anorexia, you are more likely to develop the disorder. Parents who think looks are important, diet themselves, or criticize their children's bodies are more likely to have a child with anorexia.
- **Life Changes Or Stressful Events:** Traumatic events like rape as well as stressful things like starting a new job, can lead to the onset of anorexia.
- **Personality Traits:** Someone with anorexia may not like her or himself, hate the way she or he looks, or feel hopeless. She or he often sets hard-to-reach goals for her or himself and tries to be perfect in every way.
- **Biology:** Genes, hormones, and chemicals in the brain may be factors in developing anorexia.

What are signs of anorexia?

Someone with anorexia may look very thin. She or he may use extreme measures to lose weight by using these tactics:

- Making her or himself throw up
- Taking pills to urinate or have a bowel movement
- Taking diet pills
- Not eating or eating very little
- Exercising a lot, even in bad weather or when hurt or tired

✤ It's A Fact!!

Men And Boys Are Affected By Eating Disorders

Although eating disorders primarily affect women and girls, boys and men are also vulnerable. One in four preadolescent cases of anorexia occurs in boys, and binge-eating disorder affects females and males about equally.

Like females who have eating disorders, males with the illness have a warped sense of body image and often have muscle dysmorphia, a type of disorder that is characterized by an extreme concern with becoming more muscular. Some boys with the disorder want to lose weight, while others want to gain weight or "bulk up." Boys who think they are too small are at a greater risk for using steroids or other dangerous drugs to increase muscle mass.

Boys with eating disorders exhibit the same types of emotional, physical and behavioral signs and symptoms as girls, but for a variety of reasons, boys are less likely to be diagnosed with what is often considered a stereotypically "female" disorder.

Source: Excerpted from "Eating Disorders," National Institute of Mental Health, February 11, 2009.

- Weighing food and counting calories
- Moving food around the plate instead of eating it

Someone with anorexia may also have a distorted body image, shown by thinking she or he is fat, wearing baggy clothes, weighing her or himself many times a day, and fearing weight gain.

Anorexia can also cause someone to not act like her or himself. She or he may talk about weight and food all the time, not eat in front of others, be moody or sad, or not want to go out with friends.

What happens to your body with anorexia?

With anorexia, your body doesn't get the energy from foods that it needs, so it slows down. See Figure 25.1 for to find out how anorexia affects your health.

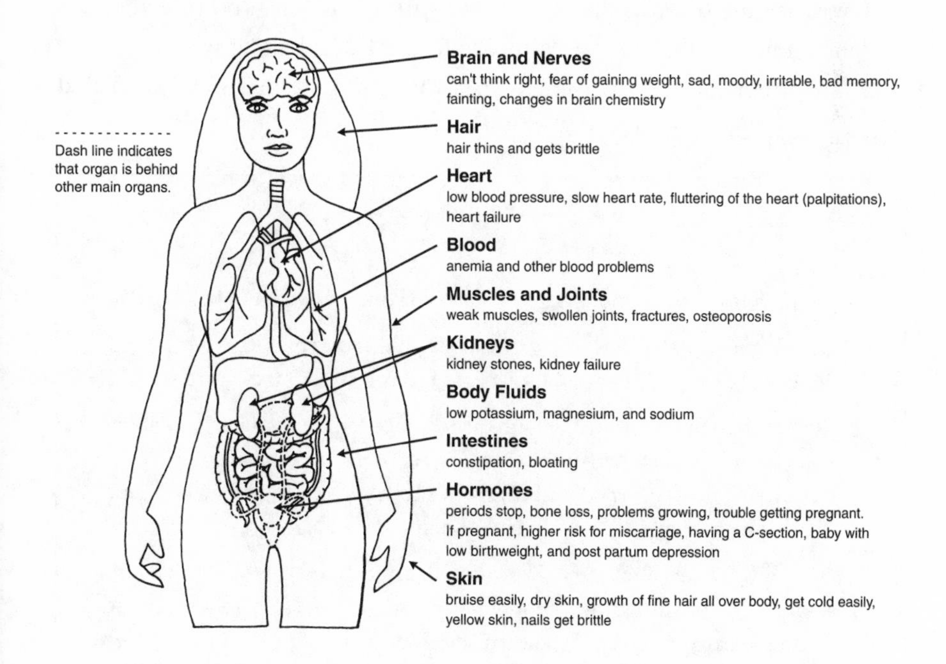

Figure 25.1. How anorexia affects your body.

Can someone with anorexia get better?

Yes. Someone with anorexia can get better. A health care team of doctors, nutritionists, and therapists will help the patient get better. They will help her or him learn healthy eating patterns, cope with thoughts and feelings, and gain weight. With outpatient care, the patient receives treatment through visits with members of their health care team. Some patients may need "partial hospitalization." This means that the person goes to the hospital during the day for treatment, but lives at home. Sometimes, the patient goes to a hospital and stays there for treatment. After leaving the hospital, the patient continues to get help from her or his health care team.

Individual counseling can also help someone with anorexia. If the patient is young, counseling may involve the whole family too. Support groups may also be a part of treatment. In support groups, patients and families meet and share what they've been through.

Often, eating disorders happen along with mental health problems such as depression and anxiety. These problems are treated along with the anorexia. Treatment may include medicines that fix hormone imbalances that play a role in these disorders.

✔ Quick Tip

If someone you know is showing signs of an eating disorder, you may be able to help.

- Set a time to talk. Set aside a time to talk privately with your friend. Make sure you talk in a quiet place where you won't be distracted.
- Tell your friend about your concerns. Be honest. Tell your friend about your worries about her or his not eating or over exercising. Tell your friend you are concerned and that you think these things may be a sign of a problem that needs professional help.
- Ask your friend to talk to a professional. Your friend can talk to a counselor or doctor who knows about eating issues. Offer to help your friend find a counselor or doctor and make an appointment, and offer to go with her or him to the appointment.

Frequently Asked Questions About Bulimia Nervosa

What is bulimia?

Bulimia (buh-LEE-me-ah) nervosa is a type of eating disorder. It is often called just bulimia. A person with bulimia eats a lot of food in a short amount of time. This is called binging. The person may fear gaining weight after a binge. Binging also can cause feelings of shame and guilt. So, the person tries to "undo" the binge by getting rid of the food. This is called purging. Purging might be done by using one or more of the following tactics:

- Making yourself throw up
- Taking laxatives (LAX-uh-tiv)—pills or liquids that speed up the movement of food through your body and lead to a bowel movement
- Exercising a lot
- Eating very little or not at all
- Taking water pills to urinate

Who becomes bulimic?

Many people think that only young, upper-class, white females get eating disorders. It is true that many more women than men have bulimia. In fact, nine

- Avoid conflicts. If your friend won't admit that she or he has a problem, don't push. Be sure to tell your friend you are always there to listen if she or he wants to talk.
- Don't place shame, blame, or guilt on your friend. Don't say, "You just need to eat." Instead, say things like, "I'm concerned about you because you won't eat breakfast or lunch." Or, "It makes me afraid to hear you throwing up."
- Don't give simple solutions. Don't say, "If you'd just stop, then things would be fine!"
- Let your friend know that you will always be there no matter what.

These tips are adapted from "What Should I Say? Tips for Talking to a Friend Who May Be Struggling with an Eating Disorder," from the National Eating Disorders Association.

Source of this text: Adapted from National Women's Information Center, July 1, 2006, and January 1, 2007.

out of ten people with bulimia are women. But bulimia can affect anyone: Men, older women, and women of color can become bulimic. It was once thought that women of color were protected from eating disorders by their cultures. These cultures tend to be more accepting of all body sizes. But research shows that as women of color are more exposed to images of thin women, they are more likely to get eating disorders. African-American, Latina, Asian/Pacific Islander, and American Indian and Alaska Native women can become bulimic.

What causes bulimia?

Bulimia is more than just a problem with food. A binge can be set off by dieting or stress. Painful emotions, like anger or sadness, also can bring on binging. Purging is how people with bulimia try to gain control and to ease stress and anxiety. There is no single known cause of bulimia. But these factors might play a role:

Culture: Women in the U.S. are under constant pressure to be very thin. This "ideal" is not realistic for most women. But seeing images of flawless, thin females everywhere can make it hard for women to feel good about their bodies. More and more, men are also feeling pressure to have a perfect body.

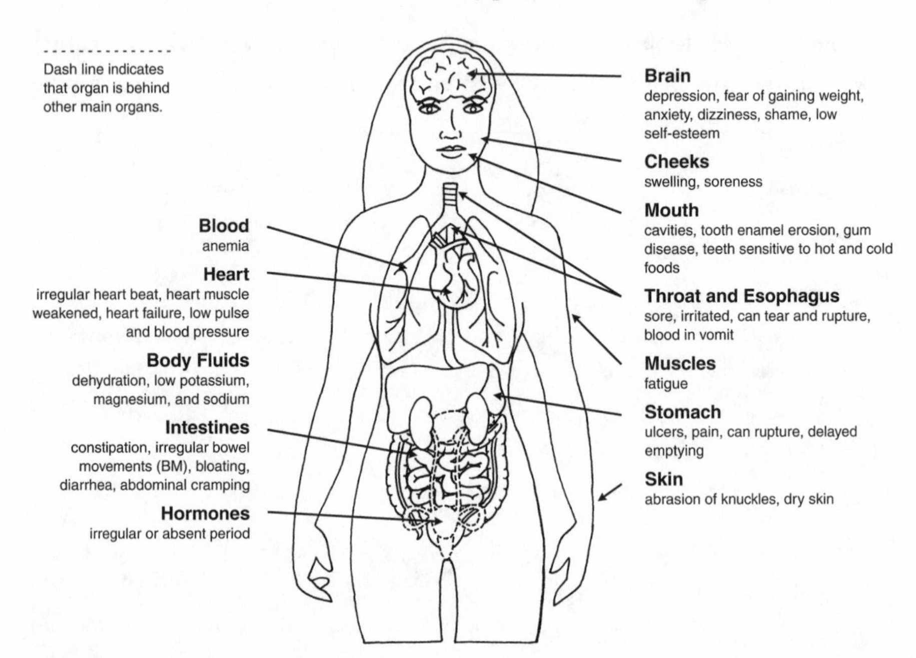

Figure 25.2. How bulimia affects your body.

Families. It is likely that bulimia runs in families. Many people with bulimia have sisters or mothers with bulimia. Parents who think looks are important, diet themselves, or judge their children's bodies are more likely to have a child with bulimia.

Life Changes Or Stressful Events: Traumatic events like rape can lead to bulimia. So can stressful events like being teased about body size.

Psychology: Having low self-esteem is common in people with bulimia. People with bulimia have higher rates of depression. They may have problems expressing anger and feelings. They might be moody or feel like they can't control impulsive behaviors.

Biology: Genes, hormones, and chemicals in the brain may be factors in getting bulimia.

What are signs of bulimia?

A person with bulimia may be thin, overweight, or normal weight. This makes it hard to know if someone has bulimia. But there are warning signs to look out for. Someone with bulimia may do extreme things to lose weight, such as the following:

- Using diet pills, or taking pills to urinate or have a bowel movement
- Going to the bathroom all the time after eating (to throw up)
- Exercising too much, even when hurt or tired

Someone with bulimia may show signs of throwing up:

- Swollen cheeks or jaw area
- Rough skin on knuckles (if using fingers to make one throw up)
- Teeth that look clear
- Broken blood vessels in the eyes

Someone with bulimia often thinks she or he is fat, even if this is not true. The person might hate his or her body. Or worry a lot about gaining weight. Bulimia can cause someone to not seem like him or herself. The person might be moody or sad. Someone with bulimia might not want to go out with friends.

What happens to someone who has bulimia?

Bulimia can hurt your body. See Figure 25.2 to find out how bulimia harms your health.

Can someone with bulimia get better?

Yes. Someone with bulimia can get better with the help of a health care team. A doctor will provide medical care. A nutritionist (noo-TRISH-un-ist) can teach healthy eating patterns. A therapist (thair-uh-pist) can help the patient learn new ways to cope with thoughts and feelings.

Therapy is an important part of any treatment plan. It might be alone, with family members, or in a group. Medicines can help some people with bulimia. These include medicines used to treat depression. Medicines work best when used with therapy.

Chances of getting better are greatest when bulimia is found out and treated early.

Frequently Asked Questions About Binge Eating Disorder

What is binge eating disorder?

People with binge eating disorder often eat an unusually large amount of food and feel out of control during the binges. People with binge eating disorder also may have the following characteristics:

- Eat more quickly than usual during binge episodes
- Eat until they are uncomfortably full
- Eat when they are not hungry
- Eat alone because of embarrassment
- Feel disgusted, depressed, or guilty after overeating

What causes binge eating disorder?

No one knows for sure what causes binge eating disorder. Researchers are looking at the following factors that may affect binge eating:

- **Depression:** As many as half of all people with binge eating disorder are depressed or have been depressed in the past.
- **Dieting:** Some people binge after skipping meals, not eating enough food each day, or avoiding certain kinds of food.
- **Coping Skills:** Studies suggest that people with binge eating may have trouble handling some of their emotions. Many people who are binge eaters say that being angry, sad, bored, worried, or stressed can cause them to binge eat.
- **Biology:** Researchers are looking into how brain chemicals and metabolism (the way the body uses calories) affect binge eating disorder. Research also suggests that genes may be involved in binge eating, since the disorder often occurs in several members of the same family.

Certain behaviors and emotional problems are more common in people with binge eating disorder. These include abusing alcohol, acting quickly without thinking (impulsive behavior), and not feeling in charge of themselves.

What are the health consequences of binge eating disorder?

People with binge eating disorder are usually very upset by their binge eating and may become depressed. Research has shown that people with binge eating disorder report more health problems, stress, trouble sleeping, and suicidal thoughts than people without an eating disorder. People with binge eating disorder often feel badly about themselves and may miss work, school, or social activities to binge eat.

People with binge eating disorder may gain weight. Weight gain can lead to obesity, and obesity raises the risk for these health problems:

- Type 2 diabetes
- High blood pressure
- High cholesterol
- Gallbladder disease
- Heart disease
- Certain types of cancer

What is the treatment for binge eating disorder?

People with binge eating disorder should get help from a health care provider, such as a psychiatrist, psychologist, or clinical social worker. There are several different ways to treat binge eating disorder:

- Cognitive-behavioral therapy teaches people how to keep track of their eating and change their unhealthy eating habits. It teaches them how to cope with stressful situations. It also helps them feel better about their body shape and weight.
- Interpersonal psychotherapy helps people look at their relationships with friends and family and make changes in problem areas.
- Drug therapy, such as antidepressants, may be helpful for some people.
- Other treatments include dialectical behavior therapy, which helps people regulate their emotions; drug therapy with the anti-seizure medication topiramate; exercise in combination with cognitive-behavioral therapy; and support groups.

Many people with binge eating disorder also have a problem with obesity. There are treatments for obesity, like weight loss surgery (gastrointestinal surgery), but these treatments will not treat the underlying problem of binge eating disorder.

✤ It's A Fact!! Working To Better Understand And Treat Eating Disorders

Researchers are working to define the basic processes of eating disorders, which should help identify better treatments. For example, is anorexia the result of skewed body image, self esteem problems, obsessive thoughts, compulsive behavior, or a combination of these? Can it be predicted or identified as a risk factor before drastic weight loss occurs, and therefore avoided?

These and other questions may be answered in the future as scientists and doctors think of eating disorders as medical illnesses with certain biological causes. Researchers are studying behavioral questions, along with genetic and brain systems information, to understand risk factors, identify biological markers and develop medications that can target specific pathways that control eating behavior. Finally, neuroimaging and genetic studies may also provide clues for how each person may respond to specific treatments.

Source: National Institute of Mental Health, February 11, 2009.

Chapter 26

Compulsive Exercise

Rachel and her cheerleading team practice three to five times a week. Rachel feels a lot of pressure to keep her weight down—as head cheerleader, she wants to set an example to the team. So she adds extra daily workouts to her regimen. But lately, she's been feeling worn out, and she has a hard time just making it through a regular team practice.

You may think you can't get too much of a good thing, but in the case of exercise, a healthy activity can sometimes turn into an unhealthy compulsion. Rachel is a good example of how an overemphasis on physical fitness or weight control can become unhealthy. Read on to find out more about compulsive exercise and its effects.

Too Much of a Good Thing?

We all know the benefits of exercise, and it seems that everywhere we turn, we hear that we should exercise more. The right kind of exercise does many great things for your body and soul: It can strengthen your heart and muscles, lower your body fat, and reduce your risk of many diseases.

Many teens who play sports have higher self-esteem than their less active pals, and exercise can even help keep the blues at bay because of the endorphin rush it can cause. Endorphins are chemicals that naturally relieve pain and lift mood. These chemicals are released in your body during and after a workout and they go a long way in helping to control stress.

So how can something with so many benefits have the potential to cause harm?

Why Do People Overexercise?

Lots of people start working out because it's fun or it makes them feel good, but exercise can become a compulsive habit when it is done for the wrong reasons.

Some people start exercising with weight loss as their main goal. Although exercise is part of a safe and healthy way to control weight, many people may have unrealistic expectations. We are bombarded with images from advertisers of the ideal body: young and thin for women; strong and muscular for men. To try to reach these unreasonable ideals, people may turn to diets, and for some, this may develop into eating disorders such as anorexia and bulimia. And some people who grow frustrated with the results from diets alone may overexercise to speed up weight loss.

Some athletes may also think that repeated exercise will help them to win an important game. Like Rachel, they add extra workouts to those regularly scheduled with their teams without consulting their coaches or trainers. The pressure to succeed may also lead these people to exercise more than is healthy. The body needs activity but it also needs rest. Overexercising can lead to injuries like fractures and muscle strains.

Are You A Healthy Exerciser?

Fitness experts recommend that teens do at least 60 minutes of moderate to vigorous physical activity every day. Most young people exercise much less than this recommended amount (which can be a problem for different reasons), but some, such as athletes, do more.

Experts say that repeatedly exercising beyond the requirements for good health is an indicator of compulsive behavior. Some people need more than the average amount of exercise, of course—such as athletes in training for a big event. But several workouts a day, every day, when a person is not in training is a sign that the person is probably overdoing it.

People who are exercise dependent also go to extremes to fit activity into their lives. If you put workouts ahead of friends, homework, and other responsibilities, you may be developing a dependence on exercise.

Signs Of Compulsive Exercise

If you are concerned about your own exercise habits or a friend's, ask yourself the following questions. Do you:

- force yourself to exercise, even if you don't feel well?
- prefer to exercise rather than being with friends?
- become very upset if you miss a workout?
- base the amount you exercise on how much you eat?
- have trouble sitting still because you think you're not burning calories?
- worry that you'll gain weight if you skip exercising for a day?

If the answer to any of these questions is yes, you or your friend may have a problem. What should you do?

How To Get Help

The first thing you should do if you suspect that you are a compulsive exerciser is get help. Talk to your parents, doctor, a teacher or counselor, a coach, or another trusted adult. Compulsive exercise, especially when it is combined with an eating disorder, can cause serious and permanent health problems, and in extreme cases, death.

Because compulsive exercise is closely related to eating disorders, help can be found at community agencies specifically set up to deal with anorexia, bulimia, and other eating problems. Your school's health or physical education department may also have support programs and nutrition advice available. Ask your teacher, coach, or counselor to recommend local organizations that may be able to help.

You should also schedule a checkup with a doctor. Because our bodies go through so many important developments during the teen years, guys and girls who have compulsive exercise problems need to see a doctor to make sure they are developing normally. This is especially true if the person also has an eating disorder. Female athlete triad, a condition that affects girls who overexercise and restrict their eating because of their sports, can cause a girl to stop having her period. Medical help is necessary to resolve the physical problems associated with overexercising before they cause long-term damage to the body.

Make A Positive Change

Changes in activity of any kind—eating or sleeping, for example—can often be a sign that something else is wrong in your life. Girls and guys who exercise compulsively may have a distorted body image and low self-esteem. They may see themselves as overweight or out of shape even when they are actually a healthy weight.

Compulsive exercisers need to get professional help for the reasons described above. But there are also some things that you can do to help you take charge again:

- Work on changing your daily self-talk. When you look in the mirror, make sure you find at least one good thing to say about yourself. Be more aware of your positive attributes.
- When you exercise, focus on the positive, mood-boosting qualities.
- Give yourself a break. Listen to your body and give yourself a day of rest after a hard workout.
- Control your weight by exercising and eating moderate portions of healthy foods. Don't try to change your body into an unrealistically lean shape. Talk with your doctor, dietitian, coach, athletic trainer, or other adult about what a healthy body weight is for you and how to develop healthy eating and exercise habits.

Remember!!

Exercise and sports are supposed to be fun and keep you healthy. Working out in moderation will do both.

Chapter 27

Self-Injury

What does hurting yourself mean?

Hurting yourself, sometimes called self-injury, is when a person deliberately hurts his or her own body. Some self-injuries can leave scars that won't go away, while others leave marks or bruises that eventually will go away. These are some forms of self-injury:

- Cutting yourself (such as using a razor blade, knife or other sharp object to cut the skin)
- Punching yourself or other objects
- Burning yourself with cigarettes, matches or candles
- Pulling out your hair
- Poking objects through body openings
- Breaking your bones or bruising yourself
- Plucking hair for hours

Why do some teens want to hurt themselves?

Many people cut themselves because it gives them a sense of relief. Some people use cutting as a means to cope with any problem. Some teens say that

About This Chapter: Text in this chapter is from "Cutting and Hurting Yourself," U.S. Department of Health and Human Services (www.girlshealth.gov), March 12, 2008.

when they hurt themselves, they are trying to stop feeling lonely, angry, or hopeless. Some teens who hurt themselves have low self-esteem, they may feel unloved by their family and friends, and they may have an eating disorder, an alcohol or drug problem, or may have been victims of abuse.

Teens who hurt themselves often keep their feelings "bottled up" inside and have a hard time letting their feelings show. Some teens who hurt themselves say that feeling the pain provides a sense of relief from intense feelings. Cutting can relieve the tension from bottled up sadness or anxiety. Others hurt themselves in order to "feel." Often people who hold back strong emotions can begin feeling numb, and cutting can be a way to cope with this because it causes them to feel something. Some teens also may hurt themselves because they want to fit in with others who do it.

If you are hurting yourself, please get help—it is possible to overcome the urge to cut. There are other ways to find relief and cope with your emotions. Please talk to your parents, your doctor, or an adult you trust, like a teacher or religious leader.

Who are the people who hurt themselves?

People who hurt themselves come from all walks of life, no matter their age, gender, race or ethnicity. About one in 100 people hurts himself or herself on purpose. More females hurt themselves than males. Teens usually hurt themselves by cutting with sharp objects.

✔ Quick Tip

Have you been pressured to cut yourself by others who do it?

If so, think about how much you value that friendship or relationship. Do you really want a friend who wants you to hurt yourself, cause you pain and put you in danger? Try to hang out with other friends who don't pressure you in this way.

What are the signs of self-injury?

These are some signs of self-injury:

- Cuts or scars on the arms or legs
- Hiding cuts or scars by wearing long sleeved shirts or pants, even in hot weather
- Making poor excuses about how the injuries happened

Self-injury can be dangerous—cutting can lead to infections, scars, numbness, and even hospitalization and death. People who share tools to cut themselves are at risk of getting and spreading diseases like HIV and hepatitis. Teens who continue to hurt themselves are less likely to learn how to cope with negative feelings.

Are you or a friend depressed, angry, or having a hard time coping with life?

If you are thinking about hurting yourself, PLEASE ASK FOR HELP! Talk with an adult you trust, like a teacher or minister or doctor. There is nothing wrong with asking for help—everyone needs help sometimes. You have a right to be strong, safe and happy.

Do you have a friend who hurts herself or himself?

Please try to get your friend to talk to a trusted adult. Your friend may need professional counseling and treatment. Help is available—counselors can teach positive ways to cope with problems without turning to self-injury.

Chapter 28

Factitious Disorders

What are factitious disorders?

Mental illness describes abnormal cognitive or emotional patterns related to how a person thinks, feels, acts, and/or relates to others and his or her surroundings. Factitious disorders are mental disorders in which a person acts as if he or she has a physical or mental illness when, in fact, he or she has consciously created his or her symptoms. (The name factitious comes from the Latin word for "artificial.")

People with factitious disorders deliberately create or exaggerate symptoms of an illness in several ways. They may lie about or mimic symptoms, hurt themselves to bring on symptoms, or alter diagnostic tests (such as contaminating a urine sample). People with factitious disorders have an inner need to be seen as ill or injured, but not to achieve a concrete benefit, such as a financial gain. People with factitious disorders are even willing to undergo painful or risky tests and operations in order to obtain the sympathy and special attention given to people who are truly ill. Factitious disorders are considered mental illnesses because they are associated with severe emotional difficulties.

About This Chapter: "Overview of Factitious Disorders," © 2008 The Cleveland Clinic Foundation, 9500 Euclid Avenue, Cleveland, OH 44195, http://my.clevelandclinic.org. Additional information is available from the Cleveland Clinic Health Information Center, 216-444-3771, toll-free 800-223-2273 extension 43771, or at http://my.clevelandclinic.org/health.

Many people with factitious disorders also suffer from other mental disorders, particularly personality disorders. People with personality disorders have long-standing patterns of thinking and acting that differ from what society considers usual or normal. People with personality disorders generally also have poor coping skills and problems forming healthy relationships.

Factitious disorders are similar to another group of mental disorders called somatoform disorders, which also involve the presence of symptoms that are not due to actual physical illnesses. The main difference between the two groups of disorders is that people with somatoform disorders do not intentionally fake symptoms or mislead others about their symptoms. Similarly, the behavior of people with factitious disorders is not malingering, a term that refers to faking illness for financial gain (such as to collect insurance money), food or shelter, or to avoid criminal prosecution or other responsibilities.

What are the symptoms of factitious disorders?

Possible warning signs of factitious disorders include the following:

- Dramatic but inconsistent medical history
- Unclear symptoms that are not controllable, become more severe, or change once treatment has begun
- Predictable relapses following improvement in the condition
- Extensive knowledge of hospitals and/or medical terminology, as well as the textbook descriptions of illness
- Presence of many surgical scars
- Appearance of new or additional symptoms following negative test results
- Presence of symptoms only when the patient is alone or not being observed
- Willingness or eagerness to have medical tests, operations, or other procedures
- History of seeking treatment at many hospitals, clinics, and doctors' offices, possibly even in different cities
- Reluctance by the patient to allow health care professionals to meet with or talk to family members, friends, and prior health care providers

✎ What's It Mean?
Types Of Factitious Disorders

The *Diagnostic and Statistical Manual of Mental Disorders, Fourth Edition* (*DSM-IV*), which is the standard reference book for recognized mental illnesses in the United States, organizes factitious disorders into four main types:

Factitious disorder with mostly psychological symptoms: As the description implies, people with this disorder mimic behavior that is typical of a mental illness, such as schizophrenia. They may appear confused, make absurd statements, and report hallucinations (the experience of sensing things that are not there; for example, hearing voices). Ganser syndrome, sometimes called prison psychosis, is a factitious disorder that was first observed in prisoners. People with Ganser syndrome have short-term episodes of bizarre behavior that appear similar to serious mental illnesses.

Factitious disorder with mostly physical symptoms: People with this disorder claim to have symptoms related to a physical illness—symptoms such as chest pain, stomach problems, or fever. This disorder is sometimes referred to as Munchausen syndrome, named for Baron von Munchausen, an 18th century German officer who was known for embellishing the stories of his life and experiences. NOTE: Although Munchausen syndrome most properly refers to a factitious disorder with physical symptoms, the term is sometimes used to refer to factitious disorders in general.

Factitious disorder with both psychological and physical symptoms: People with this disorder report symptoms of both physical and mental illness.

Factitious disorder not otherwise specified: This type includes a disorder called factitious disorder by proxy (also called Munchausen syndrome by proxy). People with this disorder produce or fabricate symptoms of illness in another person under their care. It most often occurs in mothers (although it can occur in fathers) who intentionally harm their children in order to receive attention. (The term "by proxy" means "through a substitute.")

What causes factitious disorders?

The exact cause of factitious disorders is not known, but researchers believe both biological and psychological factors play a role in the development of these disorders. Some theories suggest that a history of abuse or neglect as a child, or a history of frequent illnesses in themselves or family that required hospitalization, may be factors in the development of the disorder.

How common are factitious disorders?

There are no reliable statistics regarding the number of people in the United States who suffer from factitious disorders. Obtaining accurate statistics is difficult because dishonesty is common with this disorder. In addition, people with factitious disorders tend to seek treatment at many different health care facilities, resulting in statistics that are misleading.

While Munchausen syndrome can occur in children, it most often affects young adults.

How are factitious disorders diagnosed?

Due to the dishonesty involved, diagnosing factitious disorders is very difficult. In addition, doctors must rule out any possible physical and mental illnesses, and often use a variety of diagnostic tests and procedures before considering a diagnosis of factitious disorder.

If the health care provider finds no physical reason for the symptoms, he or she may refer the person to a psychiatrist or psychologist—mental health professionals who are specially trained to diagnose and treat mental illnesses. Psychiatrists and psychologists use thorough history, physical, laboratory tests, imagery, and psychological testing to evaluate a person for Munchausen syndrome. The doctor bases his or her diagnosis on the exclusion of actual physical or mental illness, and his or her observation of the patient's attitude and behavior.

Questions to be answered include:

- Do the patient's reported symptoms make sense in the context of all test results and assessments?
- Do we have collateral information from other sources that confirm the patient's information? (If the patient does not allow this, this is a helpful clue.)
- Is the patient more willing to take the risk for more procedures and tests than you would expect?
- Are treatments working in a predictable way?

The doctor then determines if the patient's symptoms point to Munchausen syndrome as outlined in *DSM-IV*.

How are factitious disorders treated?

The first goal of treatment is to modify the person's behavior and reduce his or her misuse or overuse of medical resources. In the case of factitious disorder by proxy, the main goal is to ensure the safety and protection of any real or potential victims. Once the initial goal is met, treatment aims to resolve any underlying psychological issues that may be causing the person's behavior or help them find solutions to housing or other social needs.

The primary treatment for factitious disorders is psychotherapy (a type of counseling). Treatment likely will focus on changing the thinking and behavior of the individual with the disorder (cognitive-behavioral therapy). Family therapy also may be helpful in teaching family members not to reward or reinforce the behavior of the person with the disorder.

There are no medications to actually treat factitious disorders. Medication may be used, however, to treat any related disorder, such as depression or anxiety. The use of medications must be carefully monitored in people with factitious disorders due to the risk that the drugs may never be picked up from the pharmacy or may be used in a harmful way.

What are the complications of factitious disorders?

People with factitious disorders are at risk for health problems associated with hurting themselves by causing symptoms. In addition, they may suffer health problems related to multiple tests, procedures, and treatments, and are at high risk for substance abuse and suicide attempts. A complication of factitious disorder by proxy is the abuse and potential death of the victims.

What is the prognosis (outlook) for people with factitious disorders?

Some people with factitious disorders suffer one or two brief episodes of symptoms. In most cases, however, factitious disorder is a chronic, or long-term, condition that can be very difficult to treat. Additionally, many people with factitious disorders deny they are faking symptoms and will not seek or follow treatment.

Can factitious disorders be prevented?

There is no known way to prevent factitious disorders. However, it may be helpful to start treatment in people as soon as they begin to have symptoms.

Chapter 29

Personality Disorders

Everyone has characteristic patterns of perceiving and relating to other people and events (personality traits). That is, people tend to cope with stresses in an individual but consistent way. For example, some people respond to a troubling situation by seeking someone else's help; others prefer to deal with problems on their own. Some people minimize problems; others exaggerate them. Regardless of their usual style, however, mentally healthy people are likely to try an alternative approach if their first response is ineffective.

In contrast, people with a personality disorder are rigid and tend to respond inappropriately to problems, to the point that relationships with family members, friends, and coworkers are affected. These maladaptive responses usually begin in adolescence or early adulthood and do not change over time. Personality disorders vary in severity. They are usually mild and rarely severe.

Most people with a personality disorder are distressed about their life and have problems with relationships at work or in social situations. Many people also have mood, anxiety, substance abuse, or eating disorders.

People with a personality disorder are unaware that their thought or behavior patterns are inappropriate; thus, they tend not to seek help on their own. Instead, they may be referred by their friends, family members, or a social agency because their behavior is causing difficulty for others. When they seek help on their own, usually because of the life stresses created by their personality disorder, or troubling symptoms (for example, anxiety, depression, or substance abuse), they tend to believe their problems are caused by other people or by circumstances beyond their control.

Until fairly recently, many psychiatrists and psychologists felt that treatment did not help people with a personality disorder. However, specific types of psychotherapy (talk therapy), sometimes with drugs, have now been shown to help many people. Choosing an experienced, understanding therapist is essential.

✎ What's It Mean?

Personality disorders are patterns of perceiving, reacting, and relating to other people and events that are relatively inflexible and that impair a person's ability to function socially.

- Behavior may be odd or eccentric, dramatic or erratic, or anxious or inhibited.
- Doctors consider the diagnosis when inappropriate thinking or behavior is repeated despite negative consequences.
- Drugs do not change people's personality traits, but psychotherapy may help people recognize their problem and change their socially undesirable behaviors.

Personality disorders are grouped into three clusters. Cluster A personality disorders involve odd or eccentric behavior; cluster B, dramatic or erratic behavior; and cluster C, anxious or inhibited behavior.

Cluster A: Odd Or Eccentric Behavior

Paranoid Personality: People with a paranoid personality are distrustful and suspicious of others. Based on little or no evidence, they suspect that others are out to harm them and usually find hostile or malicious motives behind other people's actions. Thus, people with a paranoid personality may take actions that they feel are justifiable retaliation but that others find baffling. This behavior often leads to rejection by others, which seems to justify their original feelings. They are generally cold and distant in their relationships.

People with a paranoid personality often take legal action against others, especially if they feel righteously indignant. They are unable to see their own role in a conflict. They usually work in relative isolation and may be highly efficient and conscientious.

Sometimes people who already feel alienated because of a defect or handicap (such as deafness) are more likely to suspect that other people have negative ideas or attitudes toward them. Such heightened suspicion, however, is not evidence of a paranoid personality unless it involves wrongly attributing malice to others.

Schizoid Personality: People with a schizoid personality are introverted, withdrawn, and solitary. They are emotionally cold and socially distant. They are most often absorbed with their own thoughts and feelings and are fearful of closeness and intimacy with others. They talk little, are given to daydreaming, and prefer theoretical speculation to practical action. Fantasizing is a common coping (defense) mechanism.

Schizotypal Personality: People with a schizotypal personality, like those with a schizoid personality, are socially and emotionally detached. In addition, they display oddities of thinking, perceiving, and communicating similar to those of people with schizophrenia. Although schizotypal personality is sometimes present in people with schizophrenia before they become ill, most adults with a schizotypal personality do not develop schizophrenia.

Some people with a schizotypal personality show signs of magical thinking—that is, they believe that their thoughts or actions can control something or someone. For example, people may believe that they can harm others by thinking angry thoughts. People with a schizotypal personality may also have paranoid ideas.

✤ It's A Fact!!
Did You Know...

People with a personality disorder do not know that there is anything wrong with their thinking or behavior.

Cluster B: Dramatic Or Erratic Behavior

Histrionic (Hysterical) Personality: People with a histrionic personality conspicuously seek attention, are dramatic and excessively emotional, and are overly concerned with appearance. Their lively, expressive manner results in easily established but often superficial and transient relationships. Their expression of emotions often seems exaggerated, childish, and contrived to evoke sympathy or attention (often erotic or sexual) from others.

People with a histrionic personality are prone to sexually provocative behavior or to sexualizing nonsexual relationships. However, they may not really want a sexual relationship; rather, their seductive behavior often masks their wish to be dependent and protected. Some people with a histrionic personality also are hypochondriacal and exaggerate their physical problems to get the attention they need.

Narcissistic Personality: People with a narcissistic personality have a sense of superiority, a need for admiration, and a lack of empathy. They have an exaggerated belief in their own value or importance, which is what therapists call grandiosity. They may be extremely sensitive to failure, defeat, or criticism. When confronted by a failure to fulfill their high opinion of themselves, they can easily become enraged or severely depressed. Because they believe themselves to be superior in their relationships with other people, they expect to be admired and often suspect that others envy them. They believe they are entitled to having their needs met without waiting, so they exploit others, whose needs or beliefs they deem to be less important. Their behavior is usually offensive to others, who view them as being self-centered, arrogant, or selfish. This personality disorder typically occurs in high achievers, although it may also occur in people with few achievements.

Antisocial Personality: People with an antisocial personality (previously called psychopathic or sociopathic personality), most of whom are male, show callous disregard for the rights and feelings of others. Dishonesty and deceit permeate their relationships. They exploit others for material gain or personal gratification (unlike narcissistic people, who exploit others because they think their superiority justifies it).

Characteristically, people with an antisocial personality act out their conflicts impulsively and irresponsibly. They tolerate frustration poorly, and sometimes they are hostile or violent. Often they do not anticipate the negative consequences of their antisocial behaviors and, despite the problems or harm they cause others, do not feel remorse or guilt. Rather, they glibly rationalize their behavior or blame it on others. Frustration and punishment do not motivate them to modify their behaviors or improve their judgment and foresight but, rather, usually confirm their harshly unsentimental view of the world.

People with an antisocial personality are prone to alcoholism, drug addiction, sexual deviation, promiscuity, and imprisonment. They are likely to fail at their jobs and move from one area to another. They often have a family history of antisocial behavior, substance abuse, divorce, and physical abuse. As children, many were emotionally neglected and physically abused. People with an antisocial personality have a shorter life expectancy than the general population. The disorder tends to diminish or stabilize with age.

Borderline Personality: People with a borderline personality, most of whom are women, are unstable in their self-image, moods, behavior, and interpersonal relationships. Their thought processes are more disturbed than those of people with an antisocial personality, and their aggression is more often turned against the self. They are angrier, more impulsive, and more confused about their identity than are people with a histrionic personality. Borderline personality becomes evident in early adulthood but becomes less common in older age groups.

People with a borderline personality often report being neglected or abused as children. Consequently, they feel empty, angry, and deserving of nurturing. They have far more dramatic and intense interpersonal relationships than people with cluster A personality disorders. When they fear being abandoned by a caring person, they tend to express inappropriate and intense anger. People with a borderline personality tend to see events and relationships as black or white, good or evil, but never neutral.

When people with a borderline personality feel abandoned and alone, they may wonder whether they actually exist (that is, they do not feel real). They can become desperately impulsive, engaging in reckless promiscuity, substance abuse, or self-mutilation. At times they are so out of touch with reality that they have brief episodes of psychotic thinking, paranoia, and hallucinations.

People with a borderline personality commonly visit primary care doctors. Borderline personality is also the most common personality disorder treated by therapists, because people with the disorder relentlessly seek someone to care for them. However, after repeated crises, vague unfounded complaints, and failures to comply with therapeutic recommendations, caretakers—including doctors—often become very frustrated with them and view them erroneously as people who prefer complaining to helping themselves.

Cluster C: Anxious or Inhibited Behavior

Avoidant Personality: People with an avoidant personality are overly sensitive to rejection, and they fear starting relationships or anything new. They have a strong desire for affection and acceptance but avoid intimate relationships and social situations for fear of disappointment and criticism. Unlike those with a schizoid personality, they are openly distressed by their isolation and inability to relate comfortably to others. Unlike those with a borderline personality, they do not respond to rejection with anger; instead, they withdraw and appear shy and timid. Avoidant personality is similar to generalized social phobia.

Dependent Personality: People with a dependent personality routinely surrender major decisions and responsibilities to others and permit the needs of those they depend on to supersede their own. They lack self-confidence and feel intensely insecure about their ability to take care of themselves. They often protest that they cannot make decisions and do not know what to do or how to do it. This behavior is due partly to a reluctance to express their views for fear of offending the people they need and partly to a belief that others are more capable. People with other personality disorders often have traits of a dependent personality, but the dependent traits are usually hidden by the more dominant traits of the other disorder. Sometimes adults with a prolonged illness or physical handicap develop a dependent personality.

Obsessive-Compulsive Personality: People with an obsessive-compulsive personality are preoccupied with orderliness, perfectionism, and control. They are reliable, dependable, orderly, and methodical, but their inflexibility makes them unable to adapt to change. Because they are cautious and weigh all aspects of a problem, they have difficulty making decisions. They take their responsibilities seriously, but because they cannot tolerate mistakes or imperfection, they often have trouble completing tasks. Unlike the mental health disorder called obsessive-compulsive disorder, obsessive-compulsive personality does not involve repeated, unwanted obsessions and ritualistic behavior.

People with an obsessive-compulsive personality are often high achievers, especially in the sciences and other intellectually demanding fields that require order and attention to detail. However, their responsibilities make them so anxious that they can rarely enjoy their successes. They are uncomfortable with their feelings, with relationships, and with situations in which they lack control or must rely on others or in which events are unpredictable.

Other Personality Types

Some personality types are not classified as disorders.

Passive-Aggressive (Negativistic) Personality: People with a passive-aggressive personality behave in ways that appear inept or passive. However, these behaviors are actually ways to avoid responsibility or to control or punish others. People with a passive-aggressive personality often procrastinate, perform tasks inefficiently, or claim an implausible disability. Frequently, they agree to perform tasks they do not want to perform and then subtly undermine completion of the tasks. Such behavior usually enables them to deny or conceal hostility or disagreements.

Cyclothymic Personality: People with cyclothymic personality alternate between high-spirited buoyancy and gloomy pessimism. Each mood lasts weeks or longer. Mood changes occur regularly and without any identifiable external cause. Many gifted and creative people have this personality type.

Depressive Personality: This personality type is characterized by chronic moroseness, worry, and self-consciousness. People have a pessimistic outlook, which impairs their initiative and disheartens others. To them, satisfaction seems undeserved and sinful. They may unconsciously believe their suffering is a badge of merit needed to earn the love or admiration of others.

Diagnosis

A doctor bases the diagnosis of a personality disorder on a person's history, specifically, on repetition of maladaptive thought or behavior patterns. These patterns tend to become apparent because the person tenaciously resists changing them despite their negative consequences. In addition, a doctor is likely to notice the person's immature and maladaptive use of mental coping mechanisms, which interferes with their daily functioning. A doctor may also talk with people who interact with the person.

Treatment

Relief of anxiety, depression, and other distressing symptoms (if present) is the first goal. Drug therapy can help. Drugs such as selective serotonin reuptake inhibitors (SSRIs) can help both depression and impulsivity. Anticonvulsant drugs can help reduce impulsive, angry outbursts. Other drugs such as risperidone have been helpful with both depression and feelings of depersonalization in people with borderline personality. Reducing environmental stress can also quickly relieve symptoms.

✤ It's A Fact!!

Consequences Of Personality Disorders

- People with a personality disorder are at high risk of behaviors that can lead to physical illness (such as alcohol or drug addiction); self-destructive behavior, reckless sexual behavior, hypochondriasis, and clashes with society's values.
- They may have inconsistent, detached, overemotional, abusive, or irresponsible styles of parenting, leading to medical and psychiatric problems in their children.
- They are vulnerable to mental breakdowns (a period of crisis when a person has difficulty performing even routine mental tasks) as a result of stress.
- They may develop a mental health disorder; the type (for example, anxiety, depression, or psychosis) depends in part on the type of personality disorder.
- They are less likely to follow a prescribed treatment regimen; even when they follow the regimen, they are usually less responsive to drugs than most people are.
- They often have a poor relationship with their doctor because they refuse to take responsibility for their behavior or they feel overly distrustful, deserving, or needy. The doctor may then start to blame, distrust, and ultimately reject the person.

Table 29.1. Common Coping Mechanisms

Projection: Attributing one's own feelings or thoughts to others

Result: Leads to prejudice, suspiciousness, and excessive worrying about external dangers

Personality Disorders Involved: Typical of paranoid and schizotypal personalities; used by people with borderline, antisocial, or narcissistic personality when under acute stress

Splitting: Use of black-or-white, all-or-nothing thinking to divide people into groups of idealized all-good saviors and vilified all-bad evildoers

Result: Allows a person to avoid the discomfort of having both loving and hateful feelings for the same person as well as feelings of uncertainty and helplessness

Personality Disorders Involved: Typical of borderline personality

Acting out: A direct behavioral expression of an unconscious wish or impulse that enables a person to avoid thinking about a painful situation or experiencing a painful emotion

Result: Leads to acts that are often irresponsible, reckless, and foolish. Includes many delinquent, promiscuous, and substance-abusing acts, which can become so habitual that the person remains unaware and dismissive of the feelings that initiated the acts

Personality Disorders Involved: Very common in people with antisocial or borderline personality

Turning aggression against self: Expressing the angry feelings one has toward others by hurting one's self directly (for example, through self-mutilation) or indirectly (for example, in body dysmorphic disorder); when indirect, it is called passive aggression

Result: Includes failures and illnesses that affect others more than oneself and silly, provocative clowning

Personality Disorders Involved: Dramatic in people with borderline personality

Fantasizing: Use of imaginary relationships and private belief systems to resolve conflict and to escape from painful realities, such as loneliness

Result: Is associated with eccentricity, avoidance of interpersonal intimacy, and avoidance of involvement with the outside world

Personality Disorders Involved: Used by people with an avoidant or schizoid personality, who, in contrast to people with psychoses, do not believe and thus do not act on their fantasies

Hypochondriasis: Use of health complaints to gain attention

Result: Provides a person with nurturing attention from others; may be a passive expression of anger toward others

Personality Disorders Involved: Used by people with dependent, histrionic, or borderline personality

However, drug therapy does not generally affect the personality traits themselves. Because these traits take many years to develop, treatment of the maladaptive traits may take many years as well. No short-term treatment can cure a personality disorder, although some changes may be accomplished faster than others. Behavioral changes can occur within a year; interpersonal changes take longer. For example, for people with a dependent personality, a behavioral change might be to stop stating that they cannot make decisions; the interpersonal change might be to interact with co-workers or family members in such a way that they actually seek out or at least accept some decision-making responsibilities.

Although treatments differ according to the type of personality disorder, some general principles apply to all treatments. Because people with a personality disorder usually do not see a problem with their own behavior, they must be confronted with the harmful consequences of their maladaptive thoughts and behaviors. Thus, a therapist needs to repeatedly point out the undesirable consequences of their thought and behavior patterns. Sometimes the therapist finds it necessary to set limits on behavior (for example, people might be told that they cannot raise their voice in anger). The involvement of family members is helpful and often essential because they can act in ways that either reinforce or diminish the problematic behavior or thoughts. Group and family therapy, group living in designated residential settings, and participation in therapeutic social clubs or self-help groups can all be valuable in helping to change socially undesirable behaviors.

Because personality disorders are particularly difficult to treat, choosing a therapist with experience, enthusiasm, and an understanding of the person's areas of emotional sensitivity and usual ways of coping is important. Kindness and direction alone do not change personality disorders. Psychotherapy is the cornerstone of most treatments and usually must continue for more than a year to change a person's maladaptive behavior or interpersonal patterns.

In the context of an intimate, cooperative doctor-patient relationship, people can begin to understand the sources of their distress and recognize their maladaptive behavior. Psychotherapy can help them more clearly recognize the attitudes and behaviors that lead to interpersonal problems, such as dependency, distrust, arrogance, and manipulativeness.

For maladaptive behaviors, such as recklessness, social isolation, lack of assertiveness, or temper outbursts, group therapy and behavior modification, sometimes within a day hospital or residential setting, are effective. These behaviors can be changed in months. Participation in self-help groups or family therapy can also help change maladaptive behaviors. Dialectical behavioral therapy is effective for borderline personality disorder. This therapy involves weekly individual psychotherapy and group therapy as well as telephone contact with therapists between scheduled sessions. It aims to help people understand their behaviors and teach them problem solving and adaptive behaviors. Psychodynamic therapy is also effective for people with borderline or avoidant personality disorder. These therapies help people with a personality disorder think about the effects their behaviors have on others. For some people with personality disorders, primarily those that involve maladaptive attitudes, expectations, and beliefs (such as narcissistic or obsessive-compulsive personality), psychoanalysis is recommended and is usually continued for at least three years.

Chapter 30

Borderline Personality Disorder

What Is Borderline Personality Disorder

Borderline personality disorder (BPD) is a most misunderstood, serious mental illness characterized by pervasive instability in moods, interpersonal relationships, self-image, and behavior. It is a disorder of emotion dysregulation. This instability often disrupts family and work, long-term planning, and the individual's sense of self-identity. While less well known than schizophrenia or bipolar disorder (manic-depressive illness), BPD is as common, affecting between .07 to 2% of the general population.

The disorder, characterized by intense emotions, self-destructive acts, and stormy interpersonal relationships, was officially recognized in 1980 and given the name borderline personality disorder. It was thought to occur on the border between psychotic and neurotic behavior. This is no longer considered a relevant analysis and the term itself, with its stigmatizing negative associations, has made diagnosing BPD problematic. The complex symptoms of the disorder often make patients difficult to treat and therefore may evoke feelings of anger and frustration in professionals trying to help, with the result that many professionals are often unwilling to make the diagnosis or treat persons with these symptoms. These problems have been aggravated by the lack of

About This Chapter: Text in this chapter is from "Borderline Personality Disorder," © 2006 NAMI: The Nation's Voice on Mental Illness (www.nami.org). Reprinted with permission.

appropriate insurance coverage for the extended psychosocial treatments that BPD usually requires. Nevertheless, there has been much progress and success in the past 25 years in the understanding of and specialized treatment for BPD. It is, in fact, a diagnosis that has a lot of hope for recovery.

What Are The Symptoms Of Borderline Personality Disorder?

Borderline Personality Disorder Diagnosis: *DMS-IV-TR** Diagnostic Criteria

A pervasive pattern of instability of interpersonal relationships, self-image, and affects, and marked impulsivity beginning by early adulthood ** and present in a variety of contexts, as indicated by five (or more) of the following:

1. Frantic efforts to avoid real or imagined abandonment. (Note: Do not include suicidal or self-mutilating behavior*** covered in Criterion 5.)

✤ It's A Fact!!

Different patterns of brain activity in people with borderline personality disorder were associated with disruptions in the ability to recognize social norms or modify behaviors that likely result in distrust and broken relationships, according to a study funded by the National Institute of Mental Health which was published online in the August 8, 2008 issue of *Science*.

Using brain imaging and game theory, a mathematical approach to studying social interactions, the researchers offer a potential new way to define and describe this mental illness. They conclude that people with borderline personality disorder either have a distorted sense of generally accepted social norms, or that they may not sense these norms at all. This may lead them to behave in a way that disrupts trust and cooperation with others. By not responding in a way that would repair the relationship, people with borderline personality disorder also impair the ability of others to cooperate with them.

Source: Excerpted from "Borderline Personality Disorder: Brain Differences Related to Disruptions in Cooperation in Relationships," a Science Update from the National Institute of Mental Health, August 12, 2008.

2. A pattern of unstable and intense interpersonal relationships characterized by alternating between extremes of idealization and devaluation.

3. Identity disturbance: markedly and persistently unstable self-image or sense of self.

4. Impulsivity in at least two areas that are potentially self-damaging (for example, spending, sex, substance abuse, reckless driving, binge eating). (Note: Do not include suicidal or self-mutilating behavior*** covered in Criterion 5.)

5. Recurrent suicidal behavior, gestures, or threats, or self-mutilating behavior.***

6. Affective instability due to a marked reactivity of mood (for example, intense episodic dysphoria, irritability, or anxiety usually lasting a few hours and only rarely more than a few days).

7. Chronic feelings of emptiness.

8. Inappropriate, intense anger or difficulty controlling anger (for example, frequent displays of temper, constant anger, recurrent physical fights).

9. Transient, stress-related paranoid ideation or severe dissociative symptoms.

**Diagnostic and Statistical Manual of Mental Disorders*, published by the American Psychiatric Association

** Data collected informally from many families indicate this pattern of symptoms may appear as early as the pre-teens.

***The preferred term is self-harm or self-injury.

Important Considerations About Borderline Personality Disorder

1. The five of nine criteria needed to diagnose the disorder may be present in a large number of different combinations. This results in the fact that the disorder often presents quite differently from one person to another, thus making accurate diagnosis somewhat confusing to a clinician not skilled in the area.

2. BPD rarely stands alone. There is high co-occurrence with other disorders.

3. BPD affects between .07 to 2% of the population. The highest estimation, 2%, approximates the number of persons diagnosed with schizophrenia and bipolar disorder.

4. Estimates are 10% of outpatients and 20% of inpatients who present for treatment have BPD

5. 75% are women. This number may, in part, reflect that women more often seek treatment, that anger is seen as more acceptable in men, and that men with similar symptoms often enter the penal system receiving a diagnosis of antisocial personality disorder.

6. 75% of patients self-injure.

7. Approximately 10% of individuals with BPD complete suicide attempts.

8. A chronic disorder that is resistant to change, we now know that BPD has a good prognosis when treated properly. Such treatment usually consists of medications, psychotherapy, and educational and support groups.

✤ It's A Fact!! Co-Occurring Disorders

Borderline personality disorder rarely stands alone. BPD occurs with, and complicates, other disorders. Co-morbidity with other disorders:

- Major depressive disorder: 60%
- Dysthymia (chronic, moderate to mild depression): 70%
- Eating disorders; 25%
- Substance abuse: 35%
- Bipolar disorder: 15%
- Antisocial personality disorder: 25%
- Narcissistic personality disorder: 25%

Source: © 2006 NAMI: The Nation's Voice on Mental Illness (www.nami.org).

9. In many patients with BPD, medications have been shown to be very helpful in reducing the severity of symptoms and enabling effective psychotherapy to occur. Medications are also often essential in the proper treatment of disorders that commonly co-occur with BPD.

10. There are a growing number of psychotherapeutic approaches specifically developed for people with BPD. Some of these have been in use, tested in research trials, and appear to be very effective; the newer ones are very promising.

11. These and other treatments have been shown to be effective in the treatment of BPD, and many patients do get better.

Theories Of Origins And Pathology Of Borderline Personality Disorder

At this point in time, clinical theorists believe that biogenetic and environmental components are both necessary for the disorder to develop. These factors are varied and complex. Many different environments may further contribute to the development of the disorder. Families providing reasonably nurturing and caring environments may nevertheless see their relative develop the illness. In other situations, childhood abuse has exacerbated the condition. The best explanation appears to be that there is a confluence of environmental factors and a neurobiological propensity that leads to a sensitive, emotionally labile child.

Treatment

In the past few decades, treatment for borderline personality disorder has changed radically, and, in turn, the prognosis for improvement and/or recovery has significantly improved. Unfortunately, specialized treatment for BPD is not yet widely available.

An abstract by Michael H. Stone published in *World Psychiatry*, February 2006, explained a hierarchy in therapy management for the patient with the BPD diagnosis. "Therapists must pay attention first to suicidal and self-mutilative behaviors. Next, one deals with any threats to interrupt therapy prematurely. Third in order of seriousness: non-suicidal symptoms such as (mild to moderate) depression, substance abuse, panic and other anxiety manifestations, or dissociation. Psychopharmacological treatment will often be used adjunctively to help control any target symptoms, which usually fall into such categories as cognitive-perceptual, affect dysregulation, or impulsive/behavioral dyscontrol. Therapists must then be alert to any signs of withholding, dishonesty, or antisocial tendencies, since these have an adverse effect on prognosis. When all these disruptive influences are (to the extent possible) dealt with, therapists will next take up milder symptoms such as social anxiety or lability of mood" as well as the enduring personality issues such as extreme attitudes and inappropriate anger.

One of the preliminary questions confronting families/friends is how and when to place confidence in those responsible for treating the patient. Generally speaking, the more clinical experience the treatment provider has had working with borderline patients, the better. Most often, a good "fit" with the primary therapist is the "key" to successful therapy intervention.

A discussion of hospitalization and treatment techniques, including specialized treatment for BPD, follows:

A. Hospitalization: Hospitalization in the care of those with BPD is usually restricted to the management of crises (including, but not limited to, situations where the individual's safety is at risk). It is not uncommon for medication changes to take place in the context of a hospital stay, where professionals can monitor the impact of new medications in a controlled environment. Hospitalizations are usually short in duration.

B. Medication: Medications play an important role in the comprehensive treatment of BPD. For more on this topic, refer to the section "Medications Used and Studied in the Treatment of BPD."

C. Psychotherapy: Psychotherapy is the cornerstone of most treatments for borderline personality disorder. Although development of a secure attachment to

✤ It's A Fact!! Grey Matter Changes Linked To Runaway Fear Hub

Differences in the working tissue of the brain, called grey matter, have been linked to impaired functioning of an emotion-regulating circuit in patients with borderline personality disorder (BPD). People with BPD had excess grey matter in a fear hub deep in the brain, which over-activated when they viewed scary faces. By contrast, the hub's regulator near the front of the brain was deficient in grey matter and underactive, effectively taking the brakes off a runaway fear response, suggest researchers supported in part by the National Institute of Mental Health.

The imaging studies are the first to link structural brain differences with functional impairment in the same sample of BPD patients. Similar changes in the same circuit have been implicated in mood and anxiety disorders, hinting that BPD might share common mechanisms with mental illnesses that have traditionally been viewed through the lens of biology.

Source: Excerpted from "Emotion-Regulating Circuit Weakened in Borderline Personality Disorder," a Science Update from the National Institute of Mental Health, October 2, 2008.

the therapist is generally essential for the psychotherapy to have useful effects, this does not occur easily with the BPD diagnosed individual, given the intense needs and fears about relationships. The standard recommendation for individual psychotherapy involves one to two visits a week with an experienced clinician. The symptoms of the disorder can be as difficult for professionals to experience as those experienced by family members. Some therapists are apprehensive about working with individuals with this diagnosis.

There are currently three major psychotherapeutic approaches to treatment of BPD:

1. Psychodynamic
2. Cognitive-behavioral
3. Supportive

D. Group Modalities: DBT [dialectical behavior therapy] and CBT [cognitive behavior therapy] interventions are often like classes with much focus and direction offered by the group leader(s) and with homework/practice exercises assigned between sessions based on the material presented during the session. DBT, for example has a manual that is followed each week where both the lectures and the practice exercises are put together for easy access. Some patients with BPD may be resistant to interpersonal or psychodynamic groups which require the expression of strong feelings or the need for personal disclosures. However, such forums may be useful for these very reasons. Moreover, such groups offer an opportunity for borderline patients to learn from persons with similar life experiences, which, in conjunction with the other modalities discussed here, can significantly enhance the treatment course. Many individuals with BPD find it more acceptable to join self-help groups, such as AA. Self-help groups that provide a network of supportive peers can be useful as an adjunct to treatment, but should not be relied on as the sole source of support.

E. Family Therapy: Parents, spouses, and children bear a significant burden. Often, family members are grateful to be educated about the borderline diagnosis, the likely prognosis, reasonable expectations from treatment, and how they can contribute. These interventions often improve communication, decrease alienation, and relieve family burdens. Some mental disorders, as in the treatment of schizophrenia, require close family involvement in the treatment process to be optimally effective. There are now preliminary research data that suggest that family involvement is also very important in the effective treatment of borderline disorder.

Several organizations offer education programs and/or support to families challenged with mental health issues. The National Alliance on Mental Illness (NAMI), The National Education Alliance for Borderline Personality Disorder (NEA-BPD), The Depression and Bipolar Support Association (DBSA) and the Mental Health Association (MHA) offer programs across the nation.

Family training and support programs such as NAMI's Family to Family and NEA-BPD's Family Connections (http://www.neabpd.org/) are in great demand. Nonetheless, too often many psychiatrists and other mental health clinicians continue to deny meaningful input from family members of a client with BPD. This situation is especially frustrating for family members, who often provide the sole financial support for everyday living and treatment expenses, and much of the moral support, but who receive little or no response from the treating professionals. Families are especially distressed when the treatment plan is not effective, and their loved one isolates them from their therapists. Given the importance of the family in establishing functional relationships in the lives of people with borderline disorder, families should actively seek "family friendly" treatments and/or treatment providers and investigate family classes and support groups in their communities.

Suicidality And Self-Harm Behavior

The most dangerous and fear-inducing features of BPD are the self-harm behaviors and potential for suicide. An estimated 10% kill themselves. Deliberate self-harm (cutting, burning, hitting, head banging, hair pulling) are common features of BPD, occurring in approximately 75% of cases. Individuals who self-harm report that causing themselves physical pain generates a sense of release and relief which temporarily alleviates excruciating emotional feelings. Self-injurious acts can bring relief by stimulating production of endorphins, which are naturally occurring opiates produced by the brain in response to pain. Some individuals with BPD also exhibit self-destructive acts such as promiscuity, bingeing, purging, and blackouts from substance abuse.

It is important for the client, family, and clinician to be able to draw a distinction between the intent behind suicide attempts and self-injurious behaviors (SIB). Patients and researchers frequently describe self-injurious behavior as a means of reducing intense feelings of emotional pain. The release of the endogenous opiates provides a reward to the behavior. Some data suggest that self-injurious behavior in BPD patients doubles the risk of suicide attempts. This dichotomy of intent between these two behaviors requires careful evaluation and relevant therapy to meet the needs of the patient.

In addition to substance abuse, major depression can contribute to the risk of suicide. Approximately 50% of people with BPD are experiencing an episode of major depression when they seek treatment. About 70% have a major depressive episode in their lifetimes. It is imperative that treatment providers evaluate the client's mood carefully, and treat the depression appropriately, which may include the use of medication.

Medications Studied And Used In The Treatment Of Borderline Personality Disorder

There are two reasons why medications are used in the treatment of BPD. First, they have proven to be very helpful in stabilizing the emotional reactions, reducing impulsivity, and enhancing thinking and reasoning abilities in people with the disorder. Second, medications are also effective in treating the other emotional disorders that are frequently associated with borderline disorder like depression and anxiety.

The group of medications that have been studied most for the treatment of borderline disorder are neuroleptics and atypical antipsychotic agents. At their usual doses, these medications are very effective in improving the disordered thinking, emotional responses, and behavior of people with other mental disorders, such as bipolar disorder and schizophrenia. However, at smaller doses they are helpful in decreasing the over-reactive emotional responses and impulsivity, and in improving the abilities to think and reason for people with BPD. Low doses of these medications often reduce depressed moods, anger, and anxiety, and decrease the severity and frequency of impulsive actions. In addition, clients with borderline disorder report a considerable improvement in their ability to think rationally. There's also a reduction, or elimination of, paranoid thinking, if this is a problem.

Side Effects Of Medications Used To Treat Borderline Personality Disorder

All medications have side effects. Different medications produce different side effects, and people differ in the amount and severity of side effects they experience. Side effects can often be treated by changing the dose of the medication or switching to a different medication. Antidepressants may cause dry mouth, constipation, bladder problems, sexual problems, blurred vision, dizziness, drowsiness, skin rash, or weight gain or loss. One class of antidepressants, the monoamine oxidase inhibitors (MAOIs) have strict food restrictions with the consequence of life threatening elevation of blood pressure. The selective serotonin reuptake inhibitors (SSRIs) and newer antidepressants tend to have fewer and different side effects such as nausea, nervousness, insomnia, diarrhea, rash, agitation, sexual problems, or weight gain or loss. Mood stabilizers could cause side effects of nausea, drowsiness, dizziness, and possibly tremors. Some require periodic blood tests to monitor liver function and blood cell count.

The group of medications that have been studied most for the treatment of borderline disorder are neuroleptics and atypical antipsychotic agents. The neuroleptics were the first generation of medications used to treat psychotic disorders. The atypical antipsychotics are the second generation of medications developed to treat psychotic disorders. A specific side-effect the neuroleptics may produce is called tardive dyskinesia. This is an abnormal, involuntary movement disorder that typically occurs in those receiving average to large doses of neuroleptics. The risk appears to be less with low doses of neuroleptics or the atypical antipsychotic agents. Atypical antipsychotics and/or traditional narcoleptics could have the ability to produce weight gain, drowsiness, insomnia, breast engorgement and discomfort, lactation, and restlessness. Some of the side-effects are temporary and others are persistent. Before starting on a traditional neuroleptic or atypical antipsychotic, review the side-effect profile with the treating psychiatrist.

Chapter 31

Psychosis

What Is Psychosis?

Psychosis is a severe mental condition in which there is a loss of contact with reality. There are many possible causes:

- Alcohol and certain drugs
- Brain tumors
- Dementia (including Alzheimer disease)
- Epilepsy
- Manic depression (bipolar disorder)
- Psychotic depression
- Schizophrenia
- Stroke

Symptoms

- Abnormal displays of emotion
- Confusion
- Depression and sometimes suicidal thoughts
- Disorganized thought and speech
- Extreme excitement (mania)
- False beliefs (delusions)

- Loss of touch with reality
- Mistaken perceptions (illusions)
- Seeing, hearing, feeling, or perceiving things that are not there (hallucinations)
- Unfounded fear/suspicion

What's It Mean?

Psychosis is a loss of contact with reality, usually including false ideas about what is taking place or who one is (delusions) and seeing or hearing things that aren't there (hallucinations).

Source: © 2009 A.D.A.M., Inc.

Exams And Tests

Psychological evaluation and testing are used to diagnose the cause of the psychosis. Laboratory and x-ray testing may not be needed, but sometimes can help pinpoint the exact diagnosis. Tests may include drug screens, MRI of the brain, and tests for syphilis.

Treatment

Treatment depends on the cause of the psychosis. Care in a hospital is often needed to ensure the patient's safety. Antipsychotic drugs, which reduce "hearing voices" (auditory hallucinations) and delusions, and control thinking and behavior are helpful. Group or individual therapy can also be useful.

Outlook (Prognosis): How well a person will do depends on the specific disorder. Long-term treatment can control many of the symptoms.

Possible Complications: Psychosis can prevent people from functioning normally and caring for themselves. If the condition is left untreated, people can harm themselves or others.

It's A Fact!!

Prevention

Prevention depends on the cause. For example, avoiding alcohol abuse prevents alcohol-induced psychosis.

Source: © 2009 A.D.A.M., Inc.

When To Contact A Medical Professional: Call your health care provider or mental health professional if a member of your family acts as though they have lost contact with reality. If there is any concern about safety, immediately take the person to the nearest emergency room to be checked.

Brief Reactive Psychosis

From "Brief Reactive Psychosis," © 2009 A.D.A.M., Inc. Reprinted with permission.

Brief reactive psychosis is a sudden, short-term display of psychotic behavior, such as hallucinations, that occur with a stressful event.

Brief reactive psychosis is triggered by some type of extreme stress (such as a traumatic accident or loss of a loved one), after which the person returns to the previous level of function. The person may or may not be aware of the strange behavior.

This condition most often affects people in their 20s and 30s. People who have personality disorders are at greater risk for having a brief reactive psychosis.

Symptoms

A brief reactive psychosis is defined by having one of the following:

- Disorganized behavior
- False ideas about what is taking place (delusions)
- Hallucinations
- Impaired speech or language (speech disturbances)

The symptoms are not due to alcohol or other drug abuse and last longer than a day, but less than a month.

A psychological evaluation can confirm the symptoms. A physical exam can rule out possible illness as the cause of the symptoms.

Treatment

Antipsychotic drugs can help decrease or stop the psychotic symptoms and bizarre behavior. However, symptoms should decrease on their own as long as you stay in a safe environment.

Psychotherapy may also help you cope with the emotional stress that triggered the problem.

Outlook (Prognosis): Most people with this disorder have a good outcome. Repeat episodes may occur in response to stress.

Possible Complications: As with all psychotic illnesses, this condition can severely disrupt your life and possibly lead to violence and suicide.

When To Contact A Medical Professional: Call for an appointment with a mental health professional if you have symptoms of this disorder. If you are concerned for your safety or for the safety of someone else, call the local emergency number (such as 911) or go immediately to the nearest emergency room.

> ✎ **What's It Mean?**
>
> Psychotic Disorders (also called: psychoses): Psychotic disorders are severe mental disorders that cause abnormal thinking and perceptions. People with psychoses lose touch with reality. Two of the main symptoms are delusions and hallucinations. Delusions are false beliefs, such as thinking that someone is plotting against you or that the TV is sending you secret messages. Hallucinations are false perceptions, such as hearing, seeing, or feeling something that is not there. Schizophrenia is one type of psychotic disorder.
>
> Treatment for psychotic disorders varies by disorder. It might involve drugs to control symptoms, and talk therapy. Hospitalization is an option for serious cases where a person might be dangerous to himself or others.
>
> Source: From "Psychotic Disorders," MedlinePlus, National Library of Medicine, January 14, 2009.

Shared Psychotic Disorder

"Shared Psychotic Disorder," © 2009 The Cleveland Clinic Foundation, 9500 Euclid Avenue, Cleveland, OH 44195, http://my.clevelandclinic.org. Additional information is available from the Cleveland Clinic Health Information Center, 216-444-3771, toll-free 800-223-2273 extension 43771, or at http://my.clevelandclinic.org/health.

What is a psychotic disorder?

A psychotic disorder is a mental illness that causes abnormal thinking and perceptions. Psychotic illnesses alter a person's ability to think clearly, make good judgments, respond emotionally, communicate effectively, understand reality, and behave appropriately. People with psychotic disorders have difficulty staying in touch with reality and often are unable to meet the ordinary demands of daily life.

The most obvious symptoms of a psychotic disorder are hallucinations and delusions. Hallucinations are sensory perceptions of things that aren't actually present, such as hearing voices, seeing things that aren't there, or feeling sensations on the skin even though nothing is touching the body. Delusions are false beliefs that the person refuses to give up, even in the face of contradictory facts. Schizophrenia is an example of a psychotic disorder.

What is shared psychotic disorder?

Shared psychotic disorder is also known as folie a deux ("the folly of two"). It is a rare condition in which an otherwise healthy person (secondary case) shares the delusions of a person with a psychotic disorder (primary case), such as schizophrenia, who has well-established delusions. For example: A person with a psychotic disorder believes aliens are spying on him or her. The person with shared psychotic disorder will also begin to believe in spying aliens. The delusions are induced in the secondary case and usually disappear when the people are separated. Aside from the delusions, the thoughts and behavior of the secondary case usually are fairly normal.

This disorder usually occurs only in long-term relationships in which one person is dominant and the other is passive. In most cases, the person in whom the delusions are induced is dependent on or submissive to the person with the psychotic disorder. The people involved often are reclusive or otherwise isolated from society and have close emotional links with each other. The disorder also can occur in groups of individuals who are closely involved with a person who has a psychotic disorder.

What are the symptoms of shared psychotic disorder?

The person with shared psychotic disorder has delusions that are similar to those of someone close who has a psychotic disorder.

What causes shared psychotic disorder?

The cause of shared psychotic disorder is not known; however, stress and social isolation are believed to play roles in its development.

How common is shared psychotic disorder?

The true frequency of occurrence is unknown, but shared psychotic disorder is rarely seen in clinical settings, such as hospitals, outpatient clinics, or doctors' offices. In many cases, only one of the affected individuals seeks treatment, making a diagnosis of shared psychotic disorder difficult. As a result, many cases might go undetected.

How is shared psychotic disorder diagnosed?

If symptoms are present, the doctor will perform a complete medical history and physical examination. Although there are no laboratory tests to specifically diagnose shared psychotic disorder, the doctor might use various diagnostic tests—such as x-rays or blood tests—to rule out physical illness or a drug reaction as the cause of the delusions.

If the doctor finds no physical reason for the symptoms, he or she might refer the person to a psychiatrist or psychologist, health care professionals who are specially trained to diagnose and treat mental illnesses. Psychiatrists and psychologists use specially designed interview and assessment tools to evaluate a person for a psychotic disorder.

The doctor or therapist bases his or her diagnosis on the person's report of symptoms and his or her observation of the person's attitude and behavior. The doctor or therapist then determines if the person's symptoms point to a specific disorder as outlined in the *Diagnostic and Statistical Manual of Mental Disorders* (*DSM-IV*), which is published by the American Psychiatric Association and is the standard reference book for recognized mental illnesses. According to the *DSM-IV*, shared psychotic disorder occurs when a person develops a delusion as the result of a close association with another person who has an already-established delusion.

How is shared psychotic disorder treated?

The goal of treatment is to relieve the secondary case of the induced delusion and stabilize the primary person's psychotic disorder. In most cases, treatment involves separating the secondary case from the primary case. Other approaches might be necessary if separation is not possible.

Treatment options for the person with shared psychotic disorder might include the following:

- **Psychotherapy:** Psychotherapy (a type of counseling) can help the person with shared psychotic disorder recognize the delusion and correct the underlying thinking that has become distorted. It also can address relationship issues and any emotional effects of a short-term separation from the person with a psychotic disorder.
- **Family Therapy:** Family therapy might focus on increasing exposure to outside activities and interests, as well as the development of social supports, to decrease isolation and help prevent relapse. Family therapy also might help to improve communication and family dynamics.
- **Medication:** Short-term treatment with anti-psychotic medication might be used if the delusions do not resolve after separation from the primary case. In addition, tranquilizers or sedative agents such as lorazepam (Ativan) or diazepam (Valium) can help alleviate intense symptoms that might be associated with the disorder. These symptoms include anxiety (nervousness), agitation (extreme restlessness), or insomnia (inability to sleep).

What are the complications of shared psychotic disorder?

Left untreated, shared psychotic disorder can become chronic (ongoing).

What is the outlook for people with shared psychotic disorder?

With treatment, a person with shared psychotic disorder has a good chance for recovery.

Can shared psychotic disorder be prevented?

Because the cause is unknown, there is no known way to prevent shared psychotic disorder. However, early diagnosis and treatment can help decrease the disruption to the person's life, family, and friendships.

Chapter 32

Dissociative Disorders

Understanding Dissociative Disorders

Dissociative disorders are so-called because they are marked by a dissociation from or interruption of a person's fundamental aspects of waking consciousness (such as one's personal identity, one's personal history, etc.). Dissociative disorders come in many forms, the most famous of which is dissociative identity disorder (formerly known as multiple personality disorder). All of the dissociative disorders are thought to stem from trauma experienced by the individual with this disorder. The dissociative aspect is thought to be a coping mechanism—the person literally dissociates himself from a situation or experience too traumatic to integrate with his conscious self. Symptoms of these disorders, or even one or more of the disorders themselves, are also seen in a number of other mental illnesses, including post-traumatic stress disorder, panic disorder, and obsessive compulsive disorder.

Dissociative Amnesia

This disorder is characterized by a blocking out of critical personal information, usually of a traumatic or stressful nature. Dissociative amnesia, unlike other types of amnesia, does not result from other medical trauma (for example, a blow to the head). Dissociative amnesia has several subtypes:

- Localized amnesia is present in an individual who has no memory of specific events that took place, usually traumatic. The loss of memory is localized with a specific window of time. For example, a survivor of a car wreck who has no memory of the experience until two days later is experiencing localized amnesia.
- Selective amnesia happens when a person can recall only small parts of events that took place in a defined period of time. For example, an abuse victim may recall only some parts of the series of events around the abuse.
- Generalized amnesia is diagnosed when a person's amnesia encompasses his or her entire life.
- Systematized amnesia is characterized by a loss of memory for a specific category of information. A person with this disorder might, for example, be missing all memories about one specific family member.

Dissociative Fugue

Dissociative fugue is a rare disorder. An individual with dissociative fugue suddenly and unexpectedly takes physical leave of his or her surroundings and sets off on a journey of some kind. These journeys can last hours, or even several days or months. Individuals experiencing a dissociative fugue have traveled over thousands of miles. An individual in a fugue state is unaware of or confused about his identity, and in some cases will assume a new identity (although this is the exception).

Dissociative Identity Disorder

Dissociative identity disorder (DID), which has been known as multiple personality disorder, is the most famous of the dissociative disorders. An individual suffering from DID has more than one distinct identity or personality state that surfaces in the individual on a recurring basis. This disorder is also marked by differences in memory which vary with the individual's "alters," or other personalities. For more information on this, see the information later in this chapter about dissociative identity disorder.

Depersonalization Disorder

Depersonalization disorder is marked by a feeling of detachment or distance from one's own experience, body, or self. These feelings of depersonalization are recurrent. Of the dissociative disorders, depersonalization is the one most easily identified with by the general public; one can easily relate to feeling as they are in a dream, or being "spaced out." Feeling out of control of one's actions and movements is something that people describe when intoxicated. An individual with depersonalization disorder has this experience so frequently and so severely that it interrupts his or her functioning and experience. A person's experience with depersonalization can be so severe that he or she believes the external world is unreal or distorted.

Dissociative Identity Disorder

Dissociative identity disorder (DID), previously referred to as multiple personality disorder (MPD), is a dissociative disorder involving a disturbance of identity in which two or more separate and distinct personality states (or identities) control the individual's behavior at different times. When under the control of one identity, the person is usually unable to remember some of the events that occurred while other personalities were in control. The different identities, referred to as alters, may exhibit differences in speech, mannerisms,

✤ It's A Fact!!

Treatment

Since dissociative disorders seem to be triggered as a response to trauma or abuse, treatment for individuals with such a disorder may stress psychotherapy, although a combination of psychopharmacological and psychosocial treatments is often used. Many of the symptoms of dissociative disorders occur with other disorders, such as anxiety and depression, and can be controlled by the same drugs used to treat those disorders. A person in treatment for a dissociative disorder might benefit from antidepressants or antianxiety medication.

attitudes, thoughts, and gender orientation. The alters may even differ in "physical" properties such as allergies, right-or-left handedness, or the need for eyeglass prescriptions. These differences between alters are often quite striking.

The person with DID may have as few as two alters, or as many as 100. The average number is about 10. Often alters are stable over time, continuing to play specific roles in the person's life for years. Some alters may harbor aggressive tendencies, directed toward individuals in the person's environment, or toward other alters within the person.

At the time that a person with DID first seeks professional help, he or she is usually not aware of the condition. A very common complaint in people with DID is episodes of amnesia, or time loss. These individuals may be unable to remember events in all or part of a proceeding time period. They may repeatedly encounter unfamiliar people who claim to know them, find themselves somewhere without knowing how they got there, or find items that they don't remember purchasing among their possessions.

Often people with DID are depressed or even suicidal, and self-mutilation is common in this group. Approximately one-third of patients complain of auditory or visual hallucinations. It is common for these patients to complain that they hear voices within their head.

Treatment for DID consists primarily of psychotherapy with hypnosis. The therapist seeks to make contact with as many alters as possible and to understand their roles and functions in the patient's life. In particular, the therapist seeks to form an effective relationship with any personalities that are responsible for violent or self-destructive behavior, and to curb this behavior. The therapist seeks to establish communication among the personality states and to find ones that have memories of traumatic events in the patient's past. The goal of the therapist is to enable the patient to achieve breakdown of the patient's separate identities and their unification into a single identity.

Retrieving and dealing with memories of trauma is important for the person with DID, because this disorder is believed to be caused by physical or sexual abuse in childhood. Young children have a pronounced ability to dissociate, and it is believed that those who are abused may learn to use dissociation as a defense. In effect, the child slips into a state of mind in which it seems that the abuse is not really occurring to him or her, but to somebody else. In time, such a child may begin to split off alter identities. Research has shown that the average age for the initial development of alters is 5.9 years.

Children with DID have a great variety of symptoms, including depressive tendencies, anxiety, conduct problems, episodes of amnesia, difficulty paying attention in school, and hallucinations. Often these children are misdiagnosed as having schizophrenia. By the time the child reaches adolescence, it is less difficult for a mental health professional to recognize the symptoms and make a diagnosis of DID.

Chapter 33

Schizophrenia

What is schizophrenia?

Schizophrenia is a chronic, severe, and disabling brain disorder that has been recognized throughout recorded history. It affects about one percent of Americans.

Available treatments can relieve many of the disorder's symptoms, but most people who have schizophrenia must cope with some residual symptoms as long as they live. Nevertheless, this is a time of hope for people with schizophrenia and their families. Many people with the disorder now lead rewarding and meaningful lives in their communities. Researchers are developing more effective medications and using new research tools to understand the causes of schizophrenia and to find ways to prevent and treat it.

This presents information on the symptoms of schizophrenia, when the symptoms appear, how the disease develops, current treatments, support for patients and their loved ones, and new directions in research.

What are the symptoms of schizophrenia?

The symptoms of schizophrenia fall into three broad categories:

About This Chapter: Text in this chapter is excerpted from "Schizophrenia," National Institute of Mental Health (www.nimh.nih.gov), April 2, 2009.

- Positive symptoms are unusual thoughts or perceptions, including hallucinations, delusions, thought disorder, and disorders of movement.
- Negative symptoms represent a loss or a decrease in the ability to initiate plans, speak, express emotion, or find pleasure in everyday life. These symptoms are harder to recognize as part of the disorder and can be mistaken for laziness or depression.
- Cognitive symptoms (or cognitive deficits) are problems with attention, certain types of memory, and the executive functions that allow us to plan and organize. Cognitive deficits can also be difficult to recognize as part of the disorder but are the most disabling in terms of leading a normal life.

Positive Symptoms: Positive symptoms are easy-to-spot behaviors not seen in healthy people and usually involve a loss of contact with reality. They include hallucinations, delusions, thought disorder, and disorders of movement. Positive symptoms can come and go. Sometimes they are severe and at other times hardly noticeable, depending on whether the individual is receiving treatment.

- *Hallucinations:* A hallucination is something a person sees, hears, smells, or feels that no one else can see, hear, smell, or feel. "Voices" are the

Remember!!

People with schizophrenia may hear voices other people don't hear or they may believe that others are reading their minds, controlling their thoughts, or plotting to harm them. These experiences are terrifying and can cause fearfulness, withdrawal, or extreme agitation. People with schizophrenia may not make sense when they talk, may sit for hours without moving or talking much, or may seem perfectly fine until they talk about what they are really thinking. Because many people with schizophrenia have difficulty holding a job or caring for themselves, the burden on their families and society is significant as well.

Source: Excerpted from "Schizophrenia," National Institute of Mental Health, April 2, 2009.

most common type of hallucination in schizophrenia. Many people with the disorder hear voices that may comment on their behavior, order them to do things, warn them of impending danger, or talk to each other (usually about the patient). They may hear these voices for a long time before family and friends notice that something is wrong. Other types of hallucinations include seeing people or objects that are not there, smelling odors that no one else detects (although this can also be a symptom of certain brain tumors), and feeling things like invisible fingers touching their bodies when no one is near.

- *Delusions:* Delusions are false personal beliefs that are not part of the person's culture and do not change, even when other people present proof that the beliefs are not true or logical. People with schizophrenia can have delusions that are quite bizarre, such as believing that neighbors can control their behavior with magnetic waves, people on television are directing special messages to them, or radio stations are broadcasting their thoughts aloud to others. They may also have delusions of grandeur and think they are famous historical figures. People with paranoid schizophrenia can believe that others are deliberately cheating, harassing, poisoning, spying upon, or plotting against them or the people they care about. These beliefs are called delusions of persecution.

- *Thought Disorder:* People with schizophrenia often have unusual thought processes. One dramatic form is disorganized thinking, in which the person has difficulty organizing his or her thoughts or connecting them logically. Speech may be garbled or hard to understand. Another form is "thought blocking," in which the person stops abruptly in the middle of a thought. When asked why, the person may say that it felt as if the thought had been taken out of his or her head. Finally, the individual might make up unintelligible words, or "neologisms."

- *Disorders of Movement:* People with schizophrenia can be clumsy and uncoordinated. They may also exhibit involuntary movements and may grimace or exhibit unusual mannerisms. They may repeat certain motions over and over or, in extreme cases, may become catatonic. Catatonia is a state of immobility and unresponsiveness. It was more common when treatment for schizophrenia was not available; fortunately, it is now rare.

Negative Symptoms: The term "negative symptoms" refers to reductions in normal emotional and behavioral states. These include the following:

- Flat affect (immobile facial expression, monotonous voice)
- Lack of pleasure in everyday life
- Diminished ability to initiate and sustain planned activity
- Speaking infrequently, even when forced to interact

✤ It's A Fact!!

People with schizophrenia often neglect basic hygiene and need help with everyday activities. Because it is not as obvious that negative symptoms are part of a psychiatric illness, people with schizophrenia are often perceived as lazy and unwilling to better their lives.

Source: Excerpted from "Schizophrenia," National Institute of Mental Health, April 2, 2009.

Cognitive Symptoms: Cognitive symptoms are subtle and are often detected only when neuropsychological tests are performed. They include the following:

- Poor "executive functioning" (the ability to absorb and interpret information and make decisions based on that information)
- Inability to sustain attention
- Problems with "working memory" (the ability to keep recently learned information in mind and use it right away)

Cognitive impairments often interfere with the patient's ability to lead a normal life and earn a living. They can cause great emotional distress.

When does it start and who gets it?

Psychotic symptoms (such as hallucinations and delusions) usually emerge in men in their late teens and early 20s and in women in their mid-20s to early 30s. They seldom occur after age 45 and only rarely before puberty, although cases of schizophrenia in children as young as five have been reported. In adolescents, the first signs can include a change of friends, a drop in grades, sleep problems, and irritability. Because many normal adolescents exhibit these behaviors as well, a diagnosis can be difficult to make at this stage. In young people who go on to develop the disease, this is called the "prodromal" period.

Research has shown that schizophrenia affects men and women equally and occurs at similar rates in all ethnic groups around the world.

Are people with schizophrenia violent?

People with schizophrenia are not especially prone to violence and often prefer to be left alone. Studies show that if people have no record of criminal violence before they develop schizophrenia and are not substance abusers, they are unlikely to commit crimes after they become ill. Most violent crimes are not committed by people with schizophrenia, and most people with schizophrenia do not commit violent crimes. Substance abuse always increases violent behavior, regardless of the presence of schizophrenia. If someone with paranoid schizophrenia becomes violent, the violence is most often directed at family members and takes place at home.

✤ It's A Fact!!

Schizophrenia may occur, in part, because brain development goes awry during adolescence and young adulthood, when the brain is eliminating some connections between cells as a normal part of maturation, results of a study suggest. The new report appears online July 8, 2008 in *Molecular Psychiatry*.

Comparing a group of adolescents and young adults who had recently had their first bout of schizophrenia with a group of healthy peers, researchers found that this loss of tissue began around the same time and in the same brain areas in both groups. But the rate of loss was more pronounced and covered a greater area of the brain's surface in the youth with schizophrenia.

The new finding adds to evidence that changes in brain development which lead to schizophrenia aren't limited to the prenatal stage and early childhood, but also occur during the late-teen and young-adult years—the ages when symptoms usually begin to appear.

Source: Excerpted from "Abnormal Surge in Brain Development Occurs in Teens and Young Adults with Schizophrenia," a Science Update from the National Institute of Mental Health, July 8, 2008.

What about suicide?

People with schizophrenia attempt suicide much more often than people in the general population. About 10 percent (especially young adult males) succeed. It is hard to predict which people with schizophrenia are prone to suicide, so if someone talks about or tries to commit suicide, professional help should be sought right away.

Can schizophrenia be inherited?

Scientists have long known that schizophrenia runs in families. It occurs in one percent of the general population but is seen in 10 percent of people with a first-degree relative (a parent, brother, or sister) with the disorder. People who have second-degree relatives (aunts, uncles, grandparents, or cousins) with the disease also develop schizophrenia more often than the general population. The identical twin of a person with schizophrenia is most at risk, with a 40 to 65 percent chance of developing the disorder.

✤ It's A Fact!!
Schizophrenia And Nicotine

The most common form of substance abuse in people with schizophrenia is an addiction to nicotine. People with schizophrenia are addicted to nicotine at three times the rate of the general population (75–90 percent vs. 25–30 percent).

Research has revealed that the relationship between smoking and schizophrenia is complex. People with schizophrenia seem to be driven to smoke, and researchers are exploring whether there is a biological basis for this need. In addition to its known health hazards, several studies have found that smoking interferes with the action of antipsychotic drugs. People with schizophrenia who smoke may need higher doses of their medication.

Quitting smoking may be especially difficult for people with schizophrenia since nicotine withdrawal may cause their psychotic symptoms to temporarily get worse. Smoking cessation strategies that include nicotine replacement methods may be better tolerated. Doctors who treat people with schizophrenia should carefully monitor their patient's response to antipsychotic medication if the patient decides to either start or stop smoking.

Source: National Institute of Mental Health, April 2, 2009.

✤ It's A Fact!!
Front-To-Back Wave Envelopes Brain As Child Grows Up

Growth of the brain's long distance connections, called white matter, is stunted and lopsided in children who develop psychosis before puberty, National Institute of Mental Health (NIMH) researchers have discovered. The yearly growth rate of this brain tissue was up to 2.2 percent slower than normal in such childhood onset schizophrenia (COS). The slower the rate, the worse the outcome—suggesting that this magnetic resonance imaging (MRI) measure could someday lead to development of a biomarker that could aid treatment. Nitin Gogtay, M.D., and colleagues in the NIMH Child Psychiatry Branch and UCLA's Laboratory of Neuromaging report on their findings online in the *Proceedings of the National Academy of Sciences* during the week of October 13, 2008.

Source: Excerpted from "Brain's Wiring Stunted, Lopsided in Childhood Schizophrenia," a Science Update from the National Institute of Mental Health, October 30, 2008.

Our genes are located on 23 pairs of chromosomes that are found in each cell. We inherit two copies of each gene, one from each parent. Several of these genes are thought to be associated with an increased risk of schizophrenia, but scientists believe that each gene has a very small effect and is not responsible for causing the disease by itself. It is still not possible to predict who will develop the disease by looking at genetic material.

Although there is a genetic risk for schizophrenia, it is not likely that genes alone are sufficient to cause the disorder. Interactions between genes and the environment are thought to be necessary for schizophrenia to develop. Many environmental factors have been suggested as risk factors, such as exposure to viruses or malnutrition in the womb, problems during birth, and psychosocial factors, like stressful environmental conditions.

Do people with schizophrenia have faulty brain chemistry?

It is likely that an imbalance in the complex, interrelated chemical reactions of the brain involving the neurotransmitters dopamine and glutamate (and possibly others) plays a role in schizophrenia. Neurotransmitters are substances that allow brain cells to communicate with one another. Basic knowledge about brain chemistry and its link to schizophrenia is expanding rapidly and is a promising area of research.

Do the brains of people with schizophrenia look different?

The brains of people with schizophrenia look a little different than the brains of healthy people, but the differences are small. Sometimes the fluid-filled cavities at the center of the brain, called ventricles, are larger in people with schizophrenia; overall gray matter volume is lower; and some areas of the brain have less or more metabolic activity. Microscopic studies of brain tissue after death have also revealed small changes in the distribution or characteristics of brain cells in people with schizophrenia. It appears that many of these changes were prenatal because they are not accompanied by glial cells, which are always present when a brain injury occurs after birth. One theory suggests that problems during brain development lead to faulty connections that lie dormant until puberty. The brain undergoes major changes during puberty, and these changes could trigger psychotic symptoms.

The only way to answer these questions is to conduct more research. Scientists in the United States and around the world are studying schizophrenia and trying to develop new ways to prevent and treat the disorder.

How is schizophrenia treated?

Because the causes of schizophrenia are still unknown, current treatments focus on eliminating the symptoms of the disease.

Antipsychotic Medications: Antipsychotic medications have been available since the mid-1950s. They effectively alleviate the positive symptoms of schizophrenia. While these drugs have greatly improved the lives of many patients, they do not cure schizophrenia.

Everyone responds differently to antipsychotic medication. Sometimes several different drugs must be tried before the right one is found. People with schizophrenia should work in partnership with their doctors to find the medications that control their symptoms best with the fewest side effects.

People respond individually to antipsychotic medications, although agitation and hallucinations usually improve within days and delusions usually improve within a few weeks. Many people see substantial improvement in both types of symptoms by the sixth week of treatment. No one can tell beforehand exactly how a medication will affect a particular individual, and sometimes several medications must be tried before the right one is found.

✤ It's A Fact!!

What happens to us can't change the sequence of our genetic code, or DNA, but it can affect how it gets expressed. In response to environmental factors, molecules called epigenetic marks attach to DNA in ways that silence or activate genes, resulting in enduring changes in the proteins they express—and sometimes disease. For example, depression-like behaviors that develop in experimentally stressed animals have been traced to such experienced-triggered marks or "molecular scars." Epigenetic mechanisms are also known to be involved in cancer and Rett syndrome.

Andrew Feinberg, M.D., MPH, of Johns Hopkins University, and colleagues at four other universities have turned up clues to how such epigenetic changes might affect brain development. They recently reported that epigenetic changes ebb and flow over the lifecycle, with members of families often sharing a similar pattern. Such changing gene expression could hold keys to major mysteries of schizophrenia, such as delayed onset in the late teens/early 20s—how a genetically rooted illness process that likely begins prior to birth spares the brain through childhood, only to erupt in psychotic breakdowns and profound disability at the cusp of productive life.

"Understanding schizophrenia's epigenome can reveal how factors like diet, chemicals, infections and experience impact genetic predisposition," explained Feinberg. "Since epigenetic changes are potentially reversible, our findings may lead to new ways to treat schizophrenia."

Source: Excerpted from "Study Probes Environment-Triggered Genetic Changes in Schizophrenia," a Science Update from the National Institute of Mental Health, December 24, 2008.

Length Of Treatment: Like diabetes or high blood pressure, schizophrenia is a chronic disorder that needs constant management. At the moment, it cannot be cured, but the rate of recurrence of psychotic episodes can be decreased significantly by staying on medication. Although responses vary from person to person, most people with schizophrenia need to take some type of medication for the rest of their lives as well as use other approaches, such as supportive therapy or rehabilitation.

Relapses occur most often when people with schizophrenia stop taking their antipsychotic medication because they feel better, or only take it occasionally because they forget or don't think taking it regularly is important. It is very important for people with schizophrenia to take their medication on a regular basis and for as long as their doctors recommend. If they do so, they will experience fewer psychotic symptoms.

No antipsychotic medication should be discontinued without talking to the doctor who prescribed it, and it should always be tapered off under a doctor's supervision rather than being stopped all at once.

There are a variety of reasons why people with schizophrenia do not adhere to treatment. If they don't believe they are ill, they may not think they need medication at all. If their thinking is too disorganized, they may not remember to take their medication every day. If they don't like the side effects of one medication, they may stop taking it without trying a different medication. Substance abuse can also interfere with treatment effectiveness. Doctors should ask patients how often they take their medication and be sensitive to a patient's request to change dosages or to try new medications to eliminate unwelcome side effects.

There are many strategies to help people with schizophrenia take their drugs regularly. Some medications are available in long-acting, injectable forms, which eliminate the need to take a pill every day. Medication calendars or pillboxes labeled with the days of the week can both help patients remember to take their medications and let caregivers know whether medication has been taken. Electronic timers on clocks or watches can be programmed to beep when people need to take their pills, and pairing medication with routine daily events, like meals, can help patients adhere to dosing schedules.

Medication Interactions. Antipsychotic medications can produce unpleasant or dangerous side effects when taken with certain other drugs. For this reason, the doctor who prescribes the antipsychotics should be told about all medications (over-the-counter and prescription) and all vitamins, minerals, and herbal supplements the patient takes. Alcohol or other drug use should also be discussed.

Psychosocial Treatment: Numerous studies have found that psychosocial treatments can help patients who are already stabilized on antipsychotic medications deal with certain aspects of schizophrenia, such as difficulty with communication, motivation, self-care, work, and establishing and maintaining relationships with others. Learning and using coping mechanisms to address these problems allows people with schizophrenia to attend school, work, and socialize. Patients who receive regular psychosocial treatment also adhere better to their medication schedule and have fewer relapses and hospitalizations. A positive relationship with a therapist or a case manager gives the patient a reliable source of information, sympathy, encouragement, and hope, all of which are essential for managing the disease. The therapist can help patients better understand and adjust to living with schizophrenia by educating them about the causes of the disorder, common symptoms or problems they may experience, and the importance of staying on medications.

Illness Management Skills: People with schizophrenia can take an active role in managing their own illness. Once they learn basic facts about schizophrenia and the principles of schizophrenia treatment, they can make informed decisions about their care. If they are taught how to monitor the early warning signs of relapse and make a plan to respond to these signs, they can learn to prevent relapses. Patients can also be taught more effective coping skills to deal with persistent symptoms.

Integrated Treatment for Co-occurring Substance Abuse: Substance abuse is the most common co-occurring disorder in people with schizophrenia, but ordinary substance abuse treatment programs usually do not address this population's special needs. Integrating schizophrenia treatment programs and drug treatment programs produces better outcomes.

Rehabilitation: Rehabilitation emphasizes social and vocational training to help people with schizophrenia function more effectively in their communities. Because people with schizophrenia frequently become ill during the critical career-forming years of life (ages 18 to 35) and because the disease often interferes with normal cognitive functioning, most patients do not receive the training required for skilled work. Rehabilitation programs can include vocational counseling, job training, money management counseling, assistance in learning to use public transportation, and opportunities to practice social and workplace communication skills.

Family Education: Patients with schizophrenia are often discharged from the hospital into the care of their families, so it is important that family members know as much as possible about the disease to prevent relapses. Family members should be able to use different kinds of treatment adherence programs and have an arsenal of coping strategies and problem-solving skills to manage their ill relative effectively. Knowing where to find outpatient and family services that support people with schizophrenia and their caregivers is also valuable.

Cognitive Behavioral Therapy: Cognitive behavioral therapy is useful for patients with symptoms that persist even when they take medication. The cognitive therapist teaches people with schizophrenia how to test the reality of their thoughts and perceptions, how to "not listen" to their voices, and how to shake off the apathy that often immobilizes them. This treatment appears to be effective in reducing the severity of symptoms and decreasing the risk of relapse.

Self-Help Groups: Self-help groups for people with schizophrenia and their families are becoming increasingly common. Although professional therapists are not involved, the group members are a continuing source of mutual support and comfort for each other, which is also therapeutic. People in self-help groups know that others are facing the same problems they face and no longer feel isolated by their illness or the illness of their loved one. The networking that takes place in self-help groups can also generate social action. Families working together can advocate for research and more hospital and community treatment programs, and patients acting as a group may be able to draw public attention to the discriminations many people with mental illnesses still face in today's world.

Chapter 34

Schizoaffective Disorder

Schizoaffective disorder is one of the more common, chronic, and disabling mental illnesses. As the name implies, it is characterized by a combination of symptoms of schizophrenia and an affective (mood) disorder. There has been a controversy about whether schizoaffective disorder is a type of schizophrenia or a type of mood disorder. Today, most clinicians and researchers agree that it is primarily a form of schizophrenia. Although its exact prevalence is not clear, it may range from two to five in a thousand people (that is, 0.2% to 0.5%). Schizoaffective disorder may account for one-fourth or even one-third of all persons with schizophrenia.

To diagnose schizoaffective disorder, a person needs to have primary symptoms of schizophrenia (such as delusions, hallucinations, disorganized speech, disorganized behavior) along with a period of time when he or she also has symptoms of major depression or a manic episode. Accordingly, there may be two subtypes of schizoaffective disorder:

- (a) Depressive subtype, characterized by major depressive episodes only, and
- (b) Bipolar subtype, characterized by manic episodes with or without depressive symptoms or depressive episodes.

About This Chapter: Text in this chapter is from "Schizoaffective Disorder," 2003 NAMI: The Nation's Voice on Mental Illness (www.nami.org). Reprinted with permission. Reviewed for currency by David A. Cooke, MD, FACP, October 2009.

Differentiating schizoaffective disorder from schizophrenia and from mood disorders can be difficult. The mood symptoms in schizoaffective disorder are more prominent, and last for a substantially longer time than those in schizophrenia. Schizoaffective disorder may be distinguished from a mood disorder by the fact that delusions or hallucinations must be present in persons with schizoaffective disorder for at least two weeks in the absence of prominent mood symptoms. The diagnosis of a person with schizophrenia or mood disorder may change later to that of schizoaffective disorder, or vice versa.

The most effective treatment for schizoaffective disorder is a combination of drug treatment and psychosocial interventions. The medications include antipsychotics along with antidepressants or mood stabilizers. The newer atypical antipsychotics such as clozapine, risperidone, olanzapine, quetiapine, ziprasidone, and aripiprazole are safer than the older typical or conventional antipsychotics such as haloperidol and fluphenazine in terms of parkinsonism and tardive dyskinesia. The newer drugs may also have better effects on mood symptoms. Nonetheless, these medications do have some side effects, especially at higher doses. The side effects may include excessive sleepiness, weight gain, and sometimes diabetes. Different antipsychotic drugs have somewhat different side effect profiles. Changing from one antipsychotic to another one may help if a person with schizoaffective disorder does not respond well or develops distressing side effects with the first medication. The same principle applies to the use of antidepressants or mood stabilizers (please visit www.nami.org for more details about mood disorders).

✤ It's A Fact!!

There has been much less research on psychosocial treatments for schizoaffective disorder than there has been in schizophrenia or depression. However, the available evidence suggests that cognitive behavior therapy, brief psychotherapy, and social skills training are likely to have a beneficial effect. Most people with schizoaffective disorder require long-term therapy with a combination of medications and psychosocial interventions in order to avoid relapses, and maintain an appropriate level of functioning and quality of life.

Part Four

Getting Help For Mental Illness

Chapter 35

Mental Health Professionals: What They Are And How To Find One

Mental health services are provided by several different professions, each of which has its own training and areas of expertise. Finding the right professional(s) for you or a loved one can be a critical ingredient in the process of diagnosis, treatment, and recovery when faced with serious mental illness.

Types Of Mental Health Professionals

Psychiatrist: A psychiatrist is a physician with a doctor of medicine (M.D.) degree or osteopathic (D.O.) degree, with at least four more years of specialized study and training in psychiatry. Psychiatrists are licensed as physicians to practice medicine by individual states. "Board certified" psychiatrists have passed the national examination administered by the American Board of Psychiatry and Neurology. Psychiatrists provide medical and psychiatric evaluations, treat psychiatric disorders, provide psychotherapy, and prescribe and monitor medications.

Psychologist: Some psychologists have a master's degree (M.A. or M.S.) in psychology while others have a doctoral degree (Ph.D., Psy.D., or Ed.D.)

About This Chapter: "Mental Health Professionals: What They Are and How to Find One," © 1996 NAMI: The Nation's Voice on Mental Illness (www.nami.org). Reprinted with permission. Reviewed for currency by David A. Cooke, MD, FACP, October 2009.

in clinical, educational, counseling, or research psychology. Most states license psychologists to practice psychology. They can provide psychological testing, evaluations, treat emotional and behavioral problems and mental disorders, and provide psychotherapy.

Social Worker: Social workers have either a bachelor's degree (B.A., B.S., or B.S.W.), a master's degree (M.A., M.S., M.S.W., or M.S.S.W), or doctoral degree (D.S.W. or Ph.D.). In most states, social workers take an examination to be licensed to practice social work (L.C.S.W. or L.I.C.S.W.), and the type of license depends on their level of education and practice experience. Social workers provide various services including assessment and treatment of psychiatric illnesses, case management, hospital discharge planning, and psychotherapy.

Psychiatric/Mental Health Nurse: Psychiatric/mental health nurses may have various degrees ranging from associate's to bachelor's (B.S.N.) to master's (M.S.N. or A.P.R.N) to doctoral (D.N.Sc., Ph.D.). Depending on their level of education and licensing, they provide a broad range of psychiatric and medical services, including the assessment and treatment of psychiatric illnesses, case management, and psychotherapy. In some states, some psychiatric nurses may prescribe and monitor medication.

Licensed Professional Counselors: Licensed professional counselors have a master's degree (M.A.) in psychology, counseling, or a similar discipline and typically have two years of post-graduate experience. They may provide services that include diagnosis and counseling (individual, family/group or both). They have a license issued in their state and may be certified by the National Academy of Certified Clinical Mental Health Counselors.

Resources For Locating A Mental Health Professional

The following sources may help you locate a mental health professional or treatment facility to meet your needs:

- NAMI local affiliates and support groups: Speaking with NAMI members (consumers and family members) can be a good way to exchange information about mental health professionals in your local community. (Visit www.nami.org for more information.)

- Primary Care Physician (PCP): If you are part of an HMO or other managed care insurance plan, your primary physician can refer you to a specialist or therapist.
- Your insurance provider: Contact your insurance company or "behavioral health care organization" for a list of mental health care providers included in your insurance plan.

✤ It's A Fact!!

Comprehensive Services Through Systems of Care

Some children diagnosed with severe mental health disorders may be eligible for comprehensive and community-based services through systems of care. Systems of care help children with serious emotional disturbances and their families cope with the challenges of difficult mental, emotional, or behavioral problems. To learn more about systems of care, call the National Mental Health Information Center at 800-789-2647, and request fact sheets on systems of care and serious emotional disturbances, or visit the Center's web site at http://mentalhealth.samhsa.gov.

Finding The Right Services Is Critical

To find the right services, do the following:

- Get accurate information from hotlines, libraries, or other sources
- Seek referrals from professionals.
- Ask questions about treatments and services
- Talk to other families in their communities
- Find family network organizations

It is critical that people who are not satisfied with the mental health care they receive discuss their concerns with providers, ask for information, and seek help from other sources.

Source: Excerpted from "Child and Adolescent Mental Health," National Mental Health Information Center, November 2003. Reviewed for currency by David A. Cooke, MD, FACP, October 2009.

- District Branch of the American Psychiatric Association: The APA can give you names of APA members in your area. Find your district branch online or consult your local phone book under the headings "district branch" or "psychiatric society."
- Psychiatry department at local teaching hospital or medical school.
- National Association of Social Workers (NASW) has an online directory of clinical social workers. Visit www.socialworkers.org and click on Resources.
- American Psychological Association can refer to local psychologists by calling 800-964-2000.
- The Substance Abuse and Mental Health Services Administration's (SAMHSA) Center for Mental Health Services has an online database of mental health services and facilities in each state. Visit www.mentalhealth.org and click on Services Locator.

Chapter 36

Going To A Therapist

Eric went to therapy a couple of years ago when his parents were getting divorced. Although he no longer goes, he feels the two months he spent in therapy helped him get through the tough times as his parents worked out their differences.

Melody began seeing her therapist a year ago when she was being bullied at school. She still goes every two weeks because she feels therapy is really helping to build her self-esteem.

Britt just joined a therapy group for eating disorders led by her school's psychologist, and her friend Dana said she'd go with her.

When our parents were in school, very few kids went to therapy. Now it's much more common and also more accepted. Lots of teens wonder if therapy could help them.

What Are Some Reasons That Teens Go to Therapists?

When teens are going through a rough time, such as family troubles or problems in school, they might feel more supported if they talk to a therapist.

About This Chapter: Text in this chapter is from "Going to a Therapist," August 2007, reprinted with permission from www.kidshealth.org. This information was provided by KidsHealth, one of the largest resources online for medically reviewed health information written for parents, kids, and teens. For more articles like this one, visit www.KidsHealth.org, or www.TeensHealth.org.

They may be feeling sad, angry, or overwhelmed by what's been happening—and need help sorting out their feelings, finding solutions to their problems, or just feeling better. That's when therapy can help.

Deciding to seek help for something you're going through can be really hard. It may be your idea to go to therapy or it might not. Sometimes parents or teachers bring up the idea first because they notice that someone they care about is dealing with a difficult situation, is losing weight, or seems unusually sad, worried, angry, or upset. Some people in this situation might welcome the idea or even feel relieved. Others might feel criticized or embarrassed and unsure if they'll benefit from talking to someone.

Sometimes people are told by teachers, parents, or the courts that they have to go see a therapist because they have been behaving in ways that are unacceptable, illegal, self-destructive, or dangerous. When therapy is someone else's idea, a person may at first feel like resisting the whole

✤ It's A Fact!!

Just a few examples of situations in which therapy can help are when someone:

- feels sad, depressed, worried, shy, or just stressed out;
- is dieting or overeating for too long or it becomes a problem (eating disorders);
- cuts, burns, or self-injures;
- is dealing with an attention problem (ADHD) or a learning problem;
- is coping with a chronic illness (such as diabetes or asthma) or a new diagnosis of a serious problem such as HIV, cancer, or a sexually transmitted disease (STD);
- is dealing with family changes such as separation and divorce, or family problems such as alcoholism or addiction;
- is trying to cope with a traumatic event, death of a loved one, or worry over world events;
- has a habit he or she would like to get rid of, such as nail biting, hair pulling, smoking, or spending too much money, or getting hooked on medications, drugs, or pills;
- wants to sort out problems like managing anger or coping with peer pressure;
- wants to build self-confidence or figure out ways to make more friends.

In short, therapy offers people support when they are going through difficult times.

idea. But learning a bit more about what therapy involves and what to expect can help make it seem OK.

What Is Therapy?

Therapy isn't just for mental health. You've probably heard people discussing other types of medical therapy, such as physical therapy or chemotherapy. But the word "therapy" is most often used to mean psychotherapy (sometimes called "talk therapy")—in other words, psychological help to deal with stress or problems.

Psychotherapy is a process that's a lot like learning. Through therapy, people learn about themselves. They discover ways to overcome difficulties, develop inner strengths or skills, or make changes in themselves or their situations. Often, it feels good just to have a person to vent to, and other times it's useful to learn different techniques to help deal with stress.

A psychotherapist (therapist, for short) is a person who has been professionally trained to help people deal with stress or other problems. Psychiatrists, psychologists, social workers, counselors, and school psychologists are the titles of some of the licensed professionals who work as therapists. The letters following a therapist's name (for example, MD, PhD, PsyD, EdD, MA, LCSW, LPC) refer to the particular education and degree that therapist has received.

Some therapists specialize in working with a certain age group or on a particular type of problem. Other therapists treat a mix of ages and issues. Some work in hospitals, clinics, or counseling centers. Others work in schools or in psychotherapy offices, often called a "private practice" or "group practice."

What Do Therapists Do?

Most types of therapy include talking and listening, building trust, and receiving support and guidance. Sometimes therapists may recommend books for people to read or work through. They may also suggest keeping a journal. Some people prefer to express themselves using art or drawing. Others feel more comfortable just talking.

When a person talks to a therapist about which situations might be difficult for them or what stresses them out, this helps the therapist assess what is going on. The therapist and client then usually work together to set therapy goals and figure out what will help the person feel better or get back on track.

It might take a few meetings with a therapist before people really feel like they can share personal stuff. It's natural to feel that way. Trust is an essential ingredient in therapy—after all, therapy involves being open and honest about sensitive topics like feelings, ideas, relationships, problems, disappointments, and hopes. A therapist understands that people sometimes take a while to feel comfortable sharing personal information.

Most of the time, a person meets with a therapist one on one, which is known as individual therapy. Sometimes, though, a therapist might work with a family (called family therapy) or a group of people who all are dealing with similar issues (called group therapy or a support group). Family therapy gives family members a chance to talk together with a therapist about problems that involve them all. Group therapy and support groups help people give and receive support and learn from each other and their therapist by discussing the issues they have in common.

What Happens During Therapy?

If you see a therapist, he or she will talk with you about your feelings, thoughts, relationships, and important values. At the beginning, therapy sessions are focused on discussing what you'd like to work on and setting goals. Some of the goals people in therapy may set include things like:

- improving self-esteem and gaining confidence;
- figuring out how to make more friends;
- feeling less depressed or less anxious;
- improving grades at school;
- learning to manage anger and frustration;
- making healthier choices (for example, about relationships or eating) and ending self-defeating behaviors.

During the first visit, your therapist will probably ask you to talk a bit about yourself. Depending on your age, the therapist will also likely meet with a parent or caregiver and ask you to review information regarding confidentiality.

The first meeting can last longer than the usual "therapy hour" and is often called an "intake interview." This helps the therapist understand you better, and gives you a chance to see if you feel comfortable with the therapist. The therapist will probably ask about problems, concerns, and symptoms that you may be having, or the problems that parents or teachers are concerned about.

After one or two sessions, the therapist may talk to you about his or her understanding of what is going on with you, how therapy could help, and what the process will involve. Together, you and your therapist will decide on the goals for therapy and how frequently to meet. This may be once a week, every other week, or once a month.

With a better understanding of your situation, the therapist might teach you new skills or help you to think about a situation in a new way. For example, therapists can help people develop better relationship skills or coping skills, including ways to build confidence, express feelings, or manage anger.

Sticking to the schedule you agree on with your therapist and going to your appointments will ensure you have enough time with your therapist to work out your concerns. If your therapist suggests a schedule that you don't think you'll be able to keep, be up front about it so you can work out an alternative.

✤ It's A Fact!!

How Private Is It?

Therapists respect the privacy of their clients and they keep things they're told confidential. A therapist won't tell anyone else—including parents—about what a person discusses in his or her sessions unless that person gives permission. The only exception is if therapists believe their clients may harm themselves or others.

If the issue of privacy and confidentiality worries you, be sure to ask your therapist about it during your first meeting. It's important to feel comfortable with your therapist so you can talk openly about your situation.

Does It Mean I'm Crazy?

No. In fact, many people in your class have probably seen a therapist at some point—just like students often see tutors or coaches for extra help with schoolwork or sports. Getting help in dealing with emotions and stressful situations is as important to your overall health as getting help with a medical problem like asthma or diabetes.

There's nothing wrong with getting help with problems that are hard to solve alone. In fact, it's just the opposite. It takes a lot of courage and maturity to look for solutions to problems instead of ignoring or hiding them and allowing them to become worse. If you think that therapy could help you with a problem, ask an adult you trust—like a parent, school counselor, or doctor—to help you find a therapist.

A few adults still resist the idea of therapy because they don't fully understand it or have outdated ideas about it. A couple of generations ago, people didn't know as much about the mind or the mind-body connection as they do today, and people were left to struggle with their problems on their own. It used to be that therapy was only available to those with the most serious mental health problems, but that's no longer the case.

Therapy is helpful to people of all ages and with problems that range from mild to much more serious. Some people still hold on to old beliefs about therapy, such as thinking that teens "will grow out of" their problems. If the adults in your family don't seem open to talking about therapy, mention your concerns to a school counselor, coach, or doctor.

You don't have to hide the fact that you're going to a therapist, but you also don't have to tell anyone if you'd prefer not to. Some people find that talking to a few close friends about their therapy helps them to work out their problems and feel like they're not alone. Other people choose not to tell anyone, especially if they feel that others won't understand. Either way, it's a personal decision.

What Can A Person Get Out Of Therapy?

What someone gets out of therapy depends on why that person is there. For example, some people go to therapy to solve a specific problem, others want to begin making better choices, and others want to start to heal from a loss or a difficult life situation.

Therapy can help people feel better, be stronger, and make good choices as well as discover more about themselves. Those who work with therapists might learn about motivations that lead them to behave in certain ways or about inner strengths they have. Maybe you'll learn new coping skills, develop more patience, or learn to like yourself better. Maybe you'll find new ways to handle problems that come up or new ways to handle yourself in tough situations.

People who work with therapists often find that they learn a lot about themselves and that therapy can help them grow and mature. Lots of people discover that the tools they learn in therapy when they're young make them feel stronger and better able to deal with whatever life throws at them even as adults. If you are curious about the therapy process, talk to a counselor or therapist to see if you could benefit.

Chapter 37

Counseling And Therapy: A Summary Of Mental Health Treatments

Methods of Treatment

Below are brief descriptions of the methods health professionals use and/or recommend in working with teens and their families.

Behavioral Therapy/Behavior Modification: As the name implies, this approach focuses on behavior—changing unwanted behaviors through rewards, reinforcements, and desensitization. Desensitization is a process of confronting something that arouses anxiety, discomfort, or fear and overcoming the unwanted responses. Someone whose fear of germs leads to excessive washing, for example, may be trained to relax and not wash his or her hands after touching a public doorknob. Behavioral therapy often involves the cooperation of others, especially family and close friends, to reinforce a desired behavior.

Biomedical Treatment: Medication alone, or in combination with psychotherapy, can be an effective treatment for a number of emotional, behavioral, and mental disorders. The kind of medication a psychiatrist prescribes

About This Chapter: Text in this chapter is from "Counseling and Therapy: Methods of Treatment," © 2008 Focus Adolescent Services (www.focusas.com). Reprinted with permission.

varies with the disorder and the individual being treated. For example, some people who suffer from anxiety, bipolar disorder, major depression, obsessive compulsive disorder, panic disorders, and schizophrenia find their symptoms improve dramatically through careful monitoring of appropriate medication.

Client-Centered/Person-Centered Therapy: Client-centered counseling is a well-established helping approach for a wide range of problems. Based on the teachings of Carl Rogers, it assumes that the individual is the authority of his or her life and that human nature is inherently constructive and social. The client-centered counselor believes the individual is an expert on his or her own life, even if that person sometimes can't quite believe he or she is. Without diagnoses or treatment plans, the counselor enables the individual to sort through thoughts, feelings, ideas, and choices creatively with the help of attentive, nonjudgmental, and honest listening. This atmosphere of unconditional positive regard, empathy, and trust offered by the counselor fosters clarity, self-directed growth, and genuine change. Client-centered therapy is also used in conjunction with other treatment as a way for the individual to organize and integrate his or her experiences.

Cognitive Therapy: This method aims to identify and correct distorted thinking patterns that can lead to feelings and behaviors that may be troublesome, self-defeating, or even self-destructive. The goal is to replace such thinking with a more balanced view that, in turn, leads to more fulfilling and productive behavior. Consider the person who will not apply for a promotion on the assumption that it is beyond reach, for example. With cognitive therapy, the next time a promotion comes up that person might still initially think, "I won't get that position…" but then immediately add, "unless I show my boss what a good job I would do."

Cognitive-Behavioral Therapy: A combination of cognitive and behavioral therapies, this approach helps people change negative thought patterns, beliefs, and behaviors so they can manage symptoms and enjoy more productive, less stressful lives.

Couples Counseling And Family Therapy: These two similar approaches to therapy involve discussions and problem-solving sessions facilitated by a therapist—sometimes with the couple or entire family group, sometimes with

✤ It's A Fact!!

Coping with serious mental illness is hard on marriages and families. Family therapy can help educate the individuals about the nature of the disorder and teach them skills to cope better with the effects of having a family member with a mental illness—such as how to deal with feelings of anger or guilt. In addition, family therapy can help members identify and reduce factors that may trigger or worsen the disorder.

individuals. Such therapy can help couples and family members improve their understanding of, and the way they respond to, one another. This type of therapy can resolve patterns of behavior that might lead to more severe mental illness. Family therapy may be very useful with children and adolescents who are experiencing problems.

Dialectical Behavior Therapy: Dialectical behavior therapy (DBT) is a combination of behavioral and cognitive therapy originally designed for the treatment of borderline personality disorder. It is increasingly being used with adolescents and adults who exhibit impulsive and inappropriate acting-out behaviors (for example, self-injury, eating disorders, suicidal tendencies, drug dependence). The approach integrates individual and group therapies to focus on the seemingly opposite ideas of (1) the need to accept oneself as one is and the need to change, (2) getting what one needs and giving it up to become more competent, and (3) accepting one's experience and suffering, yet gaining skills to reduce the suffering.

Electro-Convulsive Therapy: Also known as ECT, this highly controversial technique uses low voltage electrical stimulation of the brain to treat some forms of major depression, acute mania, and some forms of schizophrenia. This potentially life-saving technique is considered only when other therapies have failed, when a person is seriously medically ill and/or unable to take medication, or when a person is very likely to commit suicide. Substantial improvements in the equipment, dosing guidelines, and anesthesia have significantly reduced the possibility of side effects.

Expressive Therapies

Art Therapy: Drawing, painting, and sculpting help many people to reconcile inner conflicts, release deeply repressed emotions, and foster self-awareness as well as personal growth. Some mental health providers use art therapy as both a diagnostic tool and to help treat disorders such as depression, abuse-related trauma, and schizophrenia.

For example, in coloring therapy, the activity of coloring itself is used as a way to begin to quiet the mind, listen inwardly and open up to higher knowledge, healing, and creativity. This alternative to formal meditation practices can help people of all ages in recovery improve coping and awareness skills through an enjoyable activity.

Dance/Movement Therapy: Those who are recovering from physical, sexual, or emotional abuse may find these techniques especially helpful for gaining a sense of ease with their own bodies. The underlying premise to dance/movement therapy is that it can help a person integrate the emotional, physical, and cognitive facets of "self."

Music/Sound Therapy: Research suggests music stimulates the body's natural "feel good" chemicals (opiates and endorphins). This results in improved blood flow, blood pressure, pulse rate, breathing, and posture changes. Music/sound therapy has been used to treat disorders such as stress, grief, depression, schizophrenia, autism in children, and to diagnose mental health needs.

Eye Movement Desensitization Reprocessing: EMDR creates eye movements that mimic those of rapid eye movement (REM) sleep to create the same brain waves present during REM sleep while the individual is awake. During this period, traumatic and other issues are processed more efficiently than at normal levels of brain functioning. EMDR has shown effective results for individuals with attention deficit disorder (ADD)/attention deficit hyperactivity disorder (ADHD).

Group Therapy: Group therapy focuses on learning from the experiences of others and involves groups of usually four to 12 people who have similar problems and who meet regularly with a therapist. The therapist uses the emotional interactions of the group's members to help them get relief from distress and possibly modify their behavior.

Holistic Medicine: Holistic medicine is the art and science of healing that addresses the whole person—body, mind, and spirit. The practice of holistic medicine integrates conventional and alternative therapies (such as acupressure, yoga, gi gong, and energy medicine) to prevent and treat disease, and most importantly, to promote optimal health. This condition of holistic health is defined as the unlimited and unimpeded free flow of life force energy through body, mind, and spirit.

Holistic medicine encompasses all safe and appropriate modalities of diagnosis and treatment. It includes analysis of physical, nutritional, environmental, emotional, spiritual and lifestyle elements. Holistic medicine focuses upon patient education and participation in the healing process.

Interpersonal Psychotherapy: Through one-on-one conversations, this approach focuses on the patient's current life and relationships within the family, social, and work environments. The goal is to identify and resolve problems with insight, as well as build on strengths.

Light Therapy: Seasonal affective disorder (SAD) is a form of depression that appears related to fluctuations in the exposure to natural light. It usually strikes during autumn and often continues through the winter when natural light is reduced. Researchers have found that people who have SAD can be helped with the symptoms of their illness if they spend blocks of time bathed in light from a special full-spectrum light source, called a "light box."

Pastoral Counseling: Some people prefer to seek help for mental health problems from their pastor, rabbi, or priest rather than from therapists who are not affiliated with a religious community. Counselors working within traditional faith communities increasingly are recognizing the need to incorporate psychotherapy and/or medication, along with prayer and spirituality, to effectively help some people with mental disorders.

Play Therapy: Geared toward young children, this technique uses a variety of activities—such as painting, puppets, and dioramas—to establish communication with the therapist and resolve problems. Play allows the child to express emotions and problems that would be too difficult to discuss with another person.

Psychoanalysis: This approach focuses on past conflicts as the underpinnings to current emotional and behavioral problems. In this long-term and intensive therapy, an individual meets with a psychoanalyst three to five times a week, using "free association" to explore unconscious motivations and earlier, unproductive patterns of resolving issues.

Psychodynamic Psychotherapy: Based on the principles of psychoanalysis, this therapy is less intense, tends to occur once or twice a week, and spans a shorter time. It is based on the premise that human behavior is determined by one's past experiences, genetic factors, and current situation. This approach recognizes the significant influence that emotions and unconscious motivation can have on human behavior.

Rational Emotive Behavior Therapy: Rational emotive behavior therapy (REBT) is a humanistic, action-oriented approach to emotional growth, first articulated by Dr. Albert Ellis in 1955, which emphasizes individuals' capacity for creating their emotions; the ability to change and overcome the past by focusing on the present; and the power to choose and implement satisfying alternatives to current patterns.

Reality Therapy: The fundamental idea of reality therapy is that no matter what has happened in the past, our future is ours and success is based on the behaviors we choose. Developed by William Glasser in the 1960s, reality therapy is based on choice theory which states that almost all behavior is chosen and that we are driven to satisfy five basic needs: survival, love and belonging, power, freedom, and fun. The most important need is love and belonging, as closeness and connectedness with others is necessary for satisfying all of the needs. This counseling method emphasizes personal responsibility. It focuses on the present to empower the client to satisfy his or her needs and wants in the present and in the future.

Relaxation And Stress Reduction Techniques

Biofeedback: Learning to control muscle tension and "involuntary" body functioning, such as heart rate and skin temperature, can be a path to mastering one's fears. It is used in combination with, or as an alternative to, medication to treat disorders such as anxiety, panic, and phobias. For example, a person can learn to "retrain" his or her breathing habits in stressful situations to induce relaxation and decrease hyperventilation. Some preliminary research indicates it may offer an additional tool for treating attentional disorders (ADD/ADHD), mood disorders, personality disorders, and schizophrenia.

Guided Imagery Or Visualization: This process involves going into a state of deep relaxation and creating a mental image of recovery and wellness. Physicians, nurses, and mental health providers occasionally use this approach to treat alcohol and drug addictions, depression, panic disorders, phobias, and stress.

Massage Therapy: The underlying principle of this approach is that rubbing, kneading, brushing, and tapping a person's muscles can help release tension and pent emotions. It has been used to treat trauma-related depression and stress.

Transpersonal Psychology: Transpersonal psychologists are concerned with the development of a healthy individuality and its extension to include aspects of the higher self. This viewpoint acknowledges that behind the masks,

✤ It's A Fact!!

Self-Help: Self-help has become an integral part of treatment for mental health problems. Many people with mental illnesses find that self-help groups are an invaluable resource for recovery and for empowerment. Self-help generally refers to groups or meetings that:

- involve people who have similar needs;
- are facilitated by a consumer, survivor, or other layperson;
- assist people to deal with a "life-disrupting" event—such as a death, abuse, serious accident, addiction, and diagnosis of a physical, emotional, or mental disability for oneself or a relative;
- are operated on an informal, free-of-charge, and nonprofit basis;
- provide support and education; and
- are voluntary, anonymous, and confidential.

roles, and melodramas of one's conditioned personality lies a deeper state of being that transcends individual identity. As the transpersonal perspective unites the spiritual with the psychological aspects of human experience, it addresses the integration of the whole person—body, mind, emotion, and spirit. In doing so, transpersonal psychology draws on the world's spiritual traditions; mythology, anthropology, and the arts; research on consciousness; and Western psychological theory.

Chapter 38

Mental Health Medications

What are psychiatric medications?

Psychiatric medications treat mental disorders. Sometimes called psychotropic or psychotherapeutic medications, they have changed the lives of people with mental disorders for the better. Many people with mental disorders live fulfilling lives with the help of these medications. Without them, people with mental disorders might suffer serious and disabling symptoms.

Medications treat the symptoms of mental disorders. They cannot cure the disorder, but they make people feel better so they can function.

Medications work differently for different people. Some people get great results from medications and only need them for a short time. For example, a person with depression may feel much better after taking a medication for a few months, and may never need it again. People with disorders like schizophrenia or bipolar disorder, or people who have long-term or severe depression or anxiety may need to take medication for a much longer time.

About This Chapter: Text in this chapter is excerpted from "Mental Health Medications," National Institute of Mental Health (www.nimh.nih.gov), 2008. The information included provides only a summary of commonly used medications. It does not include dosing information, does not list all known side effects, and does not discuss all possible drug interactions. Please be sure to talk with your doctor before taking any medications or herbal remedies.

What medications are used to treat schizophrenia?

Antipsychotic medications are used to treat schizophrenia and schizophrenia-related disorders. Some of these medications have been available since the mid-1950s. They are also called conventional "typical" antipsychotics. Some of the more commonly used medications include chlorpromazine (Thorazine), haloperidol (Haldol), perphenazine, and fluphenazine.

In the 1990s, new antipsychotic medications were developed. These new medications are called second generation, or "atypical" antipsychotics. One of these medications was clozapine (Clozaril). It is a very effective medication that treats psychotic symptoms, hallucinations, and breaks with reality, such as when a person believes he or she is the president. But clozapine can sometimes cause a serious problem called agranulocytosis, which is a loss of the white blood cells that help a person fight infection. Therefore, people who take clozapine must get their white blood cell counts checked every week or two. This problem and the cost of blood tests make treatment with clozapine difficult for many people. Still, clozapine is potentially helpful for people who do not respond to other antipsychotic medications.

Other atypical antipsychotics were developed. All of them are effective, and none cause agranulocytosis. These include risperidone (Risperdal), olanzapine (Zyprexa), quetiapine (Seroquel), ziprasidone (Geodon), aripiprazole (Abilify), and paliperidone (Invega).

The antipsychotics listed here are some of the medications used to treat symptoms of schizophrenia.

What medications are used to treat depression?

Depression is commonly treated with antidepressant medications. Antidepressants work to balance some of the natural chemicals in our brains. These chemicals are called neurotransmitters, and they affect our mood and emotional responses. Antidepressants work on neurotransmitters such as serotonin, norepinephrine, and dopamine.

The most popular types of antidepressants are called selective serotonin reuptake inhibitors (SSRIs). These include fluoxetine (Prozac), citalopram (Celexa), sertraline (Zoloft), paroxetine (Paxil), and escitalopram (Lexapro).

Other types of antidepressants are serotonin and norepinephrine reuptake inhibitors (SNRIs). SNRIs are similar to SSRIs and include venlafaxine (Effexor) and duloxetine (Cymbalta). Another antidepressant that is commonly used is bupropion (Wellbutrin). Bupropion, which works on the neurotransmitter dopamine, is unique in that it does not fit into any specific drug type.

SSRIs and SNRIs are popular because they do not cause as many side effects as older classes of antidepressants. Older antidepressant medications include tricyclics, tetracyclics, and monoamine oxidase inhibitors (MAOIs). For some people, tricyclics, tetracyclics, or MAOIs may be the best medications.

The herbal medicine St. John's wort has been used for centuries in many folk and herbal remedies. Today in Europe, it is used widely to treat mild-to-moderate depression. In the United States, it is one of the top-selling botanical products.

The National Institutes of Health conducted a clinical trial to determine the effectiveness of treating adults who have major depression with St. John's wort. The study found that St. John's wort was no more effective than the placebo in treating major depression. A study currently in progress is looking at the effectiveness of St. John's wort for treating mild or minor depression.

Because St. John's wort may not mix well with other medications, people should always talk with their doctors before taking it or any herbal supplement.

✤ It's A Fact!!

The U.S. Food and Drug Administration has warned that combining the newer selective serotonin reuptake inhibitors (SSRIs) or serotonin and norepinephrine reuptake inhibitors (SNRIs) antidepressants with one of the commonly used "triptan" medications used to treat migraine headaches could cause a life-threatening illness called "serotonin syndrome." A person with serotonin syndrome may be agitated, have hallucinations (see or hear things that are not real), have a high temperature, or have unusual blood pressure changes. Serotonin syndrome is usually associated with the older antidepressants called monoamine oxidase inhibitors (MAOIs), but it can happen with the newer antidepressants as well, if they are mixed with the wrong medications.

Source: NIMH, 2008.

✤ It's A Fact!!

Antidepressant Medications For Children And Adolescents

Research has shown that, as in adults, depression in children and adolescents is treatable. Certain antidepressant medications, called selective serotonin reuptake inhibitors (SSRIs), can be beneficial to children and adolescents with major depressive disorder (MDD). Certain types of psychological therapies also have been shown to be effective. However, our knowledge of antidepressant treatments in youth, though growing substantially, is limited compared to what we know about treating depression in adults.

Recently, there has been some concern that the use of antidepressant medications themselves may induce suicidal behavior in youths. Following a thorough and comprehensive review of all the available published and unpublished controlled clinical trials of antidepressants in children and adolescents, the U.S. Food and Drug Administration (FDA) issued a public warning in October 2004 about an increased risk of suicidal thoughts or behavior (suicidality) in children and adolescents treated with SSRI antidepressant medications. In 2006, an advisory committee to the FDA recommended that the agency extend the warning to include young adults up to age 25.

More recently, results of a comprehensive review of pediatric trials conducted between 1988 and 2006 suggested that the benefits of antidepressant medications likely outweigh their risks to children and adolescents with major depression and anxiety disorders. The study, partially funded by the National Institute of Mental Health (NIMH), was published in the April 18, 2007, issue of the *Journal of the American Medical Association*.

An individual's response to a medication cannot be predicted with certainty. It is extremely difficult to determine whether SSRI medications increase the risk for completed suicide, especially because depression itself increases the risk for suicide and because completed suicides, especially among children and adolescents, are rare. Most controlled trials are too small to detect for rare events such as suicide (thousands of participants are needed). In addition, controlled trials typically exclude patients considered at high risk for suicide.

Researchers are working to better understand the relationship between antidepressant medications and suicide. So far, results are mixed.

Source: Excerpted from "Antidepressant Medications for Children and Adolescents: Information for Parents and Caregivers," National Institute of Mental Health, March 31, 2009.

What medications are used to treat bipolar disorder?

Bipolar disorder, also called manic-depressive illness, is commonly treated with mood stabilizers. Sometimes, antipsychotics and antidepressants are used along with a mood stabilizer.

People with bipolar disorder usually try mood stabilizers first. In general, people continue treatment with mood stabilizers for years. Lithium is a very effective mood stabilizer. It was the first mood stabilizer approved by the FDA in the 1970s for treating both manic and depressive episodes.

Anticonvulsant medications also are used as mood stabilizers. They were originally developed to treat seizures, but they were found to help control moods as well. One anticonvulsant commonly used as a mood stabilizer is valproic acid, also called divalproex sodium (Depakote). For some people, it may work better than lithium. Other anticonvulsants used as mood stabilizers are carbamazepine (Tegretol), lamotrigine (Lamictal) and oxcarbazepine (Trileptal).

Atypical antipsychotic medications are sometimes used to treat symptoms of bipolar disorder. Often, antipsychotics are used along with other medications. Antipsychotics used to treat people with bipolar disorder include olanzapine (Zyprexa), which helps people with severe or psychotic depression, which often is accompanied by a break with reality, hallucinations, or delusions; aripiprazole (Abilify), which can be taken as a pill or as a shot; risperidone (Risperdal); ziprasidone (Geodon); and clozapine (Clozaril), which is often used for people who do not respond to lithium or anticonvulsants.

Antidepressants are sometimes used to treat symptoms of depression in bipolar disorder. However, people with bipolar disorder should not take an antidepressant on its own. Doing so can cause the person to rapidly switch from depression to mania, which can be dangerous. To prevent this problem, doctors give patients a mood stabilizer or an antipsychotic along with an antidepressant. Research on whether antidepressants help people with bipolar depression is mixed.

What medications are used to treat anxiety disorders?

Antidepressants, anti-anxiety medications, and beta-blockers are the most common medications used for anxiety disorders.

Antidepressants were developed to treat depression, but they also help people with anxiety disorders. SSRIs such as fluoxetine (Prozac), sertraline (Zoloft), escitalopram (Lexapro), paroxetine (Paxil), and citalopram (Celexa) are commonly prescribed for panic disorder, obsessive-compulsive disorder (OCD), posttraumatic syndrome disorder (PTSD), and social phobia. The SNRI venlafaxine (Effexor) is commonly used to treat generalized anxiety disorder (GAD). The antidepressant bupropion (Wellbutrin) is also sometimes used. When treating anxiety disorders, antidepressants generally are started at low doses and increased over time.

Some tricyclic antidepressants work well for anxiety. For example, imipramine (Tofranil) is prescribed for panic disorder and GAD. Clomipramine (Anafranil) is used to treat OCD. Tricyclics are also started at low doses and increased over time.

MAOIs are also used for anxiety disorders. Doctors sometimes prescribe phenelzine (Nardil), tranylcypromine (Parnate), and isocarboxazid (Marplan). People who take MAOIs must avoid certain food and medicines that can interact with their medicine and cause dangerous increases in blood pressure.

The anti-anxiety medications called benzodiazepines can start working more quickly than antidepressants. The ones used to treat anxiety disorders include clonazepam (Klonopin), which is used for social phobia and GAD; lorazepam (Ativan), which is used for panic disorder; alprazolam (Xanax), which is used for panic disorder and GAD; and buspirone (Buspar), which is an anti-anxiety medication used to treat GAD. Unlike benzodiazepines, however, it takes at least two weeks for buspirone to begin working.

Beta-blockers control some of the physical symptoms of anxiety, such as trembling and sweating. Propranolol (Inderal) is a beta-blocker usually used to treat heart conditions and high blood pressure. The medicine also helps people who have physical problems related to anxiety. For example, when a person with social phobia must face a stressful situation, such as giving a speech, or attending an important meeting, a doctor may prescribe a beta-blocker. Taking the medicine for a short period of time can help the person keep physical symptoms under control.

✤ It's A Fact!!

The non-stimulant attention deficit/hyperactivity disorder (ADHD) medication called atomoxetine (Strattera) carries a warning. Studies show that children and teenagers with ADHD who take atomoxetine are more likely to have suicidal thoughts than children and teenagers with ADHD who do not take atomoxetine. Serious symptoms may develop suddenly, so it is important to have parents, siblings, and teachers pay attention and immediately report if they notice changes in behavior. A doctor should be called right away if any of the following symptoms are noted:

- Acting more subdued or withdrawn than usual
- Feeling helpless, hopeless, or worthless
- New or worsening depression
- Thinking or talking about hurting himself or herself
- Extreme worry
- Agitation
- Panic attacks
- Trouble sleeping
- Irritability
- Aggressive or violent behavior
- Acting without thinking
- Extreme increase in activity or talking
- Frenzied, abnormal excitement
- Any sudden or unusual changes in behavior

While taking atomoxetine, your should see a doctor often, especially at the beginning of treatment. Be sure that you keeps all appointments with your doctor.

Source: NIMH, 2008.

What medications are used to treat ADHD?

Attention deficit/hyperactivity disorder (ADHD) is commonly treated with stimulants, such as methylphenidate (Ritalin, Metadate, Concerta, Daytrana), amphetamine (Adderall), and dextroamphetamine (Dexedrine, Dextrostat). The FDA has also approved the nonstimulant medication atomoxetine (Strattera) for use as a treatment for ADHD and the stimulant lisdexamfetamine dimesylate (Vyvanse) for the treatment of ADHD in children ages 6 to 12 years.

In 2007, the FDA required that all makers of ADHD medications develop Patient Medication Guides. The guides must alert patients to possible heart and psychiatric problems related to ADHD medicine. The FDA required the Patient Medication Guides because a review of data found that ADHD patients with heart conditions had a slightly higher risk of strokes, heart attacks, and sudden death when taking the medications. The review also found a slightly higher risk (about 1 in 1,000) for medication-related psychiatric problems, such as hearing voices, having hallucinations, becoming suspicious for no reason, or becoming manic. This happened to patients who had no history of psychiatric problems.

The FDA recommends that any treatment plan for ADHD include an initial health and family history examination. This exam should look for existing heart and psychiatric problems.

Do children and adolescents have special needs when taking psychiatric medications?

Most medications used to treat young people with mental illness are safe and effective. However, many medications have not been studied or approved for use with children. Researchers are not sure how these medications affect a child's growing body. Still, a doctor can give a young person an FDA-approved medication on an "off-label" basis. This means that the doctor prescribes the medication to help the patient even though the medicine is not approved for the specific mental disorder or age.

For these reasons, it is important to watch young people who take these medications. Young people may have different reactions and side effects than adults. Also, some medications, including antidepressants and ADHD medications, carry FDA warnings about potentially dangerous side effects for young people.

In addition to medications, other treatments for young people with mental disorders should be considered. Psychotherapy, family therapy, educational courses, and behavior management techniques can help everyone involved cope with the disorder.

✔ Quick Tip

Information about medications is frequently updated. Check the U.S. Food and Drug Administration (FDA) website (www.fda.gov) for the latest information on warnings, patient medication guides, or newly approved medications.

Source: NIMH, 2008.

Chapter 39

Electroconvulsive Therapy

A Brief History Of ECT

Electroconvulsive therapy, commonly called ECT, was developed in 1938. During the period following its introduction, ECT was found effective for treating multiple psychiatric illnesses, especially depression. With the development of psychiatric medications and stigma associated with ECT in the 1960s, the use of ECT treatment declined. The use of ECT has increased since the 1970s because of improved treatment delivery methods, increased safety and comfort measures, and enhanced anesthesia management. ECT is the most effective treatment for severe mental illness and is an extremely safe treatment.

ECT is most commonly used to treat patients with severe depression who fail to respond to medications or who are unable to tolerate the side effects associated with the medications. ECT may also be the treatment of choice for patients who need a more rapid response than medications can provide. This would include those who are severely agitated, delusional, suicidal, not eating or drinking, as well as those who suffer from catatonia (a potentially life threatening trance-like state).

About This Chapter: Information in this chapter, from "Electroconvulsive Therapy Program," is reprinted with permission from the website of the University of Michigan Department of Psychiatry, www.psych.med.umich.edu/ECT.

How Does ECT Work?

Mechanisms Of ECT

Electroconvulsive therapy involves applying a brief electrical pulse to the scalp while the patient is under anesthesia. This pulse excites the brain cells causing them to fire in unison and produces a seizure.

The specific reason for the positive action of ECT is unknown, but this treatment appears to have many effects. There are multiple theories to explain why ECT is effective. One theory suggests that the seizure activity itself causes an alteration of the chemical messengers in the brain known as neurotransmitters. Another theory proposes that ECT treatments adjust the stress hormone regulation in the brain, which may affect energy, sleep, appetite, and mood.

The Number Of Treatments Needed

Treatments are normally administered three times a week on Monday, Wednesday, and Friday. A course of ECT normally ranges from six to twelve treatments. The average number of treatments is nine. The number of treatments that you need will be determined by the severity of your symptoms and how rapidly you respond.

It usually takes six treatments before major improvements in your symptoms are noted. However, family members, friends, and caregivers may begin to see mild improvements following the first three to six treatments. These improvements may include an increase in your activity level, improved sleeping patterns, and a mild increase in your appetite.

Your psychiatric care providers will monitor your response to the treatments. This information combined with your input will be used to determine how many treatments you will receive.

Common Side Effects

Common Side Effects After Treatment

Occasionally, a patient may have a headache, muscle aches, or nausea after the treatment. These side effects can be treated with medications before or after the ECT. If you experience any of these side effects please inform

> **✤ It's A Fact!!**
>
> The use of electroconvulsive therapy (ECT) is not limited to the treatment of depression. It may also be used to stabilize bipolar illness during extreme episodes of mania or depression. Additionally, ECT can be used to halt psychotic episodes associated with schizophrenia. Once these individuals are stabilized, medications are started or resumed.

your doctor and nurse. Once the staff is aware of these side effects, measures can be taken to prevent them.

Additionally, some people may exhibit mental confusion resulting from the combination of anesthesia and/or ECT treatment. Acute confusion, if it occurs, typically lasts for 30 minutes to one hour. You are closely observed by nursing staff and doctors during this time for your safety.

Possible Memory Side Effects

Memory loss is one of the greatest concerns of people who receive ECT. Two different kinds of memory loss may occur during the course of ECT treatments. The first is the loss of short-term memory during the period of time that you are having ECT treatments. Some examples of short-term memory loss include forgetting what you had for lunch or not remembering talking to someone earlier in the day. Your ability to remember new information will generally return to your normal level within a few weeks to a few months after the treatments are finished.

The second type of memory loss that may occur involves memory loss for past events. Recent past events (two to six weeks before treatment) are more sensitive to ECT. However, some patients may describe "spotty" memory loss for events that occurred as far back as six months before beginning ECT. This memory impairment is potentially permanent. Although it is rare, some patients have reported a more severe memory loss of events which date back further than the six months preceding ECT treatments.

Safety And Other Issues

The Safety Of ECT

Any medical procedure involving anesthesia carries some risks. The potential risks include cardiac or respiratory arrest. The risk of respiratory or cardiac arrest resulting in death during ECT is negligible (less than one in 10,000 cases). This risk is typically regarded as being similar to the risks of having an outpatient surgical procedure under anesthesia. ECT treatments are extremely safe and severe medical complications are rare. You will be monitored constantly during the procedure by a team of medical professionals in the event of a complication.

Maintenance ECT

Because depression is often a relapsing illness, patients may experience repeated episodes of depression even if they respond very well to ECT. Patients often have failed numerous medications prior to ECT, and their illness may be significantly resistant medications. When repeated episodes of depression occur, your doctors may recommend a taper of ECT over a course of several weeks to months. Modern clinical practice and recent research have found that maintenance ECT is often very effective in keeping patients well. A common taper of ECT is treatments once a week for a month, once every two weeks for two months, once every three weeks for two months, and once every month for two–four months. Although there is a considerable commitment by patients and families to undergo maintenance ECT, the avoidance of lengthy re-hospitalizations and undergoing more medication trials is often worth any inconveniences.

☞ Remember!!
What To Expect After ECT

Electroconvulsive therapy (ECT) is an extremely effective treatment, but ECT treatment is only one component of a complete treatment regimen. After your ECT course, medications will likely be required as maintenance therapy to prevent a return of your illness. ECT also can not resolve other problems associated with personal relationships or how an individual copes with the stressors of life. Other interventions such as psychotherapy may be recommended. Hopefully, because you are being relieved of the severe symptoms of your illness, you will be able to participate more effectively with other therapies that are recommended.

Chapter 40

Alternative Approaches To Mental Health Care

What Are Alternative Approaches To Mental Health Care?

An alternative approach to mental health care is one that emphasizes the interrelationship between mind, body, and spirit. Although some alternative approaches have a long history, many remain controversial. The National Center for Complementary and Alternative Medicine at the National Institutes of Health was created in 1992 to help evaluate alternative methods of treatment and to integrate those that are effective into mainstream health care practice. It is crucial, however, to consult with your health care providers about the approaches you are using to achieve mental wellness.

Self-Help

Many people with mental illnesses find that self-help groups are an invaluable resource for recovery and for empowerment. Self-help generally refers to groups or meetings that have characteristics such as these:

- Involve people who have similar needs
- Are facilitated by a consumer, survivor, or other layperson

About This Chapter: This chapter includes text from "Alternative Approaches to Mental Health Care," National Mental Health Information Center, 2003. The complete text of this document is available online at http://mentalhealth.samhsa.gov/publications/allpubs/ken98-0044/default.asp; accessed April 10, 2009.

- Assist people to deal with a "life-disrupting" event, such as a death, abuse, serious accident, addiction, or diagnosis of a physical, emotional, or mental disability, for oneself or a relative
- Are operated on an informal, free-of-charge, and nonprofit basis
- Provide support and education
- Are voluntary, anonymous, and confidential

Diet And Nutrition

Adjusting both diet and nutrition may help some people with mental illnesses manage their symptoms and promote recovery. For example, research

✤ It's A Fact!!
Emotions And Health

Doctors have pondered the connection between our mental and physical health for centuries. Until the 1800s, most believed that emotions were linked to disease and advised patients to visit spas or seaside resorts when they were ill. Gradually emotions lost favor as other causes of illness (such as bacteria or toxins) emerged, and new treatments such as antibiotics cured illness after illness.

More recently, scientists have speculated that even behavioral disorders, such as autism, have a biological basis. At the same time, they have been rediscovering the links between stress and health. Today, we accept that there is a powerful mind-body connection through which emotional, mental, social, spiritual, and behavioral factors can directly affect our health.

Mind-body medicine focuses on treatments that may promote health, including relaxation, hypnosis, visual imagery, meditation, yoga, and biofeedback.

Over the past 20 years, mind-body medicine has provided evidence that psychological factors can play a major role in such illnesses as heart disease, and that mind-body techniques can aid in their treatment. Clinical trials have indicated mind-body therapies to be helpful in managing arthritis and other chronic pain conditions. There is also evidence they can help to improve psychological functioning and quality of life, and may help to ease symptoms of disease.

Source: From "The Mind-Body Connection," *MedlinePlus*, a publication of the National Institutes of Health and the Friends of the National Library of Medicine, Winter 2008.

suggests that eliminating milk and wheat products can reduce the severity of symptoms for some people who have schizophrenia and some children with autism. Similarly, some holistic/natural physicians use herbal treatments, B-complex vitamins, riboflavin, magnesium, and thiamine to treat anxiety, autism, depression, drug-induced psychoses, and hyperactivity.

Pastoral Counseling

Some people prefer to seek help for mental health problems from their pastor, rabbi, or priest, rather than from therapists who are not affiliated with a religious community. Counselors working within traditional faith communities increasingly are recognizing the need to incorporate psychotherapy and/or medication, along with prayer and spirituality, to effectively help some people with mental disorders.

Animal Assisted Therapies

Working with an animal (or animals) under the guidance of a health care professional may benefit some people with mental illness by facilitating positive changes, such as increased empathy and enhanced socialization skills. Animals can be used as part of group therapy programs to encourage communication and increase the ability to focus. Developing self-esteem and reducing loneliness and anxiety are just some potential benefits of individual-animal therapy (Delta Society, 2002).

Expressive Therapies

Art Therapy: Drawing, painting, and sculpting help many people to reconcile inner conflicts, release deeply repressed emotions, and foster self-awareness, as well as personal growth. Some mental health providers use art therapy as both a diagnostic tool and as a way to help treat disorders such as depression, abuse-related trauma, and schizophrenia. You may be able to find a therapist in your area who has received special training and certification in art therapy.

Dance/Movement Therapy: Some people find that their spirits soar when they let their feet fly. Others—particularly those who prefer more structure or who feel they have "two left feet"—gain the same sense of release and inner peace from the Eastern martial arts, such as Aikido and Tai Chi. Those who are recovering from physical, sexual, or emotional abuse may find these techniques especially helpful for gaining a sense of ease with their own bodies. The underlying premise to dance/movement therapy is that it can help a person integrate the emotional, physical, and cognitive facets of "self."

Music/Sound Therapy: It is no coincidence that many people turn on soothing music to relax or snazzy tunes to help feel upbeat. Research suggests that music stimulates the body's natural "feel good" chemicals (opiates and endorphins). This stimulation results in improved blood flow, blood pressure, pulse rate, breathing, and posture changes. Music or sound therapy has been used to treat disorders such as stress, grief, depression, schizophrenia, and autism in children, and to diagnose mental health needs.

Culturally Based Healing Arts

Traditional oriental medicine (such as acupuncture, shiatsu, and Reiki), Indian systems of health care (such as Ayurveda and yoga), and Native American healing practices (such as the sweat lodge and talking circles) all incorporate the beliefs that contain these elements:

- Wellness is a state of balance between the spiritual, physical, and mental/emotional "selves."
- An imbalance of forces within the body is the cause of illness.
- Herbal/natural remedies, combined with sound nutrition, exercise, and meditation/prayer, will correct this imbalance.

Acupuncture: The Chinese practice of inserting needles into the body at specific points manipulates the body's flow of energy to balance the endocrine system. This manipulation regulates functions such as heart rate, body temperature, and respiration, as well as sleep patterns and emotional changes. Acupuncture has been used in clinics to assist people with substance abuse disorders through detoxification; to relieve stress and anxiety; to treat attention deficit and hyperactivity disorder in children; to reduce symptoms of depression; and to help people with physical ailments.

Ayurveda: Ayurvedic medicine is described as "knowledge of how to live." It incorporates an individualized regimen—such as diet, meditation, herbal preparations, or other techniques—to treat a variety of conditions, including depression, to facilitate lifestyle changes, and to teach people how to release stress and tension through yoga or transcendental meditation.

Yoga/Meditation: Practitioners of this ancient Indian system of health care use breathing exercises, posture, stretches, and meditation to balance the body's energy centers. Yoga is used in combination with other treatment for depression, anxiety, and stress-related disorders.

Native American Traditional Practices: Ceremonial dances, chants, and cleansing rituals are part of Indian Health Service programs to heal depression, stress, trauma (including those related to physical and sexual abuse), and substance abuse.

Cuentos: Based on folktales, this form of therapy originated in Puerto Rico. The stories used contain healing themes and models of behavior such as self-transformation and endurance through adversity. Cuentos is used primarily to help Hispanic children recover from depression and other mental health problems related to leaving one's homeland and living in a foreign culture.

Relaxation And Stress Reduction Techniques

Biofeedback: Learning to control muscle tension and "involuntary" body functioning, such as heart rate and skin temperature, can be a path to mastering one's fears. It is used in combination with, or as an alternative to, medication to treat disorders such as anxiety, panic, and phobias. For example, a person can learn to "retrain" his or her breathing habits in stressful situations to induce relaxation and decrease hyperventilation. Some preliminary research indicates it may offer an additional tool for treating schizophrenia and depression.

Guided Imagery Or Visualization: This process involves going into a state of deep relaxation and creating a mental image of recovery and wellness. Physicians, nurses, and mental health providers occasionally use this approach to treat alcohol and drug addictions, depression, panic disorders, phobias, and stress.

Massage Therapy: The underlying principle of this approach is that rubbing, kneading, brushing, and tapping a person's muscles can help release tension and pent emotions. It has been used to treat trauma-related depression and stress. A highly unregulated industry, certification for massage therapy varies widely from state to state. Some states have strict guidelines, while others have none.

Technology-Based Applications

The boom in electronic tools at home and in the office makes access to mental health information just a telephone call or a "mouse click" away. Technology is also making treatment more widely available in once-isolated areas.

Telemedicine: Plugging into video and computer technology is a relatively new innovation in health care. It allows both consumers and providers in remote or rural areas to gain access to mental health or specialty expertise. Telemedicine can enable consulting providers to speak to and observe patients directly. It also can be used in education and training programs for generalist clinicians.

Telephone Counseling: Active listening skills are a hallmark of telephone counselors. These also provide information and referral to interested callers. For many people telephone counseling often is a first step to receiving in-depth mental health care. Research shows that such counseling from specially trained mental health providers reaches many people who otherwise might not get the help they need. Before calling, be sure to check the telephone number for service fees; a 900 area code means you will be billed for the call, an 800 or 888 area code means the call is toll-free.

Electronic Communications: Technologies such as the internet, bulletin boards, and electronic mail lists provide access directly to consumers and the public on a wide range of information. Online consumer groups can exchange information, experiences, and views on mental health, treatment systems, alternative medicine, and other related topics.

Radio Psychiatry: Another relative newcomer to therapy, radio psychiatry was first introduced in the United States in 1976. Radio psychiatrists and psychologists provide advice, information, and referrals in response to a variety of mental health questions from callers. The American Psychiatric Association and the American Psychological Association have issued ethical guidelines for the role of psychiatrists and psychologists on radio shows.

Chapter 41

St. John's Wort

Introduction

St. John's wort is a plant with yellow flowers that has been used for centuries for health purposes, such as for depression and anxiety. This chapter answers some frequently asked questions about St. John's wort and depression, and it summarizes what the science says about its effectiveness and the research being done.

About St. John's Wort

St. John's wort (*Hypericum perforatum*) is a long-living plant with yellow flowers whose medicinal uses were first recorded in ancient Greece. It contains many chemical compounds. Some are believed to be the active ingredients that produce the herb's effects, including the compounds hypericin and hyperforin.

How these compounds actually work is not yet fully understood, but several theories have been suggested. Preliminary studies suggest that St. John's wort might work by preventing nerve cells in the brain from reabsorbing the chemical messenger serotonin or by reducing levels of a protein involved in the body's immune system functioning.

About This Chapter: Text in this chapter is from "St. John's Wort and Depression," National Center for Complementary and Alternative Medicine (http://nccam.nih.gov), December 2007.

St. John's wort has been used over the centuries for mental conditions, nerve pain, and a wide variety of other health conditions. Today, St. John's wort is used for anxiety, mild to moderate depression, and sleep disorders.

In Europe, St. John's wort is widely prescribed for depression. In the United States, there is public interest in St. John's wort as a treatment for depression, but it is not a prescription medicine.

In the United States, St. John's wort products are sold as the following:

- Capsules And Tablets
- Teas: The dried herb is added to boiling water and steeped.
- Liquid Extracts: Specific types of chemicals are removed from the herb, leaving the desired chemicals in a concentrated form.

About Depression

Depression is a medical condition that affects nearly 21 million American adults each year, according to the National Institute of Mental Health. Mood,

✤ It's A Fact!!

- Studies suggest that St. John's wort is of minimal benefit in treating major depression. A study co-funded by the National Center for Complementary and Alternative Medicine (NCCAM) found that St. John's wort was no more effective than placebo in treating major depression of moderate severity. There is some scientific evidence that St. John's wort is useful for milder forms of depression.
- St. John's wort interacts with certain drugs, and these interactions can limit the effectiveness of some prescription medicines.
- St. John's wort is not a proven therapy for depression. If depression is not adequately treated, it can become severe and, in some cases, may be associated with suicide. Consult a health care provider if you or someone you care about may be experiencing depression.
- Tell your health care providers about any complementary and alternative practices you use. Give them a full picture of what you do to manage your health. This will help ensure coordinated and safe care.

> ✎ **What's It Mean?**
>
> Conventional Medicine: Medicine as practiced by holders of M.D. (medical doctor) or D.O. (doctor of osteopathy) degrees and by their allied health professionals such as physical therapists, psychologists, and registered nurses.
>
> Herb: A plant or part of a plant—used for its flavor, scent, or potential therapeutic properties. Includes flowers, leaves, bark, fruit, seeds, stems, and roots.

thoughts, physical health, and behavior all may be affected. Symptoms of depression commonly include the following:

- Persistent sad, anxious, or "empty" feelings
- Feelings of hopelessness and/or pessimism
- Feelings of guilt, worthlessness, and/or helplessness
- Restlessness or irritability
- Loss of interest or pleasure in activities that the person once enjoyed
- Fatigue and decreased energy
- Difficulty concentrating, remembering details, and/or making decisions
- Insomnia, early–morning wakefulness, or excessive sleeping
- Overeating, or appetite loss
- Thoughts of suicide, suicide attempts
- Persistent aches or pains, headaches, cramps, or digestive problems that do not ease with treatment

Depression comes in several forms and its symptoms and severity can vary from person to person. Here are some examples:

- In major depression (also called major depressive disorder) people experience symptoms that interfere with their ability to work, study, sleep, eat, and take pleasure in activities they once enjoyed. Symptoms last for at least two weeks but frequently last for several months or longer.
- In dysthymia (also called dysthymic disorder) a less severe, but more chronic form of depression, people experience symptoms that are not as disabling but keep them from functioning well or feeling good. Symptoms last at least two years. Many people with dysthymia also have episodes of major depression.

- In bipolar disorder (also called manic-depressive illness) people have periods of depressive symptoms that alternate or may co-exist with periods of mania. Symptoms of mania include abnormally high levels of excitement and energy, racing thoughts, and behavior that is impulsive and inappropriate.

In addition, milder forms of depression exist that fall into the category of minor depression. In minor depression, people experience the same symptoms as major depression, but they are fewer in number and are less disabling. Symptoms last at least six months but less than two years continuously.

Depression can be treated effectively with conventional medicine, including antidepressants and certain types of psychotherapy.

What The Science Says About St. John's Wort For Depression

Scientific evidence regarding the effectiveness of St. John's wort for depression is inconsistent. An analysis of the results of 37 clinical trials concluded that St. John's wort may have only minimal beneficial effects on major depression. However, the analysis also found that St. John's wort may benefit people with minor depression; these benefits may be similar to those from standard antidepressants. Overall, St. John's wort appeared to produce fewer side effects than some standard antidepressants.

One of the studies included in the analysis was co-funded by NCCAM and two other components of the National Institutes of Health (NIH)—the National Institute of Mental Health and the Office of Dietary Supplements. This study found that St. John's wort was no more effective than placebo in treating major depression of moderate severity. However, the antidepressant sertraline, used in one arm of the study, also showed little difference from placebo.

Side Effects And Risks

The most common side effects of St. John's wort include dry mouth, dizziness, diarrhea, nausea, increased sensitivity to sunlight, and fatigue.

Research has shown that taking St. John's wort can limit the effectiveness of some prescription medicines, including the following:

- Antidepressant medicines
- Birth control pills
- Cyclosporine, a medicine that helps prevent the body from rejecting transplanted organs
- Digoxin, a medicine used to strengthen heart muscle contractions
- Indinavir and other medicines used to control HIV infection
- Irinotecan and other anticancer medicines
- Warfarin and related medicines used to thin the blood (known as anticoagulants)
- When combined with certain antidepressants, St. John's wort also may increase side effects such as nausea, anxiety, headache, and confusion

Herbal Products: Issues To Consider

Herbal products such as St. John's wort are classified as dietary supplements by the U.S. Food and Drug Administration (FDA). The FDA's requirements for testing and obtaining approval to sell dietary supplements are different from its requirements for drugs. Unlike drugs, herbal products can be sold without requiring studies on dosage, safety, or effectiveness.

The strength and quality of herbal products are often unpredictable. Products can differ in content not only from brand to brand, but from batch to batch. Information on labels may be misleading or inaccurate.

In addition, "natural" does not necessarily mean "safe." Many natural substances can have harmful effects—especially if they are taken in large quantities or if they interact with other supplements or with prescription medicines.

Tell your health care providers about any complementary and alternative practices you use. Give them a full picture of what you do to manage your health. This will help ensure coordinated and safe care.

Chapter 42

Meditation

Introduction

Meditation is a mind-body practice in complementary and alternative medicine (CAM). There are many types of meditation, most of which originated in ancient religious and spiritual traditions. Generally, a person who is meditating uses certain techniques, such as a specific posture, focused attention, and an open attitude toward distractions. Meditation may be practiced for many reasons, such as to increase calmness and physical relaxation, to improve psychological balance, to cope with illness, or to enhance overall wellness.

Overview

The term meditation refers to a group of techniques, such as mantra meditation, relaxation response, mindfulness meditation, and Zen Buddhist meditation. Most meditative techniques started in Eastern religious or spiritual traditions. These techniques have been used by many different cultures throughout the world for thousands of years. Today, many people use meditation outside of its traditional religious or cultural settings, for health and wellness purposes.

About This Chapter: Text in this chapter is from "Meditation: An Introduction," National Center for Complementary and Alternative Medicine (http://nccam.nih.gov), February 2009.

In meditation, a person learns to focus attention. Some forms of meditation instruct the practitioner to become mindful of thoughts, feelings, and sensations and to observe them in a nonjudgmental way. This practice is believed to result in a state of greater calmness and physical relaxation, and psychological balance. Practicing meditation can change how a person relates to the flow of emotions and thoughts in the mind.

Most types of meditation have four elements in common:

- **A Quiet Location:** Meditation is usually practiced in a quiet place with as few distractions as possible. This can be particularly helpful for beginners.
- **A Specific, Comfortable Posture:** Depending on the type being practiced, meditation can be done while sitting, lying down, standing, walking, or in other positions.
- **A Focus Of Attention:** Focusing one's attention is usually a part of meditation. For example, the meditator may focus on a mantra (a specially chosen word or set of words), an object, or the sensations of the breath. Some forms of meditation involve paying attention to whatever is the dominant content of consciousness.
- **An Open Attitude:** Having an open attitude during meditation means letting distractions come and go naturally without judging them. When the attention goes to distracting or wandering thoughts, they are not suppressed; instead, the meditator gently brings attention back to the

✤ It's A Fact!!

- People practice meditation for a number of health-related purposes.
- It is not fully known what changes occur in the body during meditation; whether they influence health; and, if so, how. Research is under way to find out more about meditation's effects, how it works, and diseases and conditions for which it may be most helpful.
- Tell your health care providers about any complementary and alternative practices you use. Give them a full picture of what you do to manage your health. This will help ensure coordinated and safe care.

focus. In some types of meditation, the meditator learns to "observe" thoughts and emotions while meditating.

Meditation used as CAM is a type of mind-body medicine. Generally, mind-body medicine focuses on these two elements:

- The interactions among the brain/mind, the rest of the body, and behavior
- The ways in which emotional, mental, social, spiritual, and behavioral factors can directly affect health

Uses Of Meditation For Health In The United States

A 2007 national government survey that asked about CAM use in a sample of 23,393 U.S. adults found that 9.4 percent of respondents (representing more than 20 million people) had used meditation in the past 12 months—compared with 7.6 percent of respondents (representing more than 15 million people) in a similar survey conducted in 2002. The 2007 survey also asked about CAM use in a sample of 9,417 children; 1 percent (representing 725,000 children) had used meditation in the past 12 months.

People use meditation for various health problems, including the following:

- Anxiety
- Pain
- Depression
- Stress
- Insomnia
- Physical or emotional symptoms that may be associated with chronic illnesses (such as heart disease, HIV/AIDS, and cancer) and their treatment.

Meditation is also used for overall wellness.

Examples Of Meditation Practices

Mindfulness meditation and transcendental meditation (also known as TM) are two common forms of meditation. National Center for Complementary and Alternative Medicine (NCCAM)-sponsored research projects are studying both of these types of meditation.

Mindfulness meditation is an essential component of Buddhism. In one common form of mindfulness meditation, the meditator is taught to bring attention to the sensation of the flow of the breath in and out of the body. The meditator learns to focus attention on what is being experienced, without reacting to or judging that experience. This is seen as helping the meditator learn to experience thoughts and emotions in normal daily life with greater balance and acceptance.

The TM technique is derived from Hindu traditions. It uses a mantra (a word, sound, or phrase repeated silently) to prevent distracting thoughts from entering the mind. The goal of TM is to achieve a state of relaxed awareness.

How Meditation Might Work

Practicing meditation has been shown to induce some changes in the body. By learning more about what goes on in the body during meditation, researchers hope to be able to identify diseases or conditions for which meditation might be useful.

Some types of meditation might work by affecting the autonomic (involuntary) nervous system. This system regulates many organs and muscles, controlling functions such as the heartbeat, sweating, breathing, and digestion. It has two major parts:

- **The Sympathetic Nervous System:** Helps mobilize the body for action. When a person is under stress, it produces the "fight-or-flight response": the heart rate and breathing rate go up and blood vessels narrow (restricting the flow of blood).
- **The Parasympathetic Nervous System:** Causes the heart rate and breathing rate to slow down, the blood vessels to dilate (improving blood flow), and digestive juices to increase.

It is thought that some types of meditation might work by reducing activity in the sympathetic nervous system and increasing activity in the parasympathetic nervous system.

In one area of research, scientists are using sophisticated tools to determine whether meditation is associated with significant changes in brain function. A number of researchers believe that these changes account for many of meditation's effects.

It is also possible that practicing meditation may work by improving the mind's ability to pay attention. Since attention is involved in performing everyday tasks and regulating mood, meditation might lead to other benefits.

A 2007 NCCAM-funded review of the scientific literature found some evidence suggesting that meditation is associated with potentially beneficial health effects. However, the overall evidence was inconclusive. The reviewers concluded that future research needs to be more rigorous before firm conclusions can be drawn.

Side Effects And Risks

Meditation is considered to be safe for healthy people. There have been rare reports that meditation could cause or worsen symptoms in people who

✔ Quick Tip

If you are thinking about using meditation practices, consider these suggestions:

- Do not use meditation as a replacement for conventional care or as a reason to postpone seeing a doctor about a medical problem.
- Ask about the training and experience of the meditation instructor you are considering.
- Look for published research studies on meditation for the health condition in which you are interested.
- Tell your health care providers about any complementary and alternative practices you use. Give them a full picture of what you do to manage your health. This will help ensure coordinated and safe care.

have certain psychiatric problems, but this question has not been fully researched. People with physical limitations may not be able to participate in certain meditative practices involving physical movement. Individuals with existing mental or physical health conditions should speak with their health care providers prior to starting a meditative practice and make their meditation instructor aware of their condition.

NCCAM-Supported Research

Some recent NCCAM-supported studies have been investigating meditation for these kinds of concerns:

- Relieving stress in caregivers for elderly patients with dementia
- Reducing the frequency and intensity of hot flashes in menopausal women
- Relieving symptoms of chronic back pain
- Improving attention-related abilities (alerting, focusing, and prioritizing)
- Relieving asthma symptoms.

Part Five

Other Issues Related To Mental Health In Teens

Chapter 43

Abuse And Neglect

What Is Abuse?

Amy's finger was so swollen that she couldn't get her ring off. She didn't think her finger was broken because she could still bend it. It had been a week since her dad shoved her into the wall, but her finger still hurt a lot.

Amy hated the way her dad called her names and accused her of all sorts of things she didn't do, especially after he had been drinking. It was the worst feeling and she just kept hoping he would stop.

Abuse can be physical, sexual, emotional, verbal, or a combination of any or all of those. Neglect—when parents or guardians don't take care of the basic needs of the children who depend on them—can also be a form of abuse.

Family violence can affect anyone. It can happen in any kind of family. Sometimes parents abuse each other, which can be hard for a child to witness. Some parents abuse their kids by using physical or verbal cruelty as a way of discipline.

About This Chapter: Text in this chapter is from "Abuse," November 2007, reprinted with permission from www.kidshealth.org. This information was provided by KidsHealth, one of the largest resources online for medically reviewed health information written for parents, kids, and teens. For more articles like this one, visit www.KidsHealth.org, or www.TeensHealth.org.

✎ What's It Mean?

Physical abuse is often the most easily spotted form of abuse. It may be any kind of hitting, shaking, burning, pinching, biting, choking, throwing, beating, and other actions that cause physical injury, leave marks, or produce significant physical pain.

Sexual abuse is any type of sexual contact between an adult and anyone younger than 18, or between a significantly older child and a younger child. If a family member sexually abuses another family member, this is called incest.

Emotional abuse can be difficult to pin down because there may not be physical signs. Emotional abuse happens when yelling and anger go too far or when parents constantly criticize, threaten, or dismiss kids or teens until their self-esteem and feelings of self-worth are damaged. Emotional abuse can hurt and cause damage just as physical abuse does.

Neglect is probably the hardest type of abuse to define. Neglect occurs when a child or teen doesn't have adequate food, housing, clothes, medical care, or supervision. Emotional neglect happens when a parent doesn't provide enough emotional support or deliberately and consistently pays very little or no attention to a child. But it's not neglect if a parent doesn't give a kid something he or she wants, like a new computer or a cell phone.

Abuse doesn't just happen in families, of course. Bullying is a form of abusive behavior. Bullying someone through intimidation, threats, or humiliation can be just as abusive as beating someone up. People who bully others may have been abused themselves. This is also true of people who abuse someone they're dating. But being abused is no excuse for abusing someone else.

Abuse can also take the form of hate crimes directed at people just because of their race, religion, abilities, gender, or sexual orientation.

Recognizing Abuse

It may sound strange, but people sometimes have trouble recognizing that they are being abused. Recognizing abuse may be especially difficult for someone who has lived with it for many years. A person might think that it's just the way things are and that there's nothing that can be done. People who are abused might mistakenly think they bring it on themselves by not acting right or by not living up to someone's expectations.

Someone growing up in a family where there is violence or abuse may not know that there are other ways for family members to treat each other. A person who has only known an abusive relationship may mistakenly think that hitting, beating, pushing, shoving, or angry name-calling are perfectly normal ways to treat someone when you're mad. Seeing parents treat each other in abusive ways might lead a child to think that's a normal relationship. But abuse is not a normal or healthy way to treat people.

If you're not sure you are being abused, or if you suspect a friend is, it's always OK to ask a trusted adult or friend.

Why Does It Happen?

If you're one of the thousands of people living in an abusive situation, it can help to understand why some people abuse—and to realize that the violence is not your fault. Sometimes abusers manipulate the people they are abusing by telling them they did something wrong or "asked for it" in some way. But that's not true.

There is no single reason why people abuse others. But some factors seem to make it more likely that a person may become abusive.

Growing up in an abusive family is one factor. Other people become abusive because they're not able to manage their feelings properly. For example, someone who is unable to control anger or can't cope with stressful personal situations (like the loss of a job or marriage problems) may lash out at others inappropriately. Alcohol or drug use also can make it difficult for some people to control their actions.

Certain types of personality disorders or mental illness might also interfere with a person's ability to relate to others in healthy ways or cause people to have problems with aggression or self-control. Of course, not everyone with a personality disorder or mental illness becomes abusive.

Fortunately, abuse can always be corrected. Everyone can learn how to stop.

What Are The Effects Of Abuse?

When people are abused, it can affect every aspect of their lives, especially self-esteem. How much abuse harms a person depends on the situation and sometimes on how severe the abuse is. Sometimes a seemingly minor thing can trigger a big reaction. Being touched inappropriately by a family member, for example, can be very confusing and traumatic.

Every family has arguments. In fact, it's rare when a family doesn't have some rough times, disagreements, and anger. Punishments and discipline—like removing privileges, grounding, or being sent to your room—are normal. Yelling and anger are normal in parent–teen relationships too—although it can feel pretty bad to have an argument with a parent or friend. But if punishments, arguments, or yelling go too far or last too long it can lead to stress and other serious problems.

Teens who are abused (or have been in the past) often have trouble sleeping, eating, and concentrating. They may not do well at school because they are angry or frightened, or because they can't concentrate or don't care.

Many people who are abused distrust others. They may feel a lot of anger toward other people and themselves, and it can be hard to make friends. Abuse is a significant cause of depression in young people. Some teens may engage in self-destructive behavior, such as cutting or abusing drugs or alcohol. They may even attempt suicide.

It's normal for people who have been abused to feel upset, angry, and confused about what happened to them. They may feel guilty and embarrassed and blame themselves. But abuse is never the fault of the person who is being abused, no matter how much the abuser tries to blame others.

Abusers may manipulate a person into keeping quiet by saying stuff like: "This is a secret between you and me," or "If you ever tell anybody, I'll hurt you or your mom," or "You're going to get in trouble if you tell. No one will believe you and you'll go to jail for lying." This is the abuser's way of making a person feel like nothing can be done so he or she won't report the abuse.

People who are abused may have trouble getting help because it means they'd be reporting on someone they love—someone who may be wonderful much of the time and awful to them only some of the time. A person might be afraid of the consequences of reporting, either because they fear the abuser or the family is financially dependent on that person. For reasons like these, abuse often goes unreported.

What Should Someone Who's Being Abused Do?

People who are being abused need to get help. Keeping the abuse a secret doesn't protect anyone from being abused—it only makes it more likely that the abuse will continue.

If you or anyone you know is being abused, talk to someone you or your friend can trust—a family member, a trusted teacher, a doctor, or a school or religious youth counselor. Many teachers and counselors have training in how to recognize and report abuse.

Telephone directories list local child abuse and family violence hotline numbers that you can call for help. There's also Childhelp USA at (800) 4-A-CHILD ([800] 422-4453).

Sometimes people who are being abused by someone in their own home need to find a safe place to live temporarily. It is never easy to have to leave home, but it's sometimes necessary to be protected from further abuse. People who need to leave home to stay safe can find local shelters listed in the phone book or they can contact an abuse helpline. Sometimes a person can stay with a relative or friend.

People who are being abused often feel afraid, numb, or lonely. Getting help and support is an important first step toward changing the situation.

Many teens who have experienced abuse find that painful emotions may linger even after the abuse stops. Working with a therapist is one way to sort through the complicated feelings and reactions that being abused creates, and the process can help to rebuild feelings of safety, confidence, and self-esteem.

Chapter 44

Addiction

The brain is the command center of your body. It weighs about three pounds, and has different centers or systems that process different kinds of information.

The brain stem is the most primitive structure at the base of your brain. The brain stem controls your heart rate, breathing, and sleeping; it does the things you never think about.

Various parts or lobes of the brain process information from your sense organs: the occipital lobe receives information from your eyes, for example. And the cerebral cortex, on top of the whole brain, is the "thinking" part of you. That's where you store and process language, math, and strategies: It's the thinking center. Buried deep within the cerebral cortex is the limbic system, which is responsible for survival: It remembers and creates an appetite for the things that keep you alive, such as good food and the company of other human beings.

The cerebellum is responsible for things you learn once and never have to think about, such as balance when walking or how to throw a ball.

About This Chapter: Text in this chapter is from "Brain and Addiction," an undated document produced by the National Institute on Drug Abuse, accessed April 13, 2009. Reviewed for currency by David A. Cooke, MD, FACP, October 2009. The complete text of this document, including references, can be found online at http://teens.drugabuse.gov/facts/facts_brain1.php.

How does your brain communicate?

The brain's job is to process information. Brain cells called neurons receive and send messages to and from other neurons. There are billions of neurons in the human brain, each with as many as a thousand threadlike branches that reach out to other neurons.

In a neuron, a message is an electrical impulse. The electrical message travels along the sending branch, or axon, of the neuron. When the message reaches the end of the axon, it causes the release of a chemical called a neurotransmitter. The chemical travels across a tiny gap, or synapse, to other neurons.

Specialized molecules called receptors on the receiving neuron pick up the chemical. The branches on the receiving end of a neuron are called dendrites. Receptors there have special shapes so they can only collect one kind of neurotransmitter.

✤ It's A Fact!!

People with manic symptoms and bipolar disorder type II are at significant risk of later developing an alcohol abuse or dependence problem, a long-term study conducted in Switzerland confirms. The study was published in the January 2008 issue of the *Archives of General Psychiatry.*

Kathleen Merikangas, Ph.D., of the National Institute of Mental Health (NIMH) Mood and Anxiety Disorders Program and colleagues found that people who showed symptoms of mania, but who did not meet criteria for bipolar disorder, were at significantly greater risk for later developing an alcohol abuse or dependence problem. Those with bipolar disorder II were even more at risk of developing an alcohol problem or benzodiazepine abuse problem. Major depression was associated only with developing a benzodiazepine abuse problem among this population.

Source: Excerpted from "Mood Disorders Predict Later Substance Abuse Problems," a Science Update from the National Institute of Mental Health, January 9, 2008.

In the dendrite, the neurotransmitter starts an electrical impulse. Its work done, the chemical is released back into the synapse. The neurotransmitter then is broken down or is reabsorbed into the sending neuron.

Neurons in your brain release many different neurotransmitters as you go about your day thinking, feeling, reacting, breathing, and digesting. When you learn new information or a new skill, your brain builds more axons and dendrites first, as a tree grows roots and branches. With more branches, neurons can communicate and send their messages more efficiently.

What do drugs do to the brain?

Some drugs work in the brain because they have a similar size and shape as natural neurotransmitters. In the brain in the right amount or dose, these drugs lock into receptors and start an unnatural chain reaction of electrical charges, causing neurons to release large amounts of their own neurotransmitter.

Some drugs lock onto the neuron and act like a pump, so the neuron releases more neurotransmitter. Other drugs block reabsorption or reuptake and cause unnatural floods of neurotransmitter.

All drugs of abuse, such as nicotine, cocaine, and marijuana, primarily affect the brain's limbic system. Scientists call this the "reward" system. Normally, the limbic system responds to pleasurable experiences by releasing the neurotransmitter dopamine, which creates feelings of pleasure.

What is drug addiction?

Drug addiction is a complex brain disease. It is characterized by compulsive, at times uncontrollable, drug craving, seeking, and use that persist even in the face of extremely negative consequences. Drug seeking becomes compulsive, in large part as a result of the effects of prolonged drug use on brain functioning and on behavior. For many people, drug addiction becomes chronic, with relapses possible even after long periods of abstinence.

How quickly can I become addicted to a drug?

There is no easy answer to this. If and how quickly you might become addicted to a drug depends on many factors including your genes (which you inherit from your parents) and the biology of your body. All drugs are potentially harmful and may have life-threatening consequences associated with their use. There are also vast differences among individuals in sensitivity to various drugs. While one person may use a drug one or many times and suffer no ill effects, another person may be particularly vulnerable and overdose with first use. There is no way of knowing in advance how someone may react.

How do I know if someone is addicted to drugs?

If a person is compulsively seeking and using a drug despite negative consequences, such as loss of job, debt, physical or mental problems brought on by drug abuse, or family problems, then he or she is probably addicted. We don't have a perfect screening tool quite yet, but health care professionals who screen for drug use often ask questions like these to detect substance abuse in their adolescent patients:

- Have you ever ridden in a car driven by someone (including yourself) who had been using alcohol or drugs?
- Do you ever use alcohol or drugs to relax, feel better about yourself, or fit in?

✎ What's It Mean?

What are dual diagnosis services?

Dual diagnosis services are treatments for people who suffer from co-occurring disorders—mental illness and substance abuse. Research has strongly indicated that to recover fully, a consumer with co-occurring disorder needs treatment for both problems—focusing on one does not ensure the other will go away. Dual diagnosis services integrate assistance for each condition, helping people recover from both in one setting, at the same time.

Dual diagnosis services include different types of assistance that go beyond standard therapy or medication: assertive outreach, job and housing assistance, family counseling, even money and relationship management. The personalized treatment is viewed as long-term and can be begun at whatever stage of recovery the consumer is in. Positivity, hope and optimism are at the foundation of integrated treatment.

Source: Excerpted from "Dual Diagnosis and Integrated Treatment of Mental Illness and Substance Abuse Disorder," © 2003 NAMI: The Nation's Voice on Mental Illness (www.nami.org). Reprinted with permission. Reviewed for currency by David A. Cooke, MD, FACP, October 2009.

- Do you ever use alcohol or drugs when you are alone?
- Do you ever forget things you did while using alcohol or drugs?
- Do your family or friends ever tell you to cut down on your drinking or drug use?
- Have you ever gotten into trouble while you were using alcohol or drugs?

What are the physical signs of abuse or addiction?

The physical signs of abuse or addiction can vary depending on the person and the drug being abused. In addition, each drug has short-term and long-term physical effects. For example, someone who abuses marijuana may have a chronic cough or worsening of asthmatic conditions. Stimulants like cocaine increase heart rate and blood pressure, whereas opioids like heroin may slow the heart rate and reduce respiration.

Are there effective treatments for drug addiction?

Drug addiction can be effectively treated with behavioral-based therapies and, for addiction to some drugs such as heroin or nicotine, medications. Treatment may vary for each person depending on the type of drug(s) being used and the individual's specific circumstances. In many cases, multiple courses of treatment may be needed to achieve success.

Isn't drug addiction a voluntary behavior?

A person may start out taking drugs voluntarily. But as times passes, and drug use continues something happens that makes a person go from being a voluntary drug user to a compulsive drug user. Why? Because the continued use of addictive drugs changes your brain—at times in dramatic, toxic ways, at others in more subtle ways, but often in ways that result in compulsive and even uncontrollable drug use.

Isn't becoming addicted to a drug just a character flaw?

Drug addiction is a brain disease. Every type of drug of abuse has its own individual mechanism for changing how the brain functions. But regardless of which drug a person is addicted to, many of the effects it has on the brain are similar: they range from changes in the molecules and cells that make up the brain, to mood changes, to changes in memory processes and thinking, and sometimes changes in motor skills such as walking and talking. And these changes have a huge influence on all aspects of a person's behavior. A drug can become the single most powerful motivator in a drug abuser's existence. He or she will do almost anything for the drug. This comes about because drug use has changed the individual's brain, their behavior, their social and other functioning in critical ways.

For drug treatment to work, doesn't the person have to really want it?

Two of the primary reasons people seek drug treatment are because the court ordered them to do so or because loved ones urged them to seek treatment. Many scientific studies have shown convincingly that those who enter drug treatment programs in which they face "high pressure" to confront and attempt to surmount their addiction can benefit from treatment, regardless of the reason they sought treatment in the first place.

Shouldn't treatment for drug addiction be a one-shot deal?

Like many other illnesses, drug addiction typically is a chronic disorder. To be sure, some people can quit drug use "cold turkey," or they can quit after receiving treatment just one time at a rehabilitation facility. But most of those who abuse drugs require longer-term treatment and, in many instances, repeated treatments.

There is no "one size fits all" form of drug treatment, much less a magic bullet that suddenly will cure addiction. Different people have different drug abuse-related problems. And they respond very differently to similar forms of treatment, even when they're abusing the same drug. As a result, drug addicts need an array of treatments and services tailored to address their unique needs.

Chapter 45

Attention Deficit Hyperactivity Disorder

What is attention deficit hyperactivity disorder?

Attention deficit hyperactivity disorder (ADHD) is one of the most common childhood disorders and can continue through adolescence and adulthood. Symptoms include difficulty staying focused and paying attention, difficulty controlling behavior, and hyperactivity.

ADHD has three subtypes:

- **Predominantly Hyperactive-Impulsive:** Most symptoms are in the hyperactivity-impulsivity categories. Fewer than six symptoms of inattention are present, although inattention may still be present to some degree.
- **Predominantly Inattentive:** The majority of symptoms are in the inattention category and fewer than six symptoms of hyperactivity-impulsivity are present, although hyperactivity-impulsivity may still be present to some degree. Children with this subtype are less likely to act out or have difficulties getting along with other children. They may sit quietly, but they are not paying attention to what they are doing. Therefore, the child may be overlooked, and parents and teachers may not notice that he or she has ADHD.

About This Chapter: Text in this chapter is excerpted from "Attention Deficit Hyperactivity Disorder (ADHD)," National Institute of Mental Health (www.nimh.nih.gov), January 22, 2009.

- **Combined Hyperactive-Impulsive And Inattentive:** Six or more symptoms of inattention and six or more symptoms of hyperactivity-impulsivity are present. Most children have the combined type of ADHD.

Treatments can relieve many of the disorder's symptoms, but there is no cure. With treatment, most people with ADHD can be successful in school and lead productive lives.

What are the symptoms of ADHD in children?

Inattention, hyperactivity, and impulsivity are the key behaviors of ADHD. It is normal for all children to be inattentive, hyperactive, or impulsive sometimes, but for children with ADHD, these behaviors are more severe and occur more often. To be diagnosed with the disorder, a child must have symptoms for six or more months and to a degree that is greater than other children of the same age.

Children who have symptoms of inattention may display these tendencies:

- Be easily distracted, miss details, forget things, and frequently switch from one activity to another
- Have difficulty focusing on one thing
- Become bored with a task after only a few minutes, unless they are doing something enjoyable
- Have difficulty focusing attention on organizing and completing a task or learning something new
- Have trouble completing or turning in homework assignments, often losing things (for example, pencils, toys, assignments) needed to complete tasks or activities
- Not seem to listen when spoken to
- Daydream, become easily confused, and move slowly
- Have difficulty processing information as quickly and accurately as others
- Struggle to follow instructions

Children who have symptoms of hyperactivity may display these tendencies:

- Fidget and squirm in their seats
- Talk nonstop
- Dash around, touching or playing with anything and everything in sight
- Have trouble sitting still during dinner, school, and story time
- Be constantly in motion
- Have difficulty doing quiet tasks or activities

Children who have symptoms of impulsivity may display these tendencies:

- Be very impatient
- Blurt out inappropriate comments, show their emotions without restraint, and act without regard for consequences
- Have difficulty waiting for things they want or waiting their turns in games
- Often interrupt conversations or others' activities

✤ It's A Fact!!

ADHD Can Be Mistaken For Other Problems

Parents and teachers can miss the fact that children with symptoms of inattention have the disorder because they are often quiet and less likely to act out. They may sit quietly, seeming to work, but they are often not paying attention to what they are doing. They may get along well with other children, compared with those with the other subtypes, who tend to have social problems. But children with the inattentive kind of ADHD are not the only ones whose disorders can be missed. For example, adults may think that children with the hyperactive and impulsive subtypes just have emotional or disciplinary problems.

What causes ADHD?

Scientists are not sure what causes ADHD, although many studies suggest that genes play a large role. Like many other illnesses, ADHD probably results from a combination of factors. In addition to genetics, researchers are looking at possible environmental factors, and are studying how brain injuries, nutrition, and the social environment might contribute to ADHD.

Genes: Inherited from our parents, genes are the "blueprints" for who we are. Results from several international studies of twins show that ADHD often runs in families. Researchers are looking at several genes that may make people more likely to develop the disorder. Knowing the genes involved may one day help researchers prevent the disorder before symptoms develop. Learning about specific genes could also lead to better treatments.

Children with ADHD who carry a particular version of a certain gene have thinner brain tissue in the areas of the brain associated with attention. This National Institute of Mental Health (NIMH) research showed that the difference was not permanent, however, and as children with this gene grew up, the brain developed to a normal level of thickness. Their ADHD symptoms also improved.

Environmental Factors: Studies suggest a potential link between cigarette smoking and alcohol use during pregnancy and ADHD in children. In addition, preschoolers who are exposed to high levels of lead, which can sometimes be found in plumbing fixtures or paint in old buildings, may have a higher risk of developing ADHD.

✤ It's A Fact!!

In their first few years of driving, teens with ADHD are involved in nearly four times as many car accidents as those who do not have ADHD. They are also more likely to cause injury in accidents, and they get three times as many speeding tickets as their peers.

Most states now use a graduated licensing system, in which young drivers, both with and without ADHD, learn about progressively more challenging driving situations. Teens, especially those with ADHD, need to understand and follow the rules of the road. Repeated driving practice under adult supervision is especially important for teens with ADHD.

Brain Injuries: Children who have suffered a brain injury may show some behaviors similar to those of ADHD. However, only a small percentage of children with ADHD have suffered a traumatic brain injury.

Sugar: The idea that refined sugar causes ADHD or makes symptoms worse is popular, but more research discounts this theory than supports it. In one study, researchers gave children foods containing either sugar or a sugar substitute every other day. The children who received sugar showed no different behavior or learning capabilities than those who received the sugar substitute. Another study in which children were given higher than average amounts of sugar or sugar substitutes showed similar results.

Food Additives: Recent British research indicates a possible link between consumption of certain food additives like artificial colors or preservatives, and an increase in activity. Research is under way to confirm the findings and to learn more about how food additives may affect hyperactivity.

How is ADHD diagnosed?

Children mature at different rates and have different personalities, temperaments, and energy levels. Most children get distracted, act impulsively, and struggle to concentrate at one time or another. Sometimes, these normal factors may be mistaken for ADHD. ADHD symptoms usually appear early in life, often between the ages of three and six, and because symptoms vary from person to person, the disorder can be hard to diagnose. Parents may first notice that their child loses interest in things sooner than other children, or seems constantly "out of control." Often, teachers notice the symptoms first, when a child has trouble following rules, or frequently "spaces out" in the classroom or on the playground.

No single test can diagnose a child as having ADHD. Instead, a licensed health professional needs to gather information about the child, and his or her behavior and environment. A family may want to first talk with the child's pediatrician. Some pediatricians can assess the child themselves, but many will refer the family to a mental health specialist with experience in childhood mental disorders such as ADHD. The pediatrician or mental health specialist will first try to rule out other possibilities for the symptoms. For example, certain situations, events, or health conditions may cause temporary behaviors in a child that seem like ADHD.

A specialist will also check school and medical records for clues, to see if the child's home or school settings appear unusually stressful or disrupted, and gather information from the child's parents and teachers. Coaches, babysitters, and other adults who know the child well also may be consulted.

The specialist would pay close attention to the child's behavior during different situations, some highly structured, some less structured. Others would require the child to keep paying attention. Most children with ADHD are better able to control their behaviors in situations where they are getting individual attention and when they are free to focus on enjoyable activities. These types of situations are less important in the assessment. A child also may be evaluated to see how he or she acts in social situations and may be given tests of intellectual ability and academic achievement to see if he or she has a learning disability.

If after gathering all this information the child meets the criteria for ADHD, he or she will be diagnosed with the disorder.

How is ADHD treated?

Currently available treatments focus on reducing the symptoms of ADHD and improving functioning. Treatments include medication, various types of psychotherapy, education or training, or a combination of treatments.

Medications: The most common type of medication used for treating ADHD is called a "stimulant." Although it may seem unusual to treat ADHD with a medication considered a stimulant, it actually has a calming effect on children with ADHD. Many types of stimulant medications are available. A few other ADHD medications are non-stimulants and work differently than stimulants. For many children, ADHD medications reduce hyperactivity and impulsivity and improve their ability to focus, work, and learn. Medication also may improve physical coordination.

However, a one-size-fits-all approach does not apply for all children with ADHD. What works for one child might not work for another. One child might have side effects with a certain medication, while another child may not. Sometimes several different medications or dosages must be tried before finding one that works for a particular child. Any child taking medications must be monitored closely and carefully by caregivers and doctors.

Stimulant medications come in different forms, such as a pill, capsule, liquid, or skin patch. Some medications also come in short-acting, long-acting, or extended release varieties. In each of these varieties, the active ingredient is the same, but it is released differently in the body. The long-acting and extended release forms often allow a child to take the medication just once a day before school, so they don't have to make a daily trip to the school nurse for another dose. Parents and doctors should decide together which medication is best for the child and whether the child needs medication only for school hours or for evenings and weekends, too.

ADHD can be diagnosed and medications prescribed by medical doctors (usually a psychiatrist) and in some states also by clinical psychologists, psychiatric nurse practitioners, and advanced psychiatric nurse specialists.

What are the side effects of stimulant medications?

The most commonly reported side effects are decreased appetite, sleep problems, anxiety, and irritability. Some children also report mild stomachaches or headaches. Most side effects are minor and disappear over time or if the dosage level is lowered.

Less common side effects include sudden, repetitive movements or sounds called tics and personality change, such as appearing "flat" or without emotion. Talk with your doctor if you experience any of these side effects.

Do medications cure ADHD?

Current medications do not cure ADHD. Rather, they control the symptoms for as long as they are taken. Medications can help a child pay attention and complete schoolwork. It is not clear, however, whether medications can help children learn or improve their academic skills. Adding behavioral therapy, counseling, and practical support can help children with ADHD and their families to better cope with everyday problems. Research funded by the National Institute of Mental Health (NIMH) has shown that medication works best when treatment is regularly monitored by the prescribing doctor and the dose is adjusted based on the child's needs.

How is psychotherapy used to treat ADHD?

Different types of psychotherapy are used for ADHD. Behavioral therapy aims to help a child change his or her behavior. It might involve practical assistance, such as help organizing tasks or completing schoolwork, or working

✔ Quick Tip

Here are some tips to help kids stay organized and follow directions.

Schedule: Keep the same routine every day, from wake-up time to bedtime. Include time for homework, outdoor play, and indoor activities. Keep the schedule on the refrigerator or on a bulletin board in the kitchen. Write changes on the schedule as far in advance as possible.

Organize Everyday Items: Have a place for everything, and keep everything in its place. This includes clothing, backpacks, and toys.

Use Homework And Notebook Organizers: Use organizers for school material and supplies. Stress to your child the importance of writing down assignments and bringing home the necessary books.

through emotionally difficult events. Behavioral therapy also teaches a child how to monitor his or her own behavior. Learning to give oneself praise or rewards for acting in a desired way, such as controlling anger or thinking before acting, is another goal of behavioral therapy. Parents and teachers also can give positive or negative feedback for certain behaviors. In addition, clear rules, chore lists, and other structured routines can help a child control his or her behavior.

Therapists may teach children social skills, such as how to wait their turn, share toys, ask for help, or respond to teasing. Learning to read facial expressions and the tone of voice in others, and how to respond appropriately can also be part of social skills training.

Chapter 46

Autism Spectrum Disorders

Introduction

All autism spectrum disorders (ASD) are characterized by varying degrees of impairment in communication skills, social interactions, and restricted, repetitive and stereotyped patterns of behavior.

The autism spectrum disorders can often be reliably detected by the age of three years and in some cases as early as 18 months. Studies suggest that many children eventually may be accurately identified by the age of one year or even younger. The appearance of any of the warning signs of ASD is reason to have a child evaluated by a professional specializing in these disorders.

Parents are usually the first to notice unusual behaviors in their child. In some cases, the baby seemed different from birth, unresponsive to people or focusing intently on one item for long periods of time. The first signs of an ASD can also appear in children who seem to have been developing normally. When an engaging, babbling toddler suddenly becomes silent, withdrawn, self-abusive, or indifferent to social overtures, something is wrong.

The pervasive developmental disorders, or autism spectrum disorders, range from a severe form, called autistic disorder, to a milder form, Asperger

About This Chapter: Text in this chapter is excerpted from "Autism Spectrum Disorders (Pervasive Developmental Disorders)," National Institute of Mental Health, February 5, 2009.

syndrome. If a child has symptoms of either of these disorders, but does not meet the specific criteria for either, the diagnosis is called pervasive developmental disorder not otherwise specified (PDD-NOS). Other rare, very severe disorders that are included in the autism spectrum disorders are Rett syndrome and childhood disintegrative disorder.

Rare Autism Spectrum Disorders

Rett Syndrome: Rett syndrome is relatively rare, affecting almost exclusively females, one out of 10,000 to 15,000. After a period of normal development, sometime between six and 18 months, autism-like symptoms begin to appear. The little girl's mental and social development regresses—she no longer responds to her parents and pulls away from any social contact. If she has been talking, she stops; she cannot control her feet; she wrings her hands. Some of the problems associated with Rett syndrome can be treated. Physical, occupational, and speech therapy can help with problems of coordination, movement, and speech.

Childhood Disintegrative Disorder: Very few children who have an autism spectrum disorder (ASD) diagnosis meet the criteria for childhood disintegrative disorder (CDD).

✤ It's A Fact!! Is autism related to vaccinations?

The Institute of Medicine (IOM) conducted a thorough review on the issue of a link between thimerosal (a mercury based preservative that is no longer used in vaccinations) and autism. The final report from IOM, "Immunization Safety Review: Vaccines and Autism," released in May 2004, stated that the committee did not find a link.

Until 1999, vaccines given to infants to protect them against diphtheria, tetanus, pertussis, *Haemophilus influenzae* type b (Hib), and hepatitis B contained thimerosal as a preservative. Today, with the exception of some flu vaccines, none of the vaccines used in the U.S. to protect preschool aged children against 12 infectious diseases contain thimerosal as a preservative. The MMR [measles, mumps, and rubella] vaccine does not and never did contain thimerosal. Varicella (chickenpox), inactivated polio (IPV), and pneumococcal conjugate vaccines have also never contained thimerosal.

A U.S. study looking at environmental factors including exposure to mercury, lead and other heavy metals is ongoing.

Symptoms may appear by age two, but the average age of onset is between three and four years. Until this time, the child has age-appropriate skills in communication and social relationships. The long period of normal development before regression helps differentiate CDD from Rett syndrome.

The loss of such skills as vocabulary are more dramatic in CDD than they are in classical autism. The diagnosis requires extensive and pronounced losses involving motor, language, and social skills. CDD is also accompanied by loss of bowel and bladder control and oftentimes seizures and a very low IQ.

What Are The Autism Spectrum Disorders?

All children with autism spectrum disorders (ASD) demonstrate deficits in social interaction, verbal and nonverbal communication, and repetitive behaviors or interests. In addition, they will often have unusual responses to sensory experiences, such as certain sounds or the way objects look. Each of these symptoms runs the gamut from mild to severe. They will present in each individual child differently. For instance, a child may have little trouble learning to read but exhibit extremely poor social interaction. Each child will display communication, social, and behavioral patterns that are individual but fit into the overall diagnosis of ASD.

Children with ASD do not follow the typical patterns of child development. In some children, hints of future problems may be apparent from birth. In most cases, the problems in communication and social skills become more noticeable as the child lags further behind other children the same age. Some other children start off well enough. Oftentimes between 12 and 36 months old, the differences in the way they react to people and other unusual behaviors become apparent. Some parents report the change as being sudden, and that their children start to reject people, act strangely, and lose language and social skills they had previously acquired. In other cases, there is a plateau, or leveling, of progress so that the difference between the child with autism and other children the same age becomes more noticeable.

Social Symptoms

From the start, typically developing infants are social beings. Early in life, they gaze at people, turn toward voices, grasp a finger, and even smile.

In contrast, most children with ASD seem to have tremendous difficulty learning to engage in the give and take of everyday human interaction. Even in the first few months of life, many do not interact and they avoid eye contact. They seem indifferent to other people, and often seem to prefer being alone. They may resist attention or passively accept hugs and cuddling. Later, they seldom seek comfort or respond to parents' displays of anger or affection in a typical way.

Children with ASD also are slower in learning to interpret what others are thinking and feeling. Subtle social cues—whether a smile, a wink, or a grimace—may have little meaning. To a child who misses these cues, "Come here" always means the same thing, whether the speaker is smiling and extending her arms for a hug or frowning and planting her fists on her hips. Without the ability to interpret gestures and facial expressions, the social world may seem bewildering. To compound the problem, people with ASD have difficulty seeing things from another person's perspective.

Although not universal, it is common for people with ASD also to have difficulty regulating their emotions. This can take the form of "immature" behavior such as crying in class or verbal outbursts that seem inappropriate to those around them. The individual with ASD might

Remember!!

Autism spectrum disorder (ASD) is defined by a certain set of behaviors that can range from the very mild to the severe. The following possible indicators of ASD were identified on the Public Health Training Network Webcast, Autism Among Us:

- Does not babble, point, or make meaningful gestures by one year of age
- Does not speak one word by 16 months
- Does not combine two words by two years
- Does not respond to name
- Loses language or social skills

Some other indicators include the following:

- Poor eye contact
- Doesn't seem to know how to play with toys
- Excessively lines up toys or other objects
- Is attached to one particular toy or object
- Doesn't smile
- At times seems to be hearing impaired

also be disruptive and physically aggressive at times, making social relationships still more difficult. They may at times break things, attack others, or hurt themselves. In their frustration, some bang their heads, pull their hair, or bite their arms.

Communication Difficulties

By age three, most children have passed predictable milestones on the path to learning language; one of the earliest is babbling. By the first birthday, a typical toddler says words, turns when he hears his name, points when he wants a toy, and when offered something distasteful, makes it clear that the answer is "no."

Some children diagnosed with ASD remain mute throughout their lives. Some infants who later show signs of ASD coo and babble during the first few months of life, but they soon stop. Others may be delayed, developing language as late as age five to nine. Some children may learn to use communication systems such as pictures or sign language.

Those who do speak often use language in unusual ways. They seem unable to combine words into meaningful sentences. Some speak only single words, while others repeat the same phrase over and over. Some ASD children parrot what they hear, a condition called echolalia. Although many children with no ASD go through a stage where they repeat what they hear, it normally passes by the time they are three.

Some children only mildly affected may exhibit slight delays in language, or even seem to have precocious language and unusually large vocabularies, but have great difficulty in sustaining a conversation. Another difficulty is often the inability to understand body language, tone of voice, or "phrases of speech." They might interpret a sarcastic expression such as "Oh, that's just great" as meaning it really IS great.

While it can be hard to understand what ASD children are saying, their body language is also difficult to understand. Facial expressions, movements, and gestures rarely match what they are saying. Also, their tone of voice fails to reflect their feelings. A high-pitched, sing-song, or flat, robot-like voice is

✤ It's A Fact!!

For every child eligible for special programs, each state guarantees special education and related services. The Individuals with Disabilities Education Act (IDEA) is a federally mandated program that assures a free and appropriate public education for children with diagnosed learning deficits.

By law, the public schools must prepare and carry out a set of instruction goals, or specific skills, for every child in a special education program. The list of skills is known as the child's Individualized Education Program (IEP). The IEP is an agreement between the school and the family on the child's goals.

common. Some children with relatively good language skills speak like little adults, failing to pick up on the "kid-speak" that is common in their peers.

Repetitive Behaviors

Although children with ASD usually appear physically normal and have good muscle control, odd repetitive motions may set them off from other children. These behaviors might be extreme and highly apparent or more subtle. Some children and older individuals spend a lot of time repeatedly flapping their arms or walking on their toes. Some suddenly freeze in position.

As children, they might spend hours lining up their cars and trains in a certain way, rather than using them for pretend play. If someone accidentally moves one of the toys, the child may be tremendously upset. ASD children need, and demand, absolute consistency in their environment. A slight change in any routine—in mealtimes, dressing, taking a bath, going to school at a certain time and by the same route—can be extremely disturbing.

Repetitive behavior sometimes takes the form of a persistent, intense preoccupation. For example, the child might be obsessed with learning all about vacuum cleaners, train schedules, or lighthouses. Often there is great interest in numbers, symbols, or science topics.

Problems That May Accompany ASD

Sensory Problems: When children's perceptions are accurate, they can learn from what they see, feel, or hear. On the other hand, if sensory information is faulty, the child's experiences of the world can be confusing. Many ASD children are highly attuned or even painfully sensitive to certain sounds, textures, tastes, and smells.

In ASD, the brain seems unable to balance the senses appropriately. Some ASD children are oblivious to extreme cold or pain. An ASD child may fall and break an arm, yet never cry. Another may bash his head against a wall and not wince, but a light touch may make the child scream with alarm.

Mental Retardation: Many children with ASD have some degree of mental impairment. When tested, some areas of ability may be normal, while others may be especially weak.

Seizures: One in four children with ASD develops seizures, often starting either in early childhood or adolescence. Sometimes a contributing factor is a lack of sleep or a high fever. An EEG (electroencephalogram—recording of the electric currents developed in the brain by means of electrodes applied to the scalp) can help confirm the seizure's presence.

In most cases, seizures can be controlled by a number of medicines called "anticonvulsants." The dosage of the medication is adjusted carefully so that the least possible amount of medication will be used to be effective.

Fragile X Syndrome: This disorder is the most common inherited form of mental retardation. It was so named because one part of the X chromosome has a defective piece that appears pinched and fragile when under a microscope. Fragile X syndrome affects about two to five percent of people with ASD. It is important to have a child with ASD checked for fragile X, especially if the parents are considering having another child. For an unknown reason, if a child with ASD also has fragile X, there is a one-in-two chance that boys born to the same parents will have the syndrome.

Tuberous Sclerosis: Tuberous sclerosis is a rare genetic disorder that causes benign tumors to grow in the brain as well as in other vital organs. It has a consistently strong association with ASD. One to four percent of people with ASD also have tuberous sclerosis.

The Adolescent Years

Adolescence is a time of stress and confusion; and it is no less so for teenagers with autism. Like all children, they need help in dealing with their budding sexuality. While some behaviors improve during the teenage years, some get worse. Increased autistic or aggressive behavior may be one way some teens express their newfound tension and confusion.

The teenage years are also a time when children become more socially sensitive. At the age that most teenagers are concerned with acne, popularity, grades, and dates, teens with autism may become painfully aware that they are different from their peers. They may notice that they lack friends. And unlike their schoolmates, they aren't dating or planning for a career. For some, the sadness that comes with such realization motivates them to learn new behaviors and acquire better social skills.

Chapter 47

Bullying

What is bullying?

A lot of young people have a good idea of what bullying is because they see it every day. Bullying happens when someone hurts or scares another person on purpose and the person being bullied has a hard time defending himself or herself. Usually, bullying happens over and over.

What is cyberbullying?

In recent years, technology has given children and youth a new means of bullying each other. Cyberbullying, which is sometimes referred to as online social cruelty or electronic bullying, can involve any of the following actions:

- Sending mean, vulgar, or threatening messages or images
- Posting sensitive, private information about another person
- Pretending to be someone else in order to make that person look bad
- Intentionally excluding someone from an online group

About This Chapter: This chapter includes text excerpting from "Cyberbullying," 2008, and "Stop Bullying! Now!" 2009, produced by the Health Resources and Services Administration, 2009. For additional information, visit http://stopbullyingnow.hrsa.gov.

Children and youth cyberbully each other with these tools:

- E-mails
- Instant messaging
- Text or digital imaging messages sent on cell phones
- Web pages
- Blogs
- Chat rooms or discussion groups
- Other information communication technologies

Although little research has been conducted on cyberbullying, recent studies have found this statistical information:

- 18% of students in grades 6–8 said they had been cyberbullied at least once in the last couple of months; and 6% said it had happened to them two or more times.
- 11% of students in grades 6–8 said they had cyberbullied another person at least once in the last couple of months, and 2% said they had done it two or more times.
- 19% of regular internet users between the ages of 10 and 17 reported being involved in online aggression; 15% had been aggressors, and 7% had been targets (3% were both aggressors and targets).
- 17% of 6–11 year-olds and 36% of 12–17-year-olds reported that someone said threatening or embarrassing things about them through e-mail, instant messages, web sites, chat rooms, or text messages.
- Cyberbullying has increased in recent years. In nationally representative surveys of 10-17 year-olds, twice as many children and youth indicated

✎ What's It Mean? Bullying

- Punching, shoving, and other acts that hurt people physically
- Spreading bad rumors about people
- Keeping certain people out of a "group"
- Teasing people in a mean way
- Getting certain people to "gang up" on others

Bullying also can happen online or electronically. Cyberbullying is when children or teens bully each other using the internet, mobile phones, or other cyber technology.

Source: Health Resources and Services Administration, 2009.

that they had been victims and perpetrators of online harassment in 2005 compared with 1999/2000.

Why do kids bully?

There are all kinds of reasons why young people bully others. Do any of these sound familiar to you?

- Because I see others doing it
- Because it's what you do if you want to hang out with the right crowd
- Because it makes me feel, stronger, smarter, or better than the person I'm bullying
- Because it's one of the best ways to keep others from bullying me

Whatever the reason, bullying is something we all need to think about. Whether we've done it ourselves, or whether friends or other people we know are doing it, we all need to recognize that bullying has a terrible effect on the lives of young people. It may not be happening to you today, but it could tomorrow. Working together, we can make the lives of young people better.

What are the effects of bullying?

If you've ever heard an adult—or anyone else—say that bullying is "just a fact of life" or "no big deal," you're not alone. Too often, people just don't take bullying seriously—or until the sad and sometimes scary stories are revealed.

- It can mess up a kid's future. Young people who bully are more likely than those who don't bully to skip school and drop out of school. They are also more likely to smoke, drink alcohol and get into fights.
- It scares some people so much that they skip school. As many as 160,000 students may stay home on any given day because they're afraid of being bullied.
- It can lead to huge problems later in life. Children who bully are more likely to get into fights, vandalize property, and drop out of school. And 60% of boys who were bullies in middle school had at least one criminal conviction by the age of 24.

What can you do if you bully others?

Let's face it, hurting and making others feel bad is NEVER cool. Just admitting that you are doing things to harm others takes some guts. But that's not enough. Trying to find out what you should do to change the way you're acting, now that's a step in the right direction!

Think about what you're doing and how it affects others. If you think calling others names is really harmless, or if you think pushing, hitting, or

✔ Quick Tip

Things You Can Do To Stay Out Of A Bully's Way

- Make friends and lots of them—there's safety in numbers. A bully is less likely to approach you if you're surrounded by pals. Try to be friendly and respectful to everyone—smile at someone if you make eye contact in the hallways.
- If a bully is talking smack about you, keep in mind all the good stuff you know about yourself. Do things that you are good at. Can you spell like a dictionary? Enter a spelling bee. Run like the wind? Join the track team. Sing like an angel? Choir is calling your name. Try something new; you may discover a talent you never knew you had. Take tennis lessons or audition for the school play. Bonus: you'll meet new people!
- Stand up for yourself! Practice what you might say if someone starts picking on you. Saying the words a couple of times will make you feet sure of yourself. One word to the wise: Never start a discussion or argue with a bully—even if you've got a zinger that's begging to be zung. You just want to get them off your back, not make them angry.
- Check out the way you act and be aware of your body language. How you carry yourself can bring on a bully. Slouching, looking at the ground or feet, and fidgeting make people think that you are afraid or nervous. Try to walk with your head up, make eye contact, and smile. A bully is less likely to single you out if you are the picture of self-confidence.
- Ignore insults or name-calling. It'll be hard, but stay calm and don't let them see you sweat. Take a deep breath and try not show that you are upset or angry. Above all, don't believe for one second what they're saying.

stealing from other kids is funny, you've forgotten what it feels like to be hurt yourself. Teasing, hitting, keeping others out of a group—all of these things harm someone. All of us have been hurt at one time or another and we all know how it feels—awful. So the next time you are about to bully someone, try these tips:

- Put yourself in their shoes.
- Think about how it must make them feel.

Bullies feed on attention and are just trying to get a reaction from you. It's easier to give them the brush off if you don't let them get under your skin. They'll get bored and move on.

- Avoid getting sucked into a scuffle, even if it means losing your stuff—your safety is way more important than your shoes. The only time you should ever fight back is when you have to defend yourself. Even then, keep eyes open for an escape route. Chances are, if someone wants to fight, they know they have a good chance of winning.
- Don't be afraid to tell an adult if you're being bullied. You are NOT a snitch if you tell an adult you know that someone is hurting you. If you have tried to stop someone from bothering you and it's not working, get someone you trust involved to help you. And if you see someone else in the same boat, find an adult to help. Get the problem out in the open. Once people know about it, the bully is no longer in control. Not telling anyone—especially because the bully told you not to—is just making him or her feel more powerful.
- Have a few one-liners in your pocket to pull out if you need them. Things like, "That's funny, but enough already, okay?" or "I don't do this to you. You should really think about that" can help defuse a tense situation and keep you out of harm's way. While you're coming up with your witty one-liners, keep in mind you're trying to take the wind out of the bully's sails, not add fuel to the fire with a major burn. Embarrassing the bully in front of everyone won't make your life any easier.

Source: From "The Bully Roundup," BAM! Body and Mind, Centers for Disease Control and Prevention, 2003.

- And just don't do it.
- Talk to an adult.

Making other people feel badly should never make you feel good. If it does, or if you're not really sure why you bully other kids, you need to talk to an adult about it. Even though you might think an adult won't understand, or that you'll get yourself into trouble, they can help. Whether it is your parent, a teacher or another trusted grown-up, you should tell an adult how you've been acting so that they help you deal with it. School counselors are also great people to talk to about how you feel and how to change the way you treat others.

Chapter 48

Dating Abuse

Dating abuse is a pattern of violent behavior—physical, emotional, or sexual—by one partner in a dating relationship toward the other partner.

You might be thinking, "I've never experienced anything as serious as being punched!" But hold on a sec.

In general, guys and girls don't usually start hitting their girlfriend or boyfriend out of the blue. It usually starts after a history of verbal and emotional abuse, which is far more likely to occur among young teens. If nothing is done about that abuse, it's likely to become more severe and start including sexual and physical abuse.

Dating Bill Of Rights And Responsibilities

You have certain rights and responsibilities in a dating relationship. Here are some examples. Personalize these for yourself, and make a commitment to stick by them.

Dating Rights

I have these rights:

- To be treated with respect always

About This Chapter: Information in this chapter is from "Choose Respect," National Center for Injury Prevention and Control (www.chooserespect.org), 2006.

- To be in a healthy relationship
- To not be abused—physically, sexually, or emotionally
- To keep my body, feelings, beliefs, and property to myself
- To have friends and activities apart from my boyfriend or girlfriend
- To set limits and values
- To say no
- To feel safe in the relationship
- To be treated as an equal
- To feel comfortable being myself
- To leave a relationship

Dating Responsibilities

I have these responsibilities:

- To determine my limits and values
- To respect my boyfriend's or girlfriend's limits, values, feelings, and beliefs
- To refuse to abuse—physically, sexually, or emotionally
- To be considerate
- To communicate clearly and honestly
- To give my boyfriend or girlfriend space to be his or her own person
- To not exert power or control in the relationship
- To compromise when needed
- To admit to being wrong when appropriate
- To ask for help from friends, family, and trusted adults

✎ What's It Mean?

Dating abuse may include components like these:

- Physical
- Pinching, shoving, slapping, grabbing, etc.
- Intimidation (blocking doors, throwing objects)
- Use of weapons
- Sexual
- Unwanted touching
- Forced sexual activities
- Pressure to have sex
- Threats to find someone who will do what he or she wants sexually
- Emotional/verbal
- Put-downs, insults, and rumors
- Threats
- Possessiveness
- Overdependency
- Huge mood swings
- Humiliation
- Accusations
- Withdrawal of attention
- Isolation from friends or activities

Dating Abuse Affects Many

Teen dating abuse is a huge issue. It is a problem that touches the lives of teens from all walks of life—black and white, rich and poor, big-city and country.

These statistics are about real people. They are scary when you consider that anyone can experience dating abuse. People like you, your brother or sister, your friend, or your classmate. Become familiar with these facts so you can talk about the issue with other people and be ready to do something.

✤ It's A Fact!!

- About one in 11 teens reports being a victim of physical dating abuse each year.
- About one in four teens reports verbal, physical, emotional, or sexual abuse each year.
- About one in five teens reports being a victim of emotional abuse.
- About one in five high school girls has been physically or sexually abused by a dating partner.
- The overall occurrence of dating violence is higher among black (13.9%) than Hispanic (9.3%) or white (7.0%) students.
- About 72% of students in 8th and 9th grade report dating. By the time they are in high school, 54% of students report dating violence among their peers.
- One in three teens report knowing a friend or peer who has been hit, punched, kicked, slapped, choked, or otherwise physically hurt by his or her partner.
- 80% of teens regard verbal abuse as a serious issue for their age group.
- Nearly 80% of girls who have been physically abused in their dating relationships continue to date their abuser.
- Nearly one in five teenage girls who have been in a relationship said a boyfriend had threatened violence or self-harm if presented with a break-up.
- Almost 70% of young women who have been raped knew their rapist either as a boyfriend, friend, or casual acquaintance.
- Teen dating abuse most often takes place in the home of one of the partners.

Impact Of Dating Abuse

Dating abuse can have serious consequences. The effects range from missing a few classes to attempting suicide. Abuse also affects future relationships. All consequences make compelling reasons to prevent abuse before it starts, or to speak up against it.

Effects On Victims

These things can happen shortly after the abuse:

- Bruises and aches
- Pregnancy
- Trouble sleeping
- Anxiety
- Guilt
- Missed classes
- Poor grades
- Distrust in people
- Lying to friends or family to hide the abuse
- Withdrawal from friends or family, or avoidance of school or social events
- Lower self-esteem
- Feelings of loneliness
- Feelings of isolation

✔ Quick Tip

Recognizing Warning Signs Of Abuse

Some of the following signs are just part of being a teen. But, when these changes happen suddenly, or without an explanation, these signs could signal abuse. Look out for these signs in your friends and classmates.

- Warning signs of an abusive relationship
- Bruises, scratches, or other injuries
- Failing grades
- Dropping out of school activities
- Avoiding friends and social events
- Indecision
- Changes in clothes or make-up
- Changes in eating or sleeping habits
- Secrecy
- Avoiding eye contact
- Crying spells or hysteria fits
- Constant thoughts about the dating partner
- Alcohol or drug use
- Anxiety and depression
- Sudden changes in mood or personality
- Fearfulness around the dating partner or when his or her name is mentioned

Dating abuse can also cause problems in the long run:

- Depression
- Suicide attempts
- Eating disorders
- Drug and alcohol abuse
- Medical problems
- Inability to succeed in school or at work later in life

Effects On Abusers

People who are abusive in dating relationships can be affected in the long run, too:

- Loss of respect from peers
- Loneliness
- Alienation from friends and family
- Suspension or expulsion from school
- Inability to keep a job
- Criminal activity

> **✔ Quick Tip**
>
> **Recognizing Warning Signs Of An Abusive Person**
>
> - Wants to get serious in the relationship quickly
> - Will not take no for an answer
> - Is jealous and possessive
> - Makes all the decisions
> - Dismisses other people's opinions and feelings
> - Wants to control a person's friends and activities
> - Puts constant pressure on someone
> - Demands to know where someone is all the time
> - Uses guilt trips—"If you really loved me, you would..."
> - Feels that he or she deserves unconditional love and support
> - Has a history of bad relationships
> - Blames the person for his or her feelings and actions—"You asked for it" or "You made me mad"
> - Apologizes for violent behavior and promises not to do it again

Why Does Abuse Happen?

Treat others with respect. This idea may seem like common sense. After all, why not give respect if you'll get it in return?

The truth is, quite a few teens are abusive in their relationships. And many think it's justified. After all, society seems to be okay with it—just look at all the TV shows and listen to popular songs these days.

Abuse is not fair, and it's not right. But there are reasons why it happens.

Abuse Is Related To Certain Risk Factors

Risks of having unhealthy relationships increase for teens who may have some of these characteristics: Believe it's okay to use threats or violence to get their way or to express frustration or anger; use alcohol or drugs; can't manage anger or frustration; hang out with violent peers; have low self-esteem or are depressed; have learning difficulties and other problems at school; don't have parental supervision and support; witness abuse at home or in the community; and have a history of aggressive behavior or bullying.

Abuse Is A Choice

No matter what excuses abusers make to themselves or their dating partners for their behaviors, abuse is still their choice. They will continue the abuse unless someone confronts them and helps them stop it.

Abuse Is About Power And Control

Abusers may feel insecure or uncertain about themselves or their lives. Or they may feel like they don't have much control over anything. So they use power and control in their relationships to make themselves feel better.

Excuses For Abuse

Excuses. People who are abusive in a dating relationship use excuses all the time to justify their hurtful behavior. People who hear them may start doubting whether their concerns about the relationship are valid, and they'll put up with the abuse.

Have you heard these excuses before? "It's not abuse." "I was having a bad day." "Jealousy is a normal part of any relationship." "You got me upset or angry." "It just happened once. It won't happen again." "You deserved it." "I was drunk or high. Drugs made me do it." "I had a bad childhood." "I deserve your trust, even if I messed up before." "I deserve unconditional love and support." "I should be more important than your friends." "My needs are more important than yours." "I didn't mean to hurt you."

Any of these sound familiar? These are signs of an unhealthy relationship. There is no excuse for abuse—excuses should not be tolerated! Abuse is always a choice. While some people will choose respect, others will choose abuse.

When you hear excuses like these, confront your dating partner about them. Or seek help from your friends or trusted adults, like your parents, about what you should do.

Why It Is So Hard To Leave?

If you or someone you know is in an unhealthy relationship, it may be very hard to leave. Some of the reasons include the following:

- **Love:** You may sincerely love your dating partner even if you may hate some of his or her behaviors.
- **Promises:** Your partner may sugarcoat his or her words and promise the abuse won't happen again.
- **Confusion:** You may be confusing genuine love and controlling love, especially if you've grown up in an abusive and unsupportive family.
- **Denial:** You may be thinking, "It could be worse." Trying to downplay abuse is a common reaction, but it still doesn't make the abuse right.
- **Guilt:** You may feel like the abuse is your fault, given that your boyfriend or girlfriend is likely to blame you for it.
- **Fear:** You may be afraid of what would happen if you told the truth. Or maybe you fear being alone and would rather be in this relationship than in none at all.
- **Belief You Can Change Your Partner:** You may cling to the hope that you can change your partner if you try hard enough or put enough time and devotion into it.
- **False Hopes:** You may think the violence will eventually stop. But, abuse is a pattern of behavior that's been established for a long time. It won't just stop on its own.
- **Peer Pressure:** The pressure to have a boyfriend or girlfriend can be extreme. You may be afraid of what your friends might think if you were single.
- **Low Self-Esteem:** If you've been abused emotionally or verbally, you may feel like you're not lovable or worthy at all. Even if you're unhappy

in the relationship, you may stay because you think you'll never find someone better who would love someone like you.

Do you use any of these reasons to stay in an abusive relationship? It's up to you to decide whether it's worth it to stay and whether your dating partner is sincerely committed to changing. But if you're positive that he or she can't change, leaving the relationship is the best choice to make before you get hurt even more.

Leaving The Relationship

If you're in an unhealthy relationship where you're not getting the respect that you deserve, leaving it is the best thing you can do for yourself. It will take a lot of courage and resolve, but you can do it with support from the people who care about you.

You will feel a lot better physically, emotionally, and mentally. You will finally be free of your ex's abusive and controlling behavior.

After The Relationship

Just because you've left an abusive relationship doesn't mean the risk of abuse is over. Your ex may start stalking you or calling you constantly. He or she may make threats or plead with you to come back.

Here are some tips to help you stay safe and have peace of mind.

- Tell your parents what's going on, especially since your ex may stop by your home and demand to know where you are.
- Talk with friends or adults you trust so they can look out for your safety.
- Talk to school officials. They can alert school security about your ex and take other measures to make you feel safe at school.
- Avoid isolated or dark areas at school and hangout spots.
- Don't walk home alone.
- If you go to parties or events where your ex might be, go with good friends.

Chapter 49

Learning Disabilities

Learning Disabilities At A Glance

Learning disabilities are real. A person can be of average or above-average intelligence, not have any major sensory problems (like blindness or hearing impairment), and yet struggle to keep up with people of the same age in learning and regular functioning.

How Can One Tell If A Person Has A Learning Disability?

Learning disabilities can affect a person's ability in the areas of: listening; speaking; reading; writing; mathematics.

Other features of a learning disability are:

- a distinct gap between the level of achievement that is expected and what is actually being achieved;
- difficulties that can become apparent in different ways with different people;
- difficulties that manifest themselves differently throughout development;
- difficulties with socio-emotional skills and behavior.

About This Chapter: Text in this chapter is from "Learning Disabilities at a Glance" and "LD at a Glance: A Quick Look," Reprinted with permission. For more information, visit LD.org.

A learning disability is not a disease, so there is no cure, but there are ways to overcome the challenges it poses through identification and accommodation.

Identification

If there is reason to think a person might have LD, it is important to collect observations by parents, teachers, doctors and others regularly in contact with that person. If there does seem to be a pattern of trouble that is more than just an isolated case of difficulty, the next step is to seek help from school or consult a learning specialist for an evaluation.

✎ What's It Mean?

What is a learning disability?

A learning disability (LD) is a neurological disorder that affects the brain's ability to receive, process, store and respond to information. The term learning disability is used to describe the seeming unexplained difficulty a person of at least average intelligence has in acquiring basic academic skills. These skills are essential for success at school and work, and for coping with life in general. LD is not a single disorder. It is a term that refers to a group of disorders.

Accommodation And Modification

Depending on the type of learning disability and its severity, as well as the person's age, different kinds of assistance can be provided. Under the Individuals with Disabilities Education Act (IDEA) of 1997 and Americans with Disabilities Act (ADA) of 1990 people of all ages with LD are protected against discrimination and have a right to different forms of assistance in the classroom and workplace.

What Causes Learning Disabilities?

Experts aren't exactly sure what causes learning disabilities. LD may be due to:

- **Heredity:** Often learning disabilities run in the family, so it's not uncommon to find that people with LD have parents or other relatives with similar difficulties.

- **Problems During Pregnancy And Birth:** LD may be caused by illness or injury during or before birth. It may also be caused by drug and alcohol use during pregnancy, low birth weight, lack of oxygen and premature or prolonged labor.
- **Incidents After Birth:** Head injuries, nutritional deprivation and exposure to toxic substances (for example, lead) can contribute to LD.

Learning disabilities are NOT caused by economic disadvantage, environmental factors, or cultural differences. In fact, there is frequently no apparent cause for LD.

Each type of strategy should be considered when planning instruction and support. A person with dysgraphia will benefit from help from both specialists and those who are closest to the person. Finding the most beneficial type of support is a process of trying different ideas and openly exchanging thoughts on what works best.

Are Learning Disabilities Common?

Currently, almost 2.9 million school-aged children in the U.S. are classified as having specific learning disabilities (SLD) and receive some kind of special education support. They are approximately 5% of all school-aged children in public schools. These numbers do not include children in private and religious schools or home-schooled children.

Studies show that learning disabilities do not fall evenly across racial and ethnic groups. For instance, in 2001, 1% of white children and 2.6% of non-Hispanic black children were receiving LD-related special education services (Executive Summary, National Research Council, 2001). The same studies suggest that this has to do with economic status and not ethnic background. LD is not caused by economic disadvantage, but the increased risk of exposure to harmful toxins (lead, tobacco, alcohol, etc.) at early stages of development are prevalent in low-income communities.

What Can One Do About Learning Disabilities?

Learning disabilities are lifelong, and although they won't go away, they don't have to stop a person from achieving goals. Help is available if they are identified. Learning disabilities affect every person differently, and the disorder can range from mild to severe. Sometimes people have more than one learning disability. In addition, approximately one third of people with LD also have attention deficit hyperactivity disorder (AD/HD), which makes it difficult for them to concentrate, stay focused or manage their attention to specific tasks.

LD And Adulthood

It is never too late to get help for a learning disability. Finding out about a learning disability can be a great relief to adults who could not explain the reason for their struggles in the past. Testing specialists are available for people of all ages, and assistance is available for every stage of life. Taking the initiative to seek out support and services than can provide help is the first step to overcoming a learning disability.

✔ Quick Tip

[Editor's Note: Here's a tip you can pass along to your parents.]

LD And Children: Early identification is vital in helping a child to succeed academically, as well as socially. If you think your child is displaying signs of a learning disability, share them with classroom teachers and others who come in contact with your child. Observe the way your child develops the language, motor coordination, and social skills and behaviors important for success in school. And remember: Early is better. Even preschoolers can show signs of risk for LD.

Don't panic. Not all children who are slow to develop skills have LD. If your child does have a learning disability, early intervention with specialized teaching strategies can help to overcome difficulties. As a parent, it is important to learn as much as you can and to help your child understand that he or she is not alone: other children struggle too, and adults are there to help.

Many adults (some of whom are unaware of their LD) have developed ways to cope with their difficulties and are able to lead successful, functioning lives. LD shouldn't hinder a person from attaining goals. Regardless of the situation, understanding the specific challenges and learning strategies to deal with LD directly at every stage can alleviate a lot of frustration and make successful living much easier.

LD At A Glance: A Quick Look

What You Should Know About Learning Disabilities (LD)

- LDs are specific neurological disorders that affect the brain's ability to store, process or communicate information.
- "Specific learning disability" (SLD) is the term used in the federal law for any LD.
- LDs can affect different aspects of learning and functioning. See the information below for specific types of learning disabilities and related disorders.
- LDs can be compensated for and even overcome through alternate ways of learning, accommodations, and modifications.
- According to the U.S. Department of Education, LDs affect approximately 5% of all children enrolled in public schools.
- LDs can occur with other disorders (AD/HD, information processing disorders).
- LDs are NOT the same as mental retardation, autism, deafness, blindness, behavioral disorders, or laziness.
- LDs are not the result of economic disadvantage, environmental factors, or cultural differences.

LD Terminology

Learning Disabilities

- Dyslexia
    - Area of difficulty: Processing language
    - Symptoms include trouble with: Reading, writing, and spelling
    - Example: Letters and words may be written or pronounced backwards
- Dyscalculia
    - Area of difficulty: Math skills

    - Symptoms include trouble with: Computation, remembering math facts, concepts of time and money
    - Example: Difficulty learning to count by 2s, 3s, 4s
- Dysgraphia
    - Area of difficulty: Written expression
    - Symptoms include trouble with: Handwriting, spelling, composition
    - Example: Illegible handwriting, difficulty organizing ideas
- Dyspraxia
    - Area of difficulty: Fine motor skills
    - Symptoms include trouble with: Coordination, manual dexterity
    - Example: Trouble with scissors, buttons, drawing

Information Processing Disorders

- Auditory Processing Disorder
    - Area of difficulty: Interpreting auditory information
    - Symptoms include trouble with: Language development, reading
    - Example: Difficulty anticipating how a speaker will end a sentence
- Visual Processing Disorder
    - Area of difficulty: Interpreting visual information
    - Symptoms include trouble with: Reading, writing, and math
    - Example: Difficulty distinguishing letters like "h" and "n"

Other Related Disorders

- Attention Deficit Hyperactivity Disorder (AD/HD)
    - Area of difficulty: Concentration and focus
    - Symptoms include trouble with: Over-activity, distractibility and impulsivity
    - Example: Can't sit still, loses interest quickly

Chapter 50

Puberty

How much will an adolescent grow?

The teenage years are also called adolescence. During this time, an adolescent will see the greatest amount of growth in height and weight. Adolescence is a time for growth spurts and puberty changes. An adolescent may expect to grow several inches in several months followed by a period of very slow growth, then will typically have another growth spurt. Changes with puberty may occur gradually or several signs may become visible at the same time.

There is a great amount of variation in the rate of changes that may occur. Some adolescents may experience these signs of maturity sooner or later than others. It is important to remember that these changes happen at different times for everyone. Being smaller or bigger than other females or males is normal as each child experiences puberty at his/her own time. On average males begin puberty between 9.5–14 years of age, and females begin puberty between 8–13 years of age.

About This Chapter: This chapter begins with information from "Puberty: Adolescent Male" and "Puberty: Adolescent Female," which is reprinted with permission from the Cincinnati Children's Hospital Medical Center website, http://www.cincinnati childrens.org. Additional information is cited separately within the chapter.

Female

What changes will occur during puberty?

Females experience puberty as a sequence of events, but their pubertal changes usually begin before boys of the same age. Each girl is different and may progress through these changes differently. The following is a list of changes that occur during puberty.

- Beginning of puberty: 8 to 13 years
- First pubertal change: breast development
- Pubic hair development: shortly after breast development
- Hair under the arms: 12 years of age
- Menstrual periods: 10 to 16.5 years of age

✤ It's A Fact!!

Some adolescents may experience signs of maturity sooner or later than others. It is important to remember that these changes happen at different times for everyone.

Source: © 2007 Cincinnati Children's Hospital Medical Center.

There are specific stages of development that females go through when developing secondary sexual characteristics. The following is a brief overview of the changes that occur:

- In girls, the initial puberty change is the development of breast buds, in which a small mound is formed by the elevation of the breast and papilla (nipple). The areola (the circle of different colored skin around the nipple) increases in size at this time.
- The breasts then continue to enlarge.

- Eventually, the nipples and the areolas will elevate again, forming another projection on the breasts.
- At the adult state, only the nipple remains elevated.
- Pubic hair development is similar for both girls and boys. The initial growth of hair produces long, soft hair that is only in a small area around the genitals. This hair then becomes darker and coarser as it continues to spread.
- The pubic hair eventually looks like adult hair, but in a smaller area. It may spread to the thighs and sometimes up the stomach.

The following are additional changes that may occur for the female as she experiences the changes of puberty:

- There may be an increase in hair growth, not only the pubic area, but also under the arms and on the legs. Some women may decide to shave this hair.
- Body shape will begin to change. There may be not only an increase in height and weight, but the hips may get wider and the waists get smaller. There may also be an increase in fat in the buttocks, legs, and stomach. These are normal changes that may occur during puberty.
- Body size will increase, with the feet, arms, legs, and hands sometimes growing faster than the rest of the body. This may cause an adolescent girl to experience a time of feeling clumsy.
- As the hormones of puberty increase, adolescents may experience an increase in oily skin and sweating. This is a normal part of growing. It is important to wash daily, including the face. Acne may develop.
- Adolescent girls will also experience menstruation, or menstrual periods. This begins when the body releases an egg from the ovaries. If the egg is fertilized with a sperm from a male, it could potentially grow into a baby inside the uterus. If the egg is not fertilized, the tissues inside the uterus are not needed and are shed through the vagina as fluid. The fluids are bloody and are usually released monthly. After a girl begins to menstruate, she is able to get pregnant.

Males

What changes will occur during puberty?

In males, it is difficult to know exactly when puberty is coming. There are changes that occur, but they occur gradually over a period of time rather than as a single event. The following is a list of changes that occur during puberty.

- First pubertal change: enlargement of the testicles
- Penis enlargement: begins approximately one year after the testicles begin enlarging
- Appearance of pubic hair
- Hair under the arms, on the face, voice change, and acne
- Ability to obtain orgasm, typically experienced as a wet dream

The following are additional changes that may occur for the male as he experiences the changes of puberty:

- Body size will increase, with the feet, arms, legs, and hands sometimes growing "faster" than the rest of the body. This may cause the adolescent boy to experience a time of feeling clumsy.
- Some may experience some swelling in the area of their breasts as a result of the hormonal changes that are occurring. This is common among teenage boys and is usually a temporary condition. Consult with your adolescent's physician if this is a concern.
- Voice changes may occur, as the voice gets deeper. Sometimes, the voice may "crack" during this time. This is a temporary condition and will improve over time.
- Not only will hair begin to grow in the genital area, but males will also experience hair growth on their face, under their arms, and on their legs.
- As the hormones of puberty increase, adolescents may experience an increase in oily skin and sweating. This is a normal part of growing. It is important to wash daily, including the face. Acne may develop.

- As the penis enlarges, the adolescent male may begin to experience erections. This is when the penis becomes hard and erect because it is filled with blood. This is due to hormonal changes and may occur when the boy fantasizes about sexual things or for no reason at all. This is a normal occurrence.
- During puberty, the male's body also begins producing sperm. Semen, which is composed of sperm and other bodily fluids, may be released during an erection. This is called ejaculation. Sometimes, this may happen while the male is sleeping. This is called a nocturnal emission or "wet dream." This is a normal part of puberty and will stop as the male gets older.

Understanding Normal Adolescent Mental Development

The adolescent years bring many changes, not only physically, but also mentally and socially. During these years, adolescents increase their ability to think abstractly and eventually make plans and set long-term goals. Each child may progress at different rates, and show a different view of the world. In general, the following are some of the abilities that may be evident:

- Developing the ability to think abstractly
- Concerns with philosophy, politics, and social issues
- Thinking long-term
- Setting goals
- Comparing oneself to one's peers

Relationships With Others

In order to achieve independence and control of one's environment, many changes may need to occur. The following are some of the issues that may be involved with your adolescent during these years:

- Independence from parents
- Peer influence and acceptance is very important

- Male-female relationships become very important
- He/she may be in love
- He/she may have long-term commitment in relationship

Questions And Answers About Puberty

Excerpted from "Questions Answered," BAM! Body and Mind, Centers for Disease Control and Prevention, 2003.

What is puberty?

Puberty is a time in your life when your body makes changes that cause you to develop into an adult. These changes affect both how you look like growing taller and developing more muscle. They also affect how you feel—one minute you want to be treated like an adult, at other times you want to be treated like a kid.

What causes these changes?

Hormones in your body increase, and these make the changes of puberty happen. For girls, these hormones are estrogen and progesterone. For boys it's testosterone. Much of what happens to your body is controlled by your hormones and the "genetic map" that your body is following. Of course, no one can control these two things.

What is that smell?

During puberty, both boys and girls sweat glands are more active. Kids will also sweat more during puberty. A lot of kids notice that they have a new smell under their arms and elsewhere on their bodies when they hit puberty, and it's not a pretty one. That smell is body odor (you may have heard people call it B.O. for short), and everyone gets it. The hormones become more active, affect the glands in your skin, and the glands make chemicals that smell bad.

So what can you do to feel less stinky? Well, keeping clean can stop you from smelling. You might want to take a shower every day, either in the morning before school or at night before bed. Showering after you've been

✔ Quick Tip

Learning To Love What You See In The Mirror

We all want to look our best, but a healthy body is not always linked to appearance. In fact, healthy bodies come in all shapes and sizes. Changing your body image means changing the way you think about your body. At the same time, healthy lifestyle choices are also key to improving body image.

- Healthy eating can promote healthy skin and hair, along with strong bones.
- Regular exercise has been shown to boost self-esteem, self-image, and energy levels.
- Plenty of rest is key to stress management.

Source: Excerpted from "Loving Your Body Inside and Out," National Women's Health Information Center, March 19, 2008.

playing sports or exercising is a really good idea. Another way to cut down on body odor is to use deodorant. If you use a deodorant with antiperspirant, it will cut down on sweat as well.

Does everyone get pimples during puberty?

About 85–90% of all kids—boys and girls—have acne during puberty. The hormonal changes that are happening inside your body cause the oil glands to become more active. It doesn't mean that you are dirty, it just means that what is happening on the inside has put your oil glands into high gear and can causes acne or pimples. You may notice pimples on your face, your upper back, or your upper chest. Pimples usually start around the beginning of puberty and can hang around for a few years as your body changes.

No one understands me. I am not in control. Why do I feel this way?

Just as suddenly as your body starts changing, your mind is also making changes. The same hormones that cause changes in your appearance can also affect your emotions, making you feel like no one understands what you're experiencing. You may feel like your emotions are all over the place. One minute you're happy and bouncing off the walls, the next minute you're losing your temper, or bawling your eyes out.

What's going on? Confusion and mixed-up feelings are normal. The different hormones in your body can send your emotions on a roller-coaster ride. Puberty makes almost everyone feel that way. Make no mistake—your body has taken control and you are along for the ride. These changes in emotions are normal and once you've gone through puberty, the emotional roller coaster should slow down. Just keep your cool. It'll gradually become easier as you get used to the new you.

In the meantime, you can control other things that affect how you look, how you feel, and how healthy you are. Taking charge of your health can help you to feel good, and in control during the changes of puberty.

Chapter 51

Running Away

"I'm afraid that my friend may run away. How can I stop it?"

It is estimated that on any given night, there are between five hundred and one thousand homeless youth on the streets of Seattle, Los Angeles, Las Vegas, and other major cities. Many of them are runaways—teens under the age of 18 who leave their home or place of legal residence without the permission of parents or a legal guardian. They come from every social class, race, and religion. And they are usually hungry, scared, desperate, and very vulnerable to crime.

If you think your friend is about to run away, ask her or him these questions:

- What else can you do to improve your home situation before you leave?
- What would make you stay at home?
- How will you survive?
- What will you do for money?
- Is running away safe?
- Who can you count on for help?

About This Chapter: This chapter includes text from "Running Away," Office on Women's Health (www.girlshealth.gov), June 11, 2008.

- Are you being realistic?
- Have you given this enough thought?
- What are your other options?
- If you end up in trouble, who will you call?
- When you return home, what will happen?
- Why run away?

The most common reason that teens run away is family problems over such issues as: curfew, behavior, dress code, grades, and the choice of friends. Teens also may choose to run away because of problems they are afraid to face, such as bullying at school, pregnancy, sexual orientation, or alcohol and drug problems.

There are a number of teens that may choose life on the street because of emotional, physical, and sexual abuse in their home. The nature of ANY kind of abuse—the shame your friend may have, and the possible involvement of parents, stepparents, or other family members—may make it extremely difficult for your friend to tell. This is not a time for your friend to run-away.

Encourage your friend to tell a teacher, counselor, babysitter,

✤ It's A Fact!!

According to the National Runaway Hotline, there are many problems of being a runaway, including the following:

- Nine out of ten teens return home or are returned to their home by the police within a month. If your friend runs away, she or he may not be one of the nine that returns home.
- A lot can happen in one month. Many runaways, who remain in the streets for two or more weeks, will become involved in theft, drugs, or pornography. One out of every three teens on the street will be lured into prostitution within 48 hours of leaving home.
- Your problems at home are replaced by more serious and dangerous problems on the street. It's not worth it.
- Being a teen is not easy. There are a whole lot of ups and downs, changes, and new experiences.
- Sometimes it may feel that your parents don't make things easier with their demands. "My parents don't listen to me!" This is the most common complaint teens and even younger children have about their parents. Parents, on the other hand, have the same complaint: "She won't listen to me."

neighbor, clergy person, or your parents. Offer to go along with your friend to give her or him support. Let your friend know that being abused is not her or his fault. Be clear to your friend—nothing about what they say, the way they look, or how they behave gives ANYONE the right to use or hurt them.

Here are some signs that your friend may run away:

- She or he has sudden and dramatic mood swings that affect eating and socializing patterns.
- Her or his school grades, attendance, and behavior suddenly drop.
- She or he suddenly starts carrying large amounts of money and even asks you to keep some of it.
- She or he gives away clothing and other valuable items.
- She or he starts talking to you about running away. "Do you think anyone would miss me if I leave home?" (Take these statements seriously.)

If you are afraid that your friend may run away, consider these suggestions:

- Let her or him know that running away will not solve anything. It will make things worse.
- Ask your friend to get permission to stay with you and your family for a couple of days.
- Encourage your friend to talk to her or his parents, grandparents, or teacher.
- If your friend says she or he is being abused, tell your parents immediately. Your friend's life may depend on it. Your parents can call the police, local child protective services, or 1-800-4-A-CHILD (Childhelp USA).

Here are some family communication tips:

- Set aside time to talk to your parents every day.
- Don't expect your parents to read your mind.

- Be specific about your expectations and requests.
- Have patience—good communication takes time and effort.
- Brainstorm ideas with your parents before making a final decision.
- Ask for input from all family members.
- Write things down. Make a list of changes you want to see.
- Be willing to compromise with your parents.
- Use community resources when you need help. Ask a teacher or school counselor for leads.

If this doesn't work, and you find yourself in a crisis with your parents, contact the **National Runaway Hotline (1-800-RUNAWAY).** They can help you work through your problems and even set-up conference calls with you and your parents. The hotline is staffed 24 hours a day. It is also confidential and free. Remember, running away doesn't solve anything. It can make things worse.

Chapter 52

Suicide

> **✤ It's A Fact!!**
>
> If you are thinking about suicide, call 800-273-TALK (800-273-8255).
>
> NOW!
>
> Source: Office on Women's Health, 2008.

Why do some teens think about suicide?

Thinking about suicide often goes along with stressful events and feeling sad. Some teens feel so overwhelmed and sad that they think they will never feel better. Some things that can cause these feelings include the following:

- Death of a loved one
- Seeing a lot of anger and violence at home
- Having parents get divorced
- Having a hard time in school, struggling with grades or having problems with other teens
- Depression or alcohol or drug problems
- Anger or heart-break over a relationship break-up
- Feeling like you don't belong, either within the family or with friends
- Feeling left out or alone

About This Chapter: Text in this chapter is from "Suicide," Office on Women's Health (http://www.girlshealth.gov), March 12, 2008.

✔ Quick Tip

Help is available anytime, anywhere.

The National Suicide Prevention Lifeline is a free and confidential service for those who are seeking help when they feel like there is nowhere to turn. 800-273-TALK (8255) can be dialed toll free from anywhere in the United States 24 hours a day, 7 days a week. Trained crisis center staff are available to listen to your needs and offer these services:

- Crisis counseling
- Suicide intervention
- Mental health referral information

You are not alone. We are here to listen and to help you find your way back to a happier, healthier life.

Source: Excerpted from "Lonely? Trapped? Hopeless? Alone? When it seems like there is no hope, there is help," Substance Abuse and Mental Health Services Administration, January 2006.

Sometimes, teens may feel very sad for no one clear reason. Every teen feels anxiety and confusion at some point, but it helps to get through tough times by turning to people you trust and love. If you don't think you have people like this in your life, talk to a school counselor, teacher, doctor, or another adult who can help you talk about your feelings. There are ways to help teens deal with these intense feelings and work on feeling better in the future.

How common is the problem of teen suicide?

Suicide is one of the leading causes of death for teens. Girls try to commit suicide more often than boys. The important thing for you to know is that it doesn't have to happen. It is also important to know that suicide is not a heroic act, even though sometimes media images can make it seem so. Often, a person who is thinking about attempting suicide isn't able to see that suicide is never the answer to problems.

Remember, there is always help—as well as support and love—out there for you or a friend.

How can you help a friend?

If you have a friend or friends who have talked about suicide, take it seriously. The first thing you should do is to tell an adult you trust—right away. You may wonder if your friend(s) will be mad at you, but telling an adult is the right thing to do. This can be someone in your family, a coach, a school nurse, counselor, or a teacher. You can call 911 or the toll-free number of a suicide crisis line. You can't help your friend(s) alone. They will need a good support system, including friends, family, teachers, and professional help. Suggest that they should talk with a trusted adult. Offer to listen and encourage them to talk about their feelings. Don't ignore their worries or tell them they will get better on their own. Listening shows that you take your friend(s) and their problems seriously and that you are there to help. If someone is in danger of hurting himself or herself, do not leave the person alone. You may need to call 911.

What about you?

If you feel suicidal, talk to an adult right away. Call 911 or 800-SUICIDE, or check in your phone book for the number of a suicide crisis center. The centers offer experts who can help callers talk through their problems and develop a plan of action. These hotlines can also tell you where to go for more help in person.

Things may seem bad at times, but those times don't last forever. Your pain right now probably feels like it is too overwhelming to cope with—suicide may feel like the only form of relief. But remember that people do make it through suicidal thoughts. Ask for help—you can feel better. Don't use alcohol or drugs, because they can't take your problems away. If you can't find someone to talk with, write down your thoughts. Try to remember and write down the things you are grateful for. List the people who are your friends and family and care for you. Write about your hopes for the future. Read what you have written when you need to remind yourself that your life is IMPORTANT!

There is no reason that you or a friend has to continue hurting. There are ways to find help and hope.

What if someone you know attempts or dies by suicide?

If someone you know attempts or dies by suicide, it's important to remember that it isn't your fault. You may feel many different emotions: anger, grief, guilt, or you may even feel numb. All of your feelings are okay; there is not a right or wrong way to feel. If you are having trouble dealing with your feelings, talk to a trusted adult or use the contact information below. It is important that you feel strong ties with people at this time.

If you are thinking about suicide these places can help you.

- National Hopeline Network: 800-SUICIDE (784-2433)
- National Suicide Prevention Lifeline: 800-273-TALK (8255)
- Suicide Awareness-Voices of Education: 612-946-7998

✔ Quick Tip
Suicide Warning Signs

Seek help as soon as possible by contacting a mental health professional or by calling the National Suicide Prevention Lifeline at 800-273-TALK if you or someone you know exhibits any of the following suicide warning signs:

- Threatening to hurt or kill oneself or talking about wanting to hurt or kill oneself
- Looking for ways to kill oneself by seeking access to firearms, available pills, or other means
- Talking or writing about death, dying, or suicide when these actions are out of the ordinary for the person
- Feeling hopeless
- Feeling rage or uncontrolled anger or seeking revenge
- Acting reckless or engaging in risky activities—seemingly without thinking
- Feeling trapped—like there's no way out
- Increasing alcohol or drug use
- Withdrawing from friends, family, and society
- Feeling anxious or agitated, being unable to sleep, or sleeping all the time
- Experiencing dramatic mood changes
- Seeing no reason for living or having no sense of purpose in life

Source: Excerpted from "Lonely? Trapped? Hopeless? Alone? When it seems like there is no hope, there is help," Substance Abuse and Mental Health Services Administration, January 2006.

Chapter 53

Tourette Syndrome

What is Tourette syndrome?

Tourette syndrome (TS) is a neurological disorder characterized by repetitive, stereotyped, involuntary movements and vocalizations called tics. The disorder is named for Dr. Georges Gilles de la Tourette, the pioneering French neurologist who in 1885 first described the condition in an 86-year-old French noblewoman.

The early symptoms of TS are almost always noticed first in childhood, with the average onset between the ages of seven and 10 years. TS occurs in people from all ethnic groups; males are affected about three to four times more often than females. It is estimated that 200,000 Americans have the most severe form of TS, and as many as one in 100 exhibit milder and less complex symptoms such as chronic motor or vocal tics or transient tics of childhood. Although TS can be a chronic condition with symptoms lasting a lifetime, most people with the condition experience their worst symptoms in their early teens, with improvement occurring in the late teens and continuing into adulthood.

What are the symptoms?

Tics are classified as either simple or complex. Simple motor tics are sudden, brief, repetitive movements that involve a limited number of muscle

About This Chapter: Text in this chapter is from "Tourette Syndrome Fact Sheet," National Institute of Neurological Disorders and Stroke (www.ninds.nih.gov), July 15, 2008.

groups. Some of the more common simple tics include eye blinking and other vision irregularities, facial grimacing, shoulder shrugging, and head or shoulder jerking. Simple vocalizations might include repetitive throat-clearing, sniffing, or grunting sounds. Complex tics are distinct, coordinated patterns of movements involving several muscle groups. Complex motor tics might include facial grimacing combined with a head twist and a shoulder shrug. Other complex motor tics may actually appear purposeful, including sniffing or touching objects, hopping, jumping, bending, or twisting. Simple vocal tics may include throat-clearing, sniffing/snorting, grunting, or barking. More complex vocal tics include words or phrases. Perhaps the most dramatic and disabling tics include motor movements that result in self-harm such as punching oneself in the face or vocal tics including coprolalia (uttering swear words) or echolalia (repeating the words or phrases of others). Some tics are preceded by an urge or sensation in the affected muscle group, commonly called a premonitory urge. Some with TS will describe a need to complete a tic in a certain way or a certain number of times in order to relieve the urge or decrease the sensation.

Tics are often worse with excitement or anxiety and better during calm, focused activities. Certain physical experiences can trigger or worsen tics, for example tight collars may trigger neck tics, or hearing another person sniff or throat-clear may trigger similar sounds. Tics do not go away during sleep but are often significantly diminished.

✤ It's A Fact!!
Can people with TS control their tics?

Although the symptoms of Tourette syndrome (TS) are involuntary, some people can sometimes suppress, camouflage, or otherwise manage their tics in an effort to minimize their impact on functioning. However, people with TS often report a substantial buildup in tension when suppressing their tics to the point where they feel that the tic must be expressed. Tics in response to an environmental trigger can appear to be voluntary or purposeful but are not.

What is the course of TS?

Tics come and go over time, varying in type, frequency, location, and severity. The first symptoms usually occur in the head and neck area and may progress to include muscles of the trunk and extremities. Motor tics generally precede the development of vocal tics and simple tics often precede complex tics. Most patients experience peak tic severity before the mid-teen years with improvement for the majority of patients in the late teen years and early adulthood. Approximately 10 percent of those affected have a progressive or disabling course that lasts into adulthood.

What causes TS?

Although the cause of TS is unknown, current research points to abnormalities in certain brain regions (including the basal ganglia, frontal lobes, and cortex), the circuits that interconnect these regions, and the neurotransmitters (dopamine, serotonin, and norepinephrine) responsible for communication among nerve cells. Given the often complex presentation of TS, the cause of the disorder is likely to be equally complex.

How is TS diagnosed?

TS is a diagnosis that doctors make after verifying that the patient has had both motor and vocal tics for at least one year. The existence of other neurological or psychiatric conditions can also help doctors arrive at a diagnosis. Common tics are not often misdiagnosed by knowledgeable clinicians. But atypical symptoms or atypical presentation (for example, onset of symptoms in adulthood) may require specific specialty expertise for diagnosis. There are no blood or laboratory tests needed for diagnosis, but neuroimaging studies, such as magnetic resonance imaging (MRI), computerized tomography (CT), and electroencephalogram (EEG) scans, or certain blood tests may be used to rule out other conditions that might be confused with TS.

It is not uncommon for patients to obtain a formal diagnosis of TS only after symptoms have been present for some time. The reasons for this are many. For families and physicians unfamiliar with TS, mild and even moderate tic symptoms may be considered inconsequential, part of a developmental phase, or the result of another condition. For example, parents may think that eye blinking is related to vision problems or that sniffing is related to seasonal allergies. Many patients are self-diagnosed after they, their parents, other relatives, or friends read or hear about TS from others.

How is TS treated?

Because tic symptoms do not often cause impairment, the majority of people with TS require no medication for tic suppression. However, effective medications are available for those whose symptoms interfere with functioning. Neuroleptics are the most consistently useful medications for tic suppression; a number are available but some are more effective than others (for example, haloperidol and pimozide). Unfortunately, there is no one medication that is helpful to all people with TS, nor does any medication completely eliminate symptoms. In addition, all medications have side effects. Most neuroleptic side effects can be managed by initiating treatment slowly and reducing the dose when side effects occur. The most common side effects of neuroleptics include sedation, weight gain, and cognitive dulling. Neurological side effects such as tremor, dystonic reactions (twisting movements or postures), parkinsonian-like symptoms, and other dyskinetic (involuntary) movements are less common and are readily managed with dose reduction. Discontinuing neuroleptics after long-term use must be done slowly to avoid rebound increases in tics and withdrawal dyskinesias. One form of withdrawal dyskinesia called tardive dyskinesia is a movement disorder distinct from TS that may result

✤ It's A Fact!!
What disorders are associated with TS?

Many with Tourette syndrome (TS) experience additional neurobehavioral problems including inattention; hyperactivity and impulsivity (attention deficit hyperactivity disorder—ADHD), and related problems with reading, writing, and arithmetic; and obsessive-compulsive symptoms such as intrusive thoughts/worries and repetitive behaviors. For example, worries about dirt and germs may be associated with repetitive hand-washing, and concerns about bad things happening may be associated with ritualistic behaviors such as counting, repeating, or ordering and arranging. People with TS have also reported problems with depression or anxiety disorders, as well as other difficulties with living, that may or may not be directly related to TS. Given the range of potential complications, people with TS are best served by receiving medical care that provides a comprehensive treatment plan.

from the chronic use of neuroleptics. The risk of this side effect can be reduced by using lower doses of neuroleptics for shorter periods of time.

Other medications may also be useful for reducing tic severity, but most have not been as extensively studied or shown to be as consistently useful as neuroleptics. Additional medications with demonstrated efficacy include alpha-adrenergic agonists such as clonidine and guanfacine. These medications are used primarily for hypertension but are also used in the treatment of tics. The most common side effect from these medications that precludes their use is sedation.

Effective medications are also available to treat some of the associated neurobehavioral disorders that can occur in patients with TS. Recent research shows that stimulant medications such as methylphenidate and dextroamphetamine can lessen ADHD symptoms in people with TS without causing tics to become more severe. However, the product labeling for stimulants currently contraindicates the use of these drugs in children with tics/TS and those with a family history of tics. Scientists hope that future studies will include a thorough discussion of the risks and benefits of stimulants in those with TS or a family history of TS and will clarify this issue. For obsessive-compulsive symptoms that significantly disrupt daily functioning, the serotonin reuptake inhibitors (clomipramine, fluoxetine, fluvoxamine, paroxetine, and sertraline) have been proven effective in some patients.

Psychotherapy may also be helpful. Although psychological problems do not cause TS, such problems may result from TS. Psychotherapy can help the person with TS better cope with the disorder and deal with the secondary social and emotional problems that sometimes occur. More recently, specific behavioral treatments that include awareness training and competing response training, such as voluntarily moving in response to a premonitory urge, have shown effectiveness in small controlled trials. Larger and more definitive NIH-funded studies are underway.

Is TS inherited?

Evidence from twin and family studies suggests that TS is an inherited disorder. Although early family studies suggested an autosomal dominant mode of inheritance (an autosomal dominant disorder is one in which only one copy of the defective gene, inherited from one parent, is necessary to produce the disorder), more recent studies suggest that the pattern of inheritance is much more complex. Although there may be a few genes with substantial effects, it is also possible that many genes with smaller effects and environmental factors may play a role in the development of TS. Genetic studies also suggest that some forms of ADHD and OCD are genetically related to TS, but there is less evidence for a genetic relationship between TS and other neurobehavioral problems that commonly co-occur with TS. It is important for families to understand that genetic predisposition may not necessarily result in full-blown TS; instead, it may express itself as a milder tic disorder or as obsessive-compulsive behaviors. It is also possible that the gene-carrying offspring will not develop any TS symptoms.

The sex of the person also plays an important role in TS gene expression. At-risk males are more likely to have tics and at-risk females are more likely to have obsessive-compulsive symptoms.

People with TS may have genetic risks for other neurobehavioral disorders such as depression or substance abuse. Genetic counseling of individuals with TS should include a full review of all potentially hereditary conditions in the family.

What is the prognosis?

Although there is no cure for TS, the condition in many individuals improves in the late teens and early 20s. As a result, some may actually become symptom-free or no longer need medication for tic suppression. Although the disorder is generally lifelong and chronic, it is not a degenerative condition. Individuals with TS have a normal life expectancy. TS does not impair intelligence. Although tic symptoms tend to decrease with age, it is possible that neurobehavioral disorders such as depression, panic attacks, mood swings, and antisocial behaviors can persist and cause impairment in adult life.

Chapter 54

Youth Violence

Youth Violence Facts

Youth violence is a widespread problem in the United States. Consider the following statistics:

- About 9% of murders in the U.S. were committed by youth under 18 in 2000. An estimated 1,561 youth under the age of 18 were arrested for homicide in 2000.
- Youth under 18 accounted for about 15% of violent crime arrests in 2001.
- One national survey found that for every teen arrested, at least 10 were engaged in violence that could have seriously injured or killed another person.
- About one in three high-school students say they have been in a physical fight in the past year, and about one in eight of those students required medical attention for their injuries.
- More than one in six students in grades 6 to 10 say they are bullied

About This Chapter: This chapter includes excerpts from the following fact sheets produced by the National Youth Violence Prevention Resource Center: "Youth Violence Facts," January 4, 2008; "Youth Gangs and Violence," January 4, 2008; and "Media Violence Facts and Statistics," February 26, 2008. The complete text of these documents, including references, is available online at www.safeyouth.org.

sometimes, and more than one in twelve say they are bullied once a week or more.

- Suicide is the third leading cause of death among teenagers.
- About one in eleven high-school students say they have made a suicide attempt in the past year.

Although youth violence has always been a problem in the United States, the number of deaths and serious injuries increased dramatically during the late 1980s and early 1990s, as more and more youth began to carry weapons.

Since then, however, the tide has begun to turn. Between 1992 and 2001, juvenile arrests on weapons charges dropped 35%; the juvenile arrest rate for murder fell 62%, dropping to its lowest level in more than two decades; and the juvenile arrest rate for violent crimes dropped by 21%. Clearly, considerable progress has been made, but youth violence does still remain a serious problem in the United States.

Risk And Protective Factors

Researchers have identified a number of factors that increase children and youths' risk for becoming involved in serious violence during adolescence. For children under 13, the most important factors include: early involvement in serious criminal behavior, early substance use, being male, a history of physical aggression toward others, low parent education levels or poverty, and parent involvement in illegal activities.

Once a child becomes an adolescent, different factors predict involvement in serious violence. Friends and peers are much more important for adolescents, and friendships with antisocial or delinquent peers, membership in a gang, and involvement in other criminal activity are the most important predictors of serious violence for adolescents.

A number of protective factors for youth violence have been proposed and researched, but at this point, only two have been found to buffer the risk of serious violence—an intolerant attitude toward deviance and commitment to school. As further research is conducted, it is likely that other protective factors will be identified.

✤ It's A Fact!!

The United States has the highest rate of youth firearm-related violence in the industrialized world. Many premature deaths and injuries are related to youth gun violence. During the late 1980s and early 1990s, youth firearm-related violence increased dramatically in the United States. Juvenile gun arrests rose sharply as more teens began to carry guns, and the number of gun homicides committed by juveniles more than doubled. Youth suicides with handguns also increased rapidly during that same time period. Since 1994, however, it appears that the tide may be turning. In recent years, we have seen significant decreases in youth suicides involving guns and in firearm-related homicides involving a juvenile offender. However, much remains to be done. Each year in the United States, many teens still illegally access firearms and harm others and themselves.

Source: Excerpted from "Youth Firearm-Related Violence Fact Sheet," National Youth Violence Prevention Resource Center, December 18, 2007.

Youth Gangs And Violence

Although once thought to be an inner-city problem, gang violence has spread to communities throughout the United States. At last count, there were more than 24,500 different youth gangs around the country, and more than 772,500 teens and young adults were members of gangs.

Teens join gangs for a variety of reasons. Some are seeking excitement; others are looking for prestige, protection, a chance to make money, or a sense of belonging. Few teens are forced to join gangs; in most cases, teens can refuse to join without fear of retaliation.

Since 1996, the overall number of gangs and gang members in the United States has decreased. However, in cities with a population over 25,000, gang involvement still remains near peak levels.

Most youth gang members are between the ages of 12 and 24, and the average age is about 17 to 18 years. Around half of youth gang members are 18 or older, and they are much more likely to be involved in serious and violent crimes than younger gang members. Only about one in four youth gang members are ages 15 to 17.

Male youth are much more likely to join gangs than female youth. It is hard to get a good estimate of the number of female gangs and gang members,

✤ It's A Fact!!

Hate Crimes

The National Incident-Based Reporting System (NIBRS) reporting requirements dictate that hate crimes be categorized according to the perceived bias motivation of the offender. Due to the difficulty in determining an offender's motivations, law enforcement agencies record hate crimes only when investigation reveals facts sufficient to conclude that the offender's actions were bias motivated.

Overall, bias crimes account for a relatively small percentage of all criminal incidents. Of the nearly 5.4 million NIBRS incidents reported by law enforcement agencies between 1997 and 1999, about 3,000 were identified as hate crimes.

Victims: The age of hate crime victims varied according to the nature of the offense, as a larger percentage of victims of violent hate crime were young. More than half of victims of violence were age 24 or under, and nearly a third were under 18.

Offenders: Among all NIBRS hate crime incidents, 33% of known offenders (which implies only that some characteristic of the suspect was identified) were age 17 or younger; 29%, age 18 to 24; 17%, age 25 to 34; and 21%, age 35 or older. Violent offenders were generally older than property offenders. Of violent offenders, 31% were age 17 or younger and 60% were age 24 or younger. Of property offenders, 46% were age 17 or younger and 71% were age 24 or younger.

Source: Excerpted from "Hate Crimes Reported in NIBRS, 1997–99," Bureau of Justice Statistics, U.S. Department of Justice, September 2001.

however, because many police jurisdictions do not count girls as gang members. While the national estimates based on police reports indicate that only about 8% of gang members are female, one 11-city survey of eighth-graders found that 38% of gang members are female. Female gangs are somewhat more likely to be found in small cities and rural areas than in large cities, and female gang members tend to be younger, on average, than male gang members.

Youth gangs are linked with serious crime problems in elementary and secondary schools in the United States. Students report much higher drug availability when gangs are active at their school. Schools with gangs have nearly double the likelihood of violent victimization at school than those without a gang presence. Teens that are gang members are much more likely than other teens to commit serious and violent crimes.

Media Violence Facts And Statistics

The Television Violence Monitoring Project examined the amount of violence on American television for three consecutive years, as well as contextual variables that may make it more likely for aggression and violence to be accepted, learned, and imitated. Here is some of the statistical information they found:

- 61 percent of television programs contain some violence, and only four percent of television programs with violent content feature an "anti-violence" theme.
- 44 percent of the violent interactions on television involve perpetrators who have some attractive qualities worthy of emulation.
- 43 percent of violent scenes involve humor either directed at the violence or used by characters involved with violence.
- Nearly 75 percent of violent scenes on television feature no immediate punishment for or condemnation of violence.
- 40 percent of programs feature "bad" characters who are never or rarely punished for their aggressive actions.

The report notes that many television programs fail to depict the harmful consequences of violence. Specifically, it finds that of all violent behavioral interactions on television, 58 percent depict no pain, 47 percent depict no harm, and 40 percent depict harm unrealistically. Of all violent scenes on television, 86 percent feature no blood or gore. Only 16 percent of violent programs feature the long-term, realistic consequences of violence.

✤ It's A Fact!!

Children And Aggression

Aggressive behavior is common in very small children. When toddlers are angry or frustrated, they often will push, shove, bite, and hit other children. As they move into their preschool years, they tend to turn to verbal aggression, yelling at other children and having temper tantrums.

Most children become less aggressive as they mature and develop more effective self-control and language and interpersonal skills. A few continue to be highly aggressive as they move into their elementary school years, getting into fights and bullying other children. These children are much more likely than other children to become involved in serious violence during their teenage years, and to continue that violence into adulthood.

It is important to realize, however, that most aggressive children do not go on to engage in serious violence as teens and adults. And, teens with no history of aggression as children can become aggressive and violent during their teenage years, often as they begin to spend time with other teens that are involved in antisocial activities.

As teens transition from adolescence into adulthood, most cease their involvement in serious violence. Only about 20 percent of serious violent offenders continue their violent careers into their twenties.

Source: Excerpted from "Children and Aggression," National Youth Violence Prevention Resource Center, December 27, 2007.

Is there a link between media violence and aggressive behavior?

There is now solid evidence to suggest a relationship between exposure to violent television and movies and aggressive behavior. Researchers have found that children are more physically and verbally aggressive immediately after watching violent television and movies. It is also clear that aggressive children and teens watch more violent television than their less aggressive peers. A few studies have found that exposure to television and movie violence in childhood is related to increased aggression years later, but further research is needed in this area.

A relatively small amount of research has focused on the impact of music videos with violent or antisocial themes. Researchers have found that exposure to violent or antisocial rap videos can increase aggressive thinking, but no research has yet tested how such exposure directly affects physical aggression.

Children's use of video games has become widespread. A 2001 review of the 70 top-selling video games found 89% contained some kind of violence. Almost half of all games (49%) contained serious violence, while 40% contained comic violence. In 41% of the games, violence was necessary for the protagonists to achieve their goals. In 17% of the games, violence was the primary focus of the game itself.

The impact of the widespread use of violent video games is a cause of concern for researchers, because they fear that the interactive nature of video games may increase the likelihood of children learning aggressive behavior and that the increasing realism might encourage greater identification with characters and more imitation of the behaviors of video game models.

To date, violent video games have not been studied as extensively as violent television or movies. The number of studies investigating the impact of such games on youth aggression is small, there have been none on serious violence, and none has been longitudinal. A recent meta-analysis of these studies found that the exposure to violent video games has a relatively small effect on physical aggression and a moderate effect on aggressive thinking. The impact of video games on violent behavior remains to be determined.

Part Six

If You Need More Information

Chapter 55

Crisis Helplines And Hotlines

Access Line

Washington D.C. Department of Mental Health
888-7-WE HELP (888-793-4357)

Al-Anon/Alateen Meetings Information Line

800-344-2666
Monday through Friday, 8:00 a.m.–6:00 p.m. EST

Alcohol and Drug Help Line

WellPlace
800-821-4357

Alcohol Hotline

Adcare Hospital
800-ALCOHOL (800-252-6465)

American Council on Alcoholism

800-527-5344
10:00–6:00 p.m. MST

About This Chapter: Information in this chapter was compiled from many sources deemed reliable. Inclusion does not constitute endorsement, and there is no implication associated with omission. All contact information was verified in December 2009.

ARK Crisis Line
800-873-TEEN (800-873-8336)

Boys Town National Hotline
800-448-3000

Center for Substance Abuse Treatment
U.S. Department of Health and Human Services
English: 800-662-HELP (800-662-4357)
TDD: 800-487-4889
Spanish: 877-767-8432
Monday–Friday, 9:00 a.m.–3:00 a.m.

Child Quest International Sighting Line
Phone: 888-818-HOPE (888-818-4673)

Distress/Suicide Help Line
800-232-7288 (Canada only)

Eating Disorder Awareness and Prevention
National Eating Disorders Association
800-931-2237
8:30 a.m.–4:30 p.m. PST

Emergency Shelter For Battered Women (And Their Children)
888-291-6228

Hope Line
800-SUICIDE (800-784-2433)

Life Line
800-273-TALK (800-273-8255)

NAMI Information Helpline
Nation's Voice on Mental Illness
800-950-NAMI (6264)
Monday–Friday 10:00 a.m.–6:00 p.m. EST

Narconon International Help Line
800-893-7060

National Center For Missing And Exploited Children
800-THE-LOST (800-843-5678)

National Center For Victims Of Crime
800-FYI-CALL (800-394-2255)
8:30 a.m.–8:30 p.m. EST

National Child Abuse Hot Line
Childhelp USA
800-4-A-CHILD (800-422-4453)

National Clearinghouse for Alcohol and Drug Information
800-729-6686

National Domestic Violence Hot Line
800-799-7233
TTY: 800-787-3224

National Organization for Victim Assistance
800-TRY-NOVA (800-879-6682)
Monday–Friday 9:00 a.m.–5:00 p.m. EST

National Runaway Switchboard
800-RUNAWAY (800-786-2929)
TDD: 800-621-0394

National Sexual Assault Hotline
RAINN
800-656-HOPE (800-656-4673)

NINELINE
Covenant House Hotline
800-999-9999
2:00 p.m.–12:00 a.m.

Operation Lookout National Center For Missing Youth
800-LOOKOUT (800-566-5688)

Stop It Now!
888-PREVENT (888-773-8368)
Monday 12:00–4:00 p.m.

Trevor Help Line
800-850-8078

United Way Information Referral Service
800-233-HELP (800-233-4357)

Chapter 56

A Directory Of Mental Health Organizations

General Mental Health Resources

American Academy of Child and Adolescent Psychiatry

3615 Wisconsin Avenue, N.W.
Washington, DC 20016-3007
Phone: 202-966-7300
Fax: 202-966-2891
Website: www.aacap.org

American Psychiatric Association

1000 Wilson Boulevard
Suite 1825
Arlington, VA 22209-3901
Phone: 703-907-7300
Fax: 703-907-1085
E-mail: apa@psych.org
Website: www.psych.org

American Psychiatric Nurses Association

1555 Wilson Boulevard
Suite 530
Arlington, VA 22209
Toll-Free: 866-243-2443
Phone: 703-243-2443
Fax: 703-243-3390
Website: www.apna.org

American Psychological Association

750 First Street, NE
Washington, DC 20002-4242
Toll-Free: 800-374-2721
Phone: 202-336-5500
Website: www.apa.org

About This Chapter: Information in this chapter was compiled from many sources deemed reliable. Inclusion does not constitute endorsement, and there is no implication associated with omission. All contact information was verified in December 2009.

American Psychotherapy Association

2750 E. Sunshine Street
Springfield, MO 65804
Phone: 417-823-0173
Toll-Free: 800-205-9165
Website:
www.americanpsychotherapy.com

American School Health Association

7263 State Route 43
P.O. Box 708
Kent, OH 44240
Phone: 330-678-1601
Fax: 330-678-4526
Website: www.ashaweb.org
E-mail: asha@ashaweb.org

Center for Mental Health Services

Substance Abuse and Mental Health Services Administration
P.O. Box 42557
Washington, DC 20015
Rockville, MD 20847
Toll-Free: 800-789-2647
Fax: 240-221-4295
Website:
mentalhealth.samhsa.gov
Mental Health Services Locator:
mentalhealth.samhsa.gov/databases

National Institute of Child Health and Human Development

P.O. Box 3006
Rockville, MD 20847
Toll-Free: 800-370-2943
Phone: 800-370-2943
TTY: 888-320-6942
Fax: 866-760-5947
Website: www.nichd.nih.gov
E-mail: NICHDInformationResource Center@mail.nih.gov

National Institute of Mental Health

6001 Executive Boulevard
Room 8184, MSC 9663
Bethesda, MD 20892-9663
Toll-Free: 866-615-NIMH (615-6464)
Phone: 301-443-4513
TTY: 301-443-8431
Toll-Free TTY: 866-415-8051
Fax: 301-443-4279
Website: www.nimh.nih.gov
E-mail: nimhinfo@nih.gov

Teen Issues And Mental Health

Al-Anon/Alateen

1600 Corporate Landing Pky.
Virginia Beach, VA 23454-5617
Toll-Free: 800-344-2666
Phone: 757-563-1600
Fax: 757-563-1655
Website:
http://www.al-anon.alateen.org
E-mail: wso@al-anon.org

American Association of Suicidology

5221 Wisconsin Avenue, NW
Washington, DC 20015
Phone: 202-237-2280
Fax: 202-237-2282
Website: www.suicidology.org
E-mail: info@suicidology.org

American Foundation for Suicide Prevention

120 Wall Street, 22nd Floor
New York, NY 10005
Toll-free: 888-333-AFSP (333-2377)
Phone: 212-363-3500
Fax: 212-363-6237
Website: www.afsp.org
E-mail: inquiry@afsp.org

Centre for Addiction and Mental Health

33 Russell Street
Toronto, ON M5S 2S1
Canada
Phone: 416-535-8501
Website: http://www.camh.net

CrisisLink

2503 D N. Harrison St.
Suite #114
Arlington, VA 22207
24-hour hot line:
703-527-4077 (in Northern VA)
Toll-Free: 800-SUICIDE (784-2433)
Phone: 703-527-6603 (Business Calls Only)
Fax: 703-516-6767
Website: http://www.crisislink.org
E-mail: info@crisislink.org

Do It Now Foundation (Drug Information)

P.O. Box 27568
Tempe, AZ 85285-7568
Phone: 480-736-0599
Fax: 480-736-0771
Website: http://www.doitnow.org
E-mail: email@doitnow.org

Feeling Blue Suicide Prevention Committee

A Non-Profit Community Service Organization
P.O. Box 7193
St. Davids, PA 19087
Phone: 610-715-0076
Website: http://www.feelingblue.org

Jason Foundation (Suicide Prevention)

18 Volunteer Dr.
Henderson, TN 37075
Toll-Free: 888-881-2323
Phone: 615-264-2323
Fax: 615-264-0188
Website: http://
www.jasonfoundation.com
E-mail: info@jasonfoundation.com

Jed Foundation (Suicide Prevention)

220 5th Ave, 9th Floor
New York, NY 10001
Phone: 212-647-7544
Fax: 212-647-7542
Website:
http://www.jedfoundation.org
E-mail: emailus@jedfoundation.org

National Association for Children of Alcoholics

11426 Rockville Pike, Suite 301
Rockville, MD 20852
Toll-Free: 888-55-4COAS (2627)
Phone: 301-468-0985
Fax: 301-468-0987
Website: http://www.childrenofalcoholics.org
E-mail: nacoa@nacoa.org

National Center for Victims of Crime

2000 M Street NW, Suite 480
Washington, DC 20036
Phone: 202-467-8700
Fax: (202) 467-8701
Website: http://www.ncvc.org

National Center on Addiction and Substance Abuse at Columbia University

633 Third Ave., 19th Floor
New York, NY 10017-6706
Phone: 212-841-5200
Website: http://www.casacolumbia.org

National Clearinghouse for Alcohol and Drug Information

P.O. Box 2345
Rockville, MD 20847-2345
Toll Free: 800-729-6686
Linea gratis en Español: 877-767-8432
Phone: 301-468-2600
TDD: 800-487-4889
Fax: 301-468-6433
Website: www.health.org
E-mail: info@health.org

National Coalition Against Domestic Violence

1120 Lincoln Street, Suite 1603
Denver, CO 80203
Phone: 303-839-1852
Fax: 303-831-9251
TTY: 303-839-1681
Website: http://www.ncadv.org

National Council on Alcoholism and Drug Dependence, Inc.

244 E. 58th St. 4th Floor
New York, NY 10022
Toll-Free: 800-622-2255
or 800-475-4673
Phone: 212-269-7797
Fax: 212-269-7510
Website: http://www.ncadd.org
E-mail: national@ncadd.org

National Institute on Alcohol Abuse and Alcoholism

5635 Fishers Lane, MSC 9304
Bethesda, MD 20892-9304
Phone: 301-443-3860
Website: http://www.niaaa.nih.gov
E-mail: niaaweb-r@exchange.nih.gov

National Institute on Drug Abuse

6001 Executive Boulevard
Room 5213
Bethesda, MD 20892-9561
Toll-Free: 1-800-662-HELP
(1-800-662-4357
Phone: 301-443-1124
Website: www.nida.nih.gov
E-mail: information@nida.nih.gov

National Organization for People of Color Against Suicide

P.O. Box 75571
Washington, DC 20013
Toll-Free: 866-899-5317
Phone: 202-549-6039
Website: http://www.nopcas.org
E-mail: info@nopcas.org

National Organization for Victim Assistance

510 King Street
Suite 424
Alexandria, VA 22314
Toll-Free: 800-879-6682
Phone: 703-535-6682
Fax: 703-535-5500
Website: http://www.try-nova.org
E-mail: nova@try-nova.org

Office for Victims of Crime Resource Center

National Criminal Justice Reference Service
P.O. Box 6000
Rockville, MD 20850
Toll-Free: 800-851-3420
Toll-Free TTY: 877-712-9279
Phone: 301-519-5500
Fax: 301-519-5212
Website: http://www.ncjrs.org
E-mail: askncjrs@ncjrs.org

Safe and Drug-Free Schools

550 12th St. SW. 10th Floor
Washington, DC 20202-6450
Phone: 202-245-7896
Fax 202-485-0013
Website: http://www.ed.gov/offices/OESE/SDFS
E-mail: safeschl@ed.gov

Samaritans of NY

P.O. Box 1259
Madison Square Station
New York, NY 10159
Suicide Prevention Hot Line: 212-673-3000
Website: http://www.samaritansnyc.org/samhome.html

SAVE—Suicide Awareness Voices of Education

8120 Penn Ave. S.
Suite 470
Bloomington, MN 55431
Phone: 952-946-7998
Fax: 952-829-0841
Website: http://www.save.org
E-mail: save@save.org

Substance Abuse and Mental Health Services Administration

1 Choke Cherry Road
Rockville, MD 20857
Phone: 877-726-4727
Website: http://www.samhsa.gov

Suicide Prevention Action Network

1010 Vermont Ave., NW, Suite 408
Washington, DC 20005
Phone: 202-449-3600
Fax: 202-449-3601
Website: http://www.spanusa.org
E-mail: info@spanusa.org

Suicide Prevention Resource Center

55 Chapel Street
Newton, MA 02458-1060
Toll-Free: 877-GET-SPRC (438-7772)
TTY: 617-964-5448
Website: http://www.sprc.org
E-mail: info@sprc.org

Yellow Ribbon Suicide Prevention Program

P.O. Box 644
Westminster, CO 80036
Phone: 303-429-3530
Fax: 303-426-4496
Website: http://www.yellowribbon.org
E-mail: ask4help@yellowribbon.org

Mood And Anxiety Disorders

Anxiety Disorders Association of America

8730 Georgia Ave., Suite 600
Silver Spring, MD 20910
Phone: 240-485-1001
Fax: 240-485-1035
Website: http://www.adaa.org

Child and Adolescent Bipolar Foundation

1000 Skokie Blvd., Suite 425
Willmette, IL 60091
Phone: 847-256-8525
Fax: 847-920-9498
Website: http://www.bpkids.org
E-mail: cabf@bpkids.org

Depressed Anonymous

P.O. Box 17414
Louisville, KY 40217
Phone: 502-569-1989
Website: www.depressedanon.com
E-mail: info@depressedanon.com

Depression and Bipolar Support Alliance

730 N. Franklin St.
Suite 501
Chicago, IL 60610-7224
Toll-Free: 800-826-3632
Phone: 312-642-0049
Fax: 312-642-7243
Website: http://www.dbsalliance.org
E-mail: questions@dbsalliance.org

Families for Depression Awareness

395 Totten Pond Road
Suite 404
Waltham, MA 02472-4808
Phone: 781-890-0220
Fax: 781-890-2411
Website: www.familyaware.org
E-mail: info@familyaware.org

Freedom from Fear

308 Seaview Ave.
Staten Island, NY 10305
Phone: 718-351-1717
Fax: 718-980-5022
Website: http://
www.freedomfromfear.org
E-mail: help@freedomfromfear.org

Gift from Within

16 Cobb Hill Road
Camden, ME 04843
Phone: 207-236-8858
Fax: 207-236-2818
Website: www.giftfromwithin.org

International Society for Traumatic Stress Studies

60 Revere Dr.
Suite 500
Northbrook, IL 60062
Phone: 847-480-9028
Fax: 847-480-9282
Website: http://www.istss.org
E-mail: istss@istss.org

Mood Disorders Support Group

P.O. Box 30377
New York, NY 10011
Phone: 212-533-6374
Fax: 212-675-0218
24 Hour Suicide Hotline:
212-673-3000
Website: http://www.mdsg.org
E-mail: info@mdsg.org

National Anxiety Foundation

3135 Custer Drive
Lexington, KY 40517-4001
Website:
http://www.lexington-on-line.com/
naf.html

National Center for Crisis Management and American Academy of Experts in Traumatic Stress

368 Veterans Memorial Highway
Commack, NY 11725
Phone: 631-543-2217
Fax: 631-543-6977
Website: http://www.aaets.org
E-mail: info@aaets.org

National Center for Post Traumatic Stress Disorder

VA Medical Center (116D)
215 N. Main Street
White River Junction, VT 05009
Phone: 802-296-6300
Phone: 802-296-5132
Fax: 802-296-5135
Website: http://www.ncptsd.org
E-mail: ncptsd@ncptsd.org

Social Phobia/Social Anxiety Association

Website: http://www.socialphobia.org

Behavioral, Personality, and Psychotic Disorders

Attention Deficit Disorder Association

P.O. Box 7557
Wilmington, DE 19803-9997
Toll-Free: 800-939-1019
E-mail: info@add.org

Behavioral Institute for Children and Adolescents

1711 West County Road B, Suite 110S
Roseville, MN 55113
Phone: (651) 484-5510
Fax: (651) 483-3879
Website: www.BehavioralInstitute.org

Borderline Personality Disorder Resource Center

New York-Presbyterian Hospital-Westchester Division
21 Bloomingdale Rd., Room 103
White Plains, NY 10605
Phone: 888-694-2273
Website: http://www.bpdresourcecenter.org

Children and Adults with AD/HD

CHADD National Office
8181 Professional Place, Suite 150
Landover, MD 20785
Toll-Free: 800-233-4050 (National Resource Center on AD/HD and CHADD)
Phone: 301-306-7070
Fax: 301-306-7090
Website: www.chadd.org

Council for Children with Behavioral Disorders

P.O. Box 24246
Stanley, KS 66283
Phone: 913-239-0550
Website: www.ccbd.net

Eating Disorder Referral and Information Center

Website: www.edreferral.com

National Association of Anorexia Nervosa and Associated Disorders

P.O. Box 7
Highland Park, IL 60035
Phone: 630-577-1330
Website: http://www.anad.org

National Eating Disorders Association

603 Stewart St., Suite 803
Seattle, WA 98101
Toll Free: 800-931-2237 (hotline)
Phone: 206-382-3587
Website: http://www.nationaleatingdisorders.org
E-mail: info@NationalEatingDisorders.org

National Resource Center on AD/HD

Toll-Free: 800-233-4050
Website: http://www.help4adhd.org

Obsessive Compulsive Foundation

676 State Street
New Haven, CT 06511
Phone: 203-401-2070
Fax: 203-401-2076
Website: http://www.ocfoundation.org
E-mail: info@ocfoundation.org

SAFE (Self-Abuse Finally Ends) Alternatives

800-DONT-CUT (800-366-8288)
Website: http://www.selfinjury.com

Schizophrenia Home Page

Website: http://www.schizophrenia.com

Sidran Institute (Dissociative Disorders)

200 E. Joppa Road, Suite 207
Towson, MD 21286
Phone: 410-825-8888
Fax: 410-337-0747
Website: http://www.sidran.org
E-mail: help@sidran.org

Trichotillomania Learning Center

207 McPherson St. Suite H
Santa Cruz, CA 95060
Phone: 831-457-1004
Fax: 831-426-4383
Website: www.trich.org
E-mail: info@trich.org

World Fellowship for Schizophrenia and Allied Disorders

124 Merton Street, Suite 507
Toronto, Ontario, M4S 2Z2
Canada
Phone: 416-961-2855
Fax: 416-961-1948
Website: http://www.world-schizophrenia.org
E-mail: info@world-schizophrenia.org

Getting Help For Mental Illness

Abraham Low Self-Help Systems

Recovery, Inc.
105 W. Adams St., Ste. 2940
Chicago, Illinois 60603
Phone: 866-221-0302
Fax: 312-726-4446
Website: www.recovery-inc.com

American Art Therapy Association

225 N. Fairfax St.
Alexandria, VA 22314
Toll-Free: 888-290-0878
Website: www.arttherapy.org
E-mail: info@arttherapy.org

American Association for Marriage and Family Therapy

112 South Alfred Street
Alexandria, VA 22314-3061
Phone: 703-838-9808
Fax: 703-838-9805
Website: http://www.aamft.org

American Association of Pastoral Counselors

9504-A Lee Highway
Fairfax, VA 22031-2303
Phone: 703-385-6967
Fax: 703-352-7725
Website: http://www.aapc.org
E-mail: info@aapc.org

American Counseling Association

5999 Stevenson Ave.
Alexandria, VA 22304
Toll-Free: 800-347-6647
Fax: 800-473-2329
TDD: 703-823-6862
Website: http://www.counseling.org

American Group Psychotherapy Association

25 East 21st Street, Sixth Floor
New York, NY 10010
Toll-Free: 877-668-2472
Phone: 212-477-2677
Fax: 212-979-6627
Website: http://www.agpa.org
E-mail: info@agpa.org

Association for Behavioral and Cognitive Therapies

305 7th Avenue, 16th Floor
New York, NY 10001-60008
Phone: 212-647-1890
Fax: 212-647-1865
Website: http://www.aabt.org

National Empowerment Center (Recovery from Mental Illness)

599 Canal Street, 5th Floor East
Lawrence, MA 01840
Toll-Free: 800-POWER-2-U
(800-769-3728)
Phone: 978-685-1494
Fax: 978-681-6426
Website: http://www.power2u.org
E-mail: info4@power2u.org

Treatment Advocacy Center

3300 N. Fairfax Drive, Suite 220
Arlington, VA 22201
Phone: 703-294-6001
Fax: 703-294-6010
Website: http://www.psychlaws.org
E-mail: info@psychlaws.org

Chapter 57

Additional Reading About Mental Wellness And Mental Illness

Books

Abuse and Violence Information for Teens, edited by Sandra Augustyn Lawton, published by Omnigraphics, 2007.

Alcohol Information for Teens, Second Edition, edited by Lisa Bakewell, published by Omnigraphics, 2009.

Anxiety and Phobia Workbook, Fourth Edition, by Edmund J. Bourne, published by New Harbinger Publications, 2005.

Behind Happy Faces: Taking Charge of Your Mental Health, by Ross Szabo and Melanie Hall, published by National Book Network, 2007.

Bipolar Disorder, Depression, and Other Mood Disorders, by Helen A. Demetriades, published by Enslow Publishers, 2002.

About This Chapter: There is a lot of reference material about a myriad of topics related to mental health. The books and other items listed in this chapter were compiled from many resources and recommendations. The list is far from comprehensive; it is illustrative only and intended to serve merely as a starting point for further research. Inclusion does not constitute endorsement, and there is no implication associated with omission. All website information was verified in October 2009. To make topics easier to identify, documents within each category are listed alphabetically by title.

Body Blues: Weight and Depression, by Laura Weeldreyer, published by Rosen Publishing Group, 1998.

Bullying: How to Deal with Taunting, Teasing, and Tormenting, by Kathleen Winkler, published by Enslow Publishers, 2005.

Depression: What You Need to Know, by Margaret O. Hyde and Elizabeth H. Forsyth, published by Scholastic, 2002.

Eating Disorders Information for Teens, Second Edition, edited by Sandra Augustyn Lawton, published by Omnigraphics, 2009.

The Feelings Book: The Care and Keeping of Your Emotions, by Lynda Madison, published by American Girl Publishing, 2002.

Healing a Teen's Grieving Heart: 100 Practical Ideas for Families, Friends, and Caregivers, by Alan D. Wolfelt, published by Companion Press, 2001.

My Kind of Sad: What It's Like to Be Young and Depressed, by Kate Scowen, published by Firefly Books, 2006.

Odd Girl Out: The Hidden Culture of Aggression in Girls, by Rachel Simmons, published by Houghton Mifflin, 2003.

Relaxation and Stress Reduction Workbook, Sixth Edition, by Martha Davis, Elizabeth Robbins Eshelman, and Matthew McKay, published by New Harbinger Publications, 2008.

Sleep Information for Teens, edited by Karen Bellenir, published by Omnigraphics, 2008.

Stress Information for Teens, edited by Sandra Augustyn Lawton, published by Omnigraphics, 2008.

Stress 101: An Overview for Teens, by Margaret O. Hyde and Elizabeth H. Forsyth, published by Twenty-First Century Books, 2008

Suicide Information for Teens, edited by Joyce Brennfleck Shannon, published by Omnigraphics, 2005.

Teens, Depression and the Blues, by Kathleen Winkler, published by Enslow Publishers, 2000.

Where's Your Head? Teenage Psychology, by Dale Carlson and Hannah Carlson, published by Bick Publishing, 1998.

Youth with Eating Disorders: When Food Is an Enemy, by Noa Flynn, published by Mason Crest Publishers, 2008.

Web-Based Documents

Anxiety Disorders

National Institute of Mental Health
http://www.nimh.nih.gov/health/topics/anxiety-disorders/index.shtml

Body Image and Self-Esteem

Nemours Foundation
http://kidshealth.org/teen/your_mind/body_image/body_image.html

Children and Adolescents with Mental, Emotional, and Behavioral Disorders

National Mental Health Information Center
http://mentalhealth.samhsa.gov/publications/allpubs/CA-0006/default.asp

Controlling Anger—Before It Controls You

American Psychological Association
http://apahelpcenter.org/articles/article.php?id=29

Depression

National Institute of Mental Health
http://www.nimh.nih.gov/health/topics/depression/index.shtml

Eliminate Disparities in Mental Health

Office of Minority Health and Health Disparities
http://www.cdc.gov/omhd/AMH/factsheets/mental.htm

Exercise Helps Keep Your Psyche Fit

American Psychological Association
http://www.psychologymatters.org/exercise.html

How Your Emotions Affect Your Health

American Academy of Family Physicians
http://familydoctor.org/online/famdocen/home/healthy/mental/782.html

Making and Keeping Friends—A Self-Help Guide

Substance Abuse and Mental Health Services Administration
http://mentalhealth.samhsa.gov/publications/allpubs/SMA-3716/introduction.asp

Painful Shyness

American Psychological Association
http://apahelpcenter.org/featuredtopics/feature.php?id=5

Psychotherapies for Children and Adolescents

American Academy of Child and Adolescent Psychiatry
http://www.aacap.org/page.ww?name=Psychotherapies+For+Children+And+Adolescents§ion=Facts+for+Families

Rights and Protection and Advocacy

National Mental Health Information Center
http://mentalhealth.samhsa.gov/publications/allpubs/p&a/

The Science of Mental Illness

BSCS: Center for Curriculum Development
http://science-education.nih.gov/Supplements/NIH5/Mental/guide/nih_mental_curr-supp.pdf

Suicide and Depression

SAVE: Suicide Awareness Voices of Education
http://www.save.org/index.cfm

Talk to Teens about Healthy Relationships

Centers for Disease Control and Prevention
http://www.cdc.gov/features/chooserespect

Teen Mental Health Problems: What Are the Warning Signs?

National Mental Health Information Center
http://mentalhealth.samhsa.gov/publications/allpubs/Ca-0023/default.asp

Teen Suicide

American Psychiatric Association
http://healthyminds.org/Document-Library/Brochure-Library/Teen-Suicide.aspx

Use of Mental Health Services in the Past 12 Months by Children Aged 4–17

National Center for Health Statistics
http://www.cdc.gov/nchs/data/databriefs/db08.htm

What a Difference a Friend Makes

Substance Abuse and Mental Health Services Administration
http://www.whatadifference.org/

Why Am I in Such a Bad Mood?

Nemours Foundation
http://kidshealth.org/teen/your_mind/feeling_sad/bad_mood.html

Selected Recent Research

Community violence: a meta-analysis on the effect of exposure and mental health outcomes of children and adolescents. Fowler PJ, Tompsett CJ, Braciszewski JM, Jacques-Tiura AJ, Baltes BB. *Dev Psychopathol.* 2009 Winter;21(1):227-59.

A good-quality breakfast is associated with better mental health in adolescence. O'Sullivan TA, Robinson M, Kendall GE, Miller M, Jacoby P, Silburn SR, Oddy WH. *Public Health Nutr.* 2009 Feb;12(2):249-58. Epub 2008 Nov 25.

The hidden crisis in mental health and education: the gap between student needs and existing supports. Malti T, Noam GG. *New Dir Youth Dev.* 2008 Winter;(120):13-29,

Impact of school-based health centers on students with mental health problems. Guo JJ, Wade TJ, Keller KN. *Public Health Rep.* 2008 Nov-Dec; 123(6):768-80.

Mental health consequences of child sexual abuse. Mullers ES, Dowling M. *Br J Nurs.* 2008 Dec 11-2009 Jan 7;17(22):1428-30, 1432-3.

Obesity and mental health. Talen MR, Mann MM. *Prim Care.* 2009 Jun;36(2):287-305.

Parents' work patterns and adolescent mental health. Dockery A, Li J, Kendall G. *Soc Sci Med.* 2009 Feb;68(4):689-98. Epub 2008 Dec 10.

Poverty and adolescent mental health. Dashiff C, DiMicco W, Myers B, Sheppard K. *J Child* Adolesc Psychiatr Nurs. 2009 Feb;22(1):23-32.

Relations among gender, violence exposure, and mental health: the national survey of adolescents. Hanson RF, Borntrager C, Self-Brown S, Kilpatrick DG, Saunders BE, Resnick HS, Amstadter A. *Am J Orthopsychiatry.* 2008 Jul;78(3):313-21.

Throughout Today's Industrial societies, huge numbers of children and adolescents suffer from mental health problems. Malti T, Noam GG. *New Dir Youth Dev.* 2008 Winter;(120):1-5.

Why youth mental health is so important. Kutcher S, Venn D. Medscape *J Med.* 2008;10(12):275. Epub 2008 Dec 8.

Index

Index

Page numbers that appear in *Italics* refer to illustrations. Page numbers that have a small 'n' after the page number refer to information shown as Notes at the beginning of each chapter. Page numbers that appear in **Bold** refer to information contained in boxes on that page (except Notes information at the beginning of each chapter).

A

C

D

G

H

O

Q

R

T

U

V

W

X

Y

Z